Introduction to Communication Sciences and Disorders

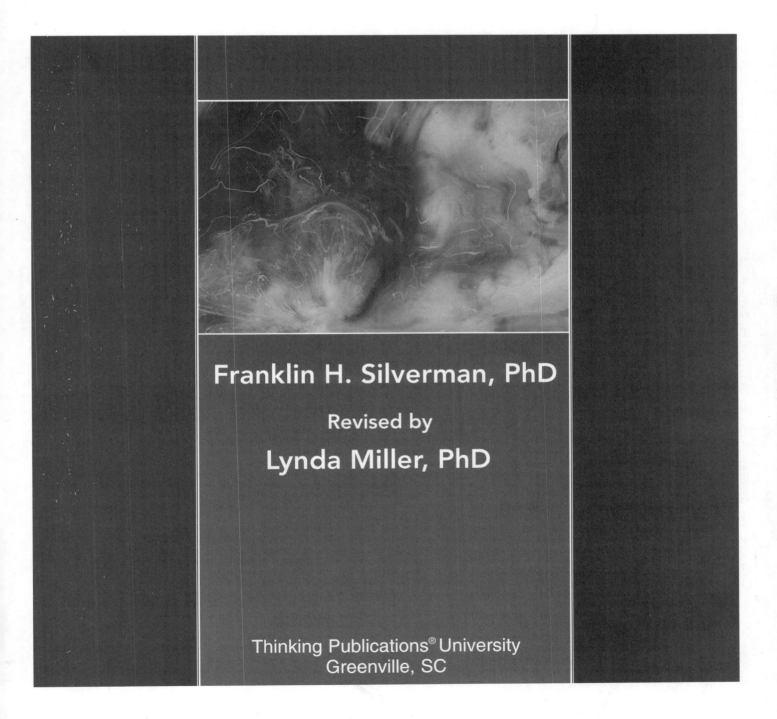

Franklin H. Silverman, PhD

Revised by

Lynda Miller, PhD

Thinking Publications® University
Greenville, SC

11   10   09   08   07   06   8   7   6   5   4   3   2   1

Library of Congress Cataloging-in-Publication Data

Silverman, Franklin H., date
   Introduction to communication sciences and disorders / Franklin H. Silverman ; revised
by Lynda Miller
      p. cm.
   Revision of: Introduction to speech, language, and hearing disorders / Franklin H.
Silverman. 3rd ed. (Cincinnati, Oh : Atomic Dog Pub., c2004).
   Includes bibliographical references and index
   ISBN 1-932054-50-2 (pbk.)
      1. Communicative disorders. I. Silverman, Franklin H., date Introduction to speech,
language, and hearing disorders. II. Miller, Lynda. III. Title

RC423.S5185 2006
616.85'5—dc22
                                                                        2005046651

Printed in the United States of America

Cover design by Nate Engen

Trademarks: All brand names and product names used in this book are the trade names, service marks, trademarks, or
              registered trademarks of their respective owners.

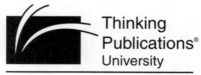

Thinking
Publications®
University

A Division of Super Duper® Inc.

P. O. Box 24997 • Greenville, SC 29616 USA
www.superduperinc.com
1-800-277-8737 • FAX 1-800-978-7379

To Nancy McKinley, who truly cared

About the Authors

Franklin H. Silverman

Dr. Fanklin H. Silverman, ASHA Fellow and pioneer in the field of augmentative and alternative communication, had been a member of the Marquette speech-language-pathology faculty for more than 30 years at the time of his death. He was the author of more than a dozen professional books and 150 articles in professional journals. He taught the Introductory Speech and Hearing Disorders course at Marquette University twice a year for more than 25 years and was the recipient of the University's annual faculty award for Teaching Excellence.

Dr. Silverman treated children and adults who have speech and language disorders for more than 40 years and was certified by both ASHA and the State of Wisconsin. His clinical advice had been sought both nationally and internationally, including by the Saudi royal family.

Dr. Silverman had more than 60 years of personal experience with speech disorders because he had stuttered since early childhood. Dr. Silverman will be greatly missed by his colleagues and friends.

Lynda Miller

Dr. Lynda Miller has been a speech-language pathologist for over 35 years and has worked in a variety of settings with people of all ages. She has taught in the public schools and at universities in Colorado, Montana, Illinois, and Texas. Dr. Miller is the author of numerous books and articles on cognition, learning, communication, language development, and learning disabilities. Her most recent publications include coauthoring a pragmatics language skills inventory and a book describing Section 504 in the public schools.

Dr. Miller has founded and directed two preschool programs for children with language disorders. She also developed a company devoted to the dissemination of innovative ideas in education and a company that provided continuing education to professional speech-language pathologists. Throughout her career, she has been active in providing continuing education for speech-language pathologists and audiologists.

Dr. Miller currently writes books, intervention materials, and tests for professionals in communication sciences and disorders. Her most recent contribution is designing and providing content for online continuing education courses for speech-language pathologists.

Contents

Contents

Preface

In 2004 Franklin H. Silverman authored the third edition of *Introduction to Speech, Language, and Hearing Disorders.* In his preface to that edition, Frank said that his primary objective was to "provide users with essential information for understanding 'at a gut level' the symptomatology, phenomenology, and etiology of speech, language, and hearing disorders as impairments, disabilities, and handicaps." I have three objectives in writing this revision of Frank's text: (1) to retain his original objective of providing readers with the essential information they need to understand and help people with communication disorders, (2) to shift the orientation of the contents to reflect more fully the profession of communication sciences and disorders today, and (3) to update and expand the contents to include a description of communication, language development, children's language disorders, multicultural issues, and concerns regarding communication and communication disorders.

Because this is an introductory text aimed at students who are enrolled in their first course in communication sciences and disorders, I have included a wide range of topics related to communication, language, speech, and hearing disorders. For each topic, I have chosen to include the information necessary to come away with an overview, rather than a complete understanding. My hope is that this book will stimulate students' interest in particular topics, which they can then pursue in more depth in additional coursework or on their own.

I have organized this revision into five parts that follow a logical progression: (1) Introduction; (2) Language Development and Disorders; (3) Speech Disorders; (4) Hearing Disorders; and (5) Communication Sciences and Disorders: The Profession.

Key vocabulary terms are highlighted and defined in several ways in this textbook. The first time a key term is mentioned in text, it is written in boldface type and its definition appears in the side margin on the same page or the adjacent page. If the same term appears in subsequent chapters, it is written in boldface but the definition does not appear in the margins. A glossary is also included, which includes all boldface terms.

Throughout this book you will be directed to audio samples, video samples, and online websites that reinforce the concepts taught. These samples and website addresses can be found on the accompanying CD-ROM.

Within this book, I have used language that reflects the fact that people have disorders. In other words, I refer to people with disorders (e.g., "adult with aphasia," "student with a language disorder") rather than to disorders attached to people (e.g., "the aphasic," "language disordered student"). My intention is to retain the focus on the human aspect of having a communication disorder. Although the field of communication sciences and disorders is based on understanding the science of communication and its disorders, at bottom the profession rests on the abilities of speech-language pathologists and audiologists to provide services in a way that is caring, humane, and professional.

Without Frank Silverman's impetus over 25 years ago when he began teaching an introductory course in communication disorders, this book would not exist. Frank's introductory text served as the framework around which I built this revision. In spite of the fact that I made substantial revisions and expanded the book considerably, I owe a tremendous debt to Frank's ideas, experiences, and clinical acumen.

I am also indebted to Nancy McKinley, who first suggested I revise this book. Had she not urged me to do it, I most likely would not have thought of it on my own! In spite of some unique challenges associated with this book, Nancy remained unflappable and dedicated to making it happen.

Vicki Lord Larson was instrumental in providing me with the feedback I needed as I worked out how to reorganize and expand the book into its current incarnation. As always, Vicki's ideas and orientation are aimed at making the book eminently usable and attractive to those students who will be our next generation of professionals.

Many thanks to Laura Hurd for her sleuth work in tracking down the often difficult-to-track permissions information.

Thanks, too, to Marietta Plummer, whose sharp editorial eye improved the book in ways both major and particular.

I must thank Linda Schreiber for her commitment to this book during a major transition at Thinking Publications. Like everyone I've ever met at Thinking Publications, Linda is focused on publishing the best possible clinical materials, and I appreciate her regarding this book in that light.

There were four authors that we were not able to locate in order to secure permission for use of information in Study Mores. These include R. Creech and J. Viggiano (1981) for use of *Consumers Speak Out on the Life of the Non-speaker,* W. Johnson (1946) for use of *People in Quandaries,* and C. Pedrey (1950) for use of a *Letter to the Editor.* We acknowledge their work and thank them for their contributions to this book.

Part 1

Introduction

The two chapters in Part 1 serve as an introduction and orientation to communication, communication disorders, and the field of communication sciences and disorders. In Chapter 1 you will learn about communication, language, speech, and hearing; how they are related; and some of their primary characteristics.

In Chapter 2, communication, language, speech, and hearing disorders are all defined. A description of how different cultural groups view these various disorders and how a communication disorder can affect a person's self-image and interpersonal relationships is also given. The following section on multicultural issues and concerns points out that the United States is becoming ever more diverse, requiring professionals to have considerable knowledge and expertise in providing services to linguistically and culturally diverse populations. The purposes of assessment of communication disorders; types of assessments used in the field; and the benefits and limitations of assessment are explored. The chapter also includes a discussion of the purposes of intervention, types of goals used by professionals, and the importance of measuring progress throughout the intervention process. This chapter ends with a brief description of the professions included in the field of communication sciences and disorders, typical work roles, and professional organizations.

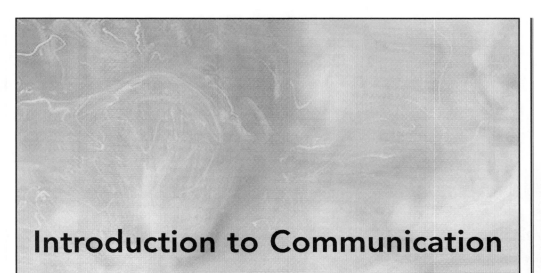

Introduction to Communication

Chapter 1

Learning Objectives

- Define *communication.*

- Describe the different types of communication.

- Define *language.*

- Define *speech.*

- Define *hearing.*

- Describe how communication, language, speech, and hearing are related.

- Develop an awareness of how cultural norms and traditions affect communication.

1

Chapter

Introduction

At its core, the professions of communication sciences and disorders are based on communication, language, speech, and hearing. This chapter will briefly define each of these topics and explain their relationships. How communication is affected by culture is also introduced.

Communication
Any exchange of information between people using a common code, or symbol system, understood by those involved.

What Is Communication?

Communication is any exchange of information between people using a common code, which may involve words, gestures, behaviors, signs, symbols, or sounds—in short, any symbol system understood by those involved. More specifically, communication is the interchange of ideas, feelings, stories, actions, events, and experiences. Human communication relies on a variety of modes, including speech, print, sign language, Braille, codes (e.g., Morse code or semaphore signals), silence, facial expressions, body postures, and gestures. Art forms such as drama, music, literature, poetry, and dance are examples of communication, albeit not always understood or agreed upon by everyone.

Communication always takes place within some sort of context, which can range from the immediacy of face-to-face conversation to the distance of reading a text written hundreds of years ago. Each communicative context influences such things as:

- How close to stand to another person when conversing (this varies by social situation and the relationship between the participants)

- The degree of formality to use during the communicative interchange (this is influenced by the mode of communication used and by the relationship between the participants)

- The purpose of the communicative interchange

- The intent of the participants

- The number of participants and their relationships

Communication in every cultural group depends on what Bates (1976), in a well-known book describing the social underpinnings of communication, described as a conversational code of conduct, or an unspoken system that seems to govern communication. This conversational code is summarized in Study More 1.1. In her research, Bates determined that,

Study More 1.1	**Conversational Code of Conduct**
• Cooperate with your conversational partner. • Tell the truth. • Offer only information you assume to be new and relevant to your listener. • Request only information you sincerely want to have.	• Provide your listener with just the right amount of background information so he or she will understand your point. • Be unambiguous. • Change your language to fit the current social situation.

Source: Bates (1976)

across cultures, communication depends on people following this code of conduct, while at the same time systematically violating it.

Although this code of conduct exists across cultural groups, each group interprets it in its own unique way, which carries implications for what is considered a communication disorder, a topic addressed in later chapters. For instance, if a person from a culture in which conversational partners stand closer than 18 inches were to stand that close to a person from a culture in which the partners stand farther away, each might think the other is violating what they perceive as the socially accepted "distance" rule. Similarly, if a person from a cultural group that uses informal address for elders addresses an older person by his or her first name, the elder might think the other person is violating the socially accepted polite form for addressing an elder.

Communication also involves violating the code, again depending on practices the cultural group has developed throughout its history. For instance, engaging in a debate violates the dictum "Cooperate with your conversational partner." Saying "Fine" when someone asks how you are and you feel terrible violates the dictum "Tell the truth." So does telling what are called "white lies," lies considered unimportant and used to be tactful or polite. You'll see in later chapters how, when they are first learning language, children act as if the code is inviolate, and they only gradually develop the ability to use the socially appropriate violations practiced by their cultural group.

Gestural Communication

Gestural communication usually refers to the facial expressions and the body postures, poses, and movements people use to impart information. (*Information* is used here to mean ideas, feelings, thoughts, emotions, facts, hypotheses, experiences, etc.) In English speakers, tilting one's head a certain way, for instance, might be used to convey doubt or humor, especially when combined with raised eyebrows and pursed lips. Romance language speakers indicate slight differences of meaning through the tilt of their heads and the thrusting of their chins.

One way to think about gestural communication is to examine the list of gestures associated with various parts of the body, shown in Study More 1.2. Although cultural groups vary significantly in the meanings they assign to gestures, all groups incorporate the body in communicative interchanges. Combined with vocal inflections, tone of voice, loudness, speech rate, and pitch, gestural communication contributes significantly—approximately 70 percent—to every communicative interchange.

It is important to note that sign languages are not simply gestural—they rely on postures; movements; and orientations of the head, face, arms, shoulders, trunk, arms, and hands. That is, they use gestures, but the gestures are codified into a symbol system just like a spoken language is codified into a symbol system. For this reason, sign languages are considered languages rather than forms of gestural communication.

Oral Communication

Oral communication, often referred to as spoken language, refers to the speech sounds people combine into the larger units we recognize as words and sentences. These speech sounds are

Study More 1.2	Gestures Associated with the Body

Head

    Head tilt

    Chin tilt

    Head shaking

    Head nodding

Face

    Forehead wrinkling

    Eyebrow raising/lowering

    Eyes narrowing/widening

    Nose wrinkling

    Nose wriggling

Mouth

    Lips compressing

    Lips pulled upward at the edges (smile, grin, laugh)

    Lips pursing

    Lips folded inward

    Upper lip raised on one side (sneering)

    Lips pulled downward at the edges

    Lips used to make "raspberry" sound

Chin

    Chin wrinkled

    Chin thrust upward

    Chin pulled inward and down

    Chin wagged side to side

    Chin wagged front to back

Neck

    Neck tensing

    Neck bent to one side (sometimes with raised shoulder)

Shoulders

    Shoulders raised

    Shoulders drooped

    One shoulder raised

    Shoulder(s) moved forward/backward

Trunk

    Chest puffed out

    Chest pulled in

    Trunk turned toward/away from listener

    Trunk bent forward/backward/sideways at waist

    Pelvis tilted forward/backward/sideways

Legs

    Hip cocked

    Knees straight/bent

    Ankles straight/bent

    If sitting: knees together/apart

    If sitting: legs crossed at knee/ankle on knee

Feet

    Foot (feet) still/tapping

    Feet parallel/at an angle to each other

    If sitting: still/tapping/circling

    If sitting: ankles straight/bent

ordered in particular ways—differently in each spoken language—so that those speaking any given language can extract particular meanings. For instance, Spanish speakers know that *curandera* means *shaman* (feminine), while for Yup'ik speakers (people living in the village of Tuntutuliak, in southwestern Alaska) the word for *shaman* is *angalkut*. In French, *shaman* is *sorcier* or *invocateur*. All three languages include a word that means roughly the same thing, yet the speech sounds used in each are significantly different.

Ideographic
A set of written characters that symbolize ideas without indicating the pronunciation of the words represented.

Syllabary
A set of written symbols that represent syllables.

Pictographic
Symbols that somewhat resemble the units of experience they represent.

Written Communication

Written communication, a more recent development historically than spoken communication, refers to the written or printed symbols used to represent spoken language. The symbol systems used in written communication include the alphabetic system used in English; the **ideographic** system used in Chinese and some other Asian languages; the **syllabary** systems used in the hiragana and katakana syllabic scripts of Japanese; and **pictographic** systems, such as those represented along the Rio Grande river in New Mexico and Utah. These written communication systems emerged from spoken language and are used in correspondence with the spoken languages they represent.

Written communication systems have also been invented to assist people who cannot speak. Some severely communicatively impaired children and adults use such symbols in communication boards. An example of one such system is Blissymbolics, which uses symbols that are both ideographic and pictographic. Both symbol types are illustrated in Figure 1.1.

Codes

Codes are symbol systems based on numbers, letters, symbols, icons, pictures, and/or sounds. The most common codes used today are alphanumeric. Alphanumeric codes combine numbers and letters and are often used as computer and Internet passwords. Computer encryption systems usually use random number strings of varying lengths, longer ones being more difficult to decode. Morse code is an example of a sound-based communication code, while football

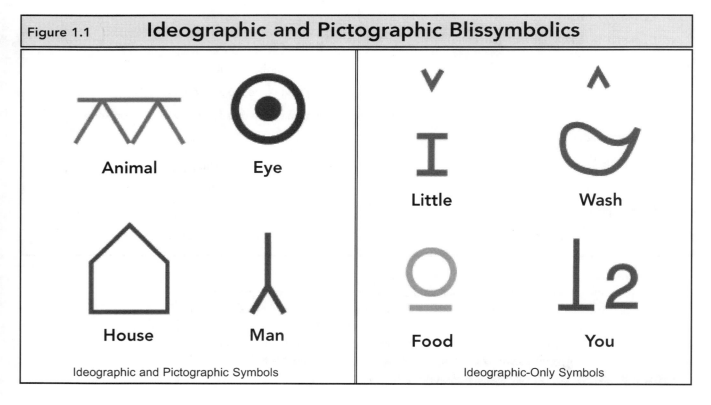

| Figure 1.1 | **Ideographic and Pictographic Blissymbolics** |

Ideographic and Pictographic Symbols — Animal, Eye, House, Man

Ideographic-Only Symbols — Little, Wash, Food, You

referees use a signal system based on body gestures and poses. Bar codes use optical patterns; Braille is a tactile code representing letters and numbers.

Codes often require a key, or a translation between the code and ordinary language, although some codes are accessible only to those who have memorized them or who have access to the technological equipment necessary to decode them. E-mail and instant messaging have produced a steady stream of communication codes in the form of acronyms and emoticons used to represent phrases or feelings. For people new to e-mail or text messaging, breaking the code can be difficult without a key.

What Is Language?

Language is the code used for communicating ideas with others. Although individual languages vary significantly, every language is based on an arbitrary set of abstract symbols people use to communicate with each other. These symbols are governed by rules for which sounds are used (humans are capable of producing many more sounds than they actually use in any given language); how those sounds are ordered; what constitutes a word; how words are modified to alter meaning; how words are strung together into sentences in certain ways to convey specific meanings; and how sounds, words, and sentences are modified in differing social contexts.

What Is Speech?

Speech is the production of **phonemes** by the **vocal tract.** It is supplied with air from the **respiratory system** and provided with voice by the vocal folds in the **larynx.** The vocal tract, which is illustrated in Figure 1.2 on page 10, consists of three main cavities (i.e., air-filled passages): the **pharyngeal cavity,** the **oral cavity,** and the **nasal cavity.**

During speech, air from the lungs passes through the vocal tract and is changed into phonemes. Air from the lungs passes through the larynx and causes the vocal folds to vibrate to produce most speech sounds—all vowel sounds and the majority of consonants—which are referred to as voiced phonemes. For the voiceless phonemes, the exhaled air is set into vibration in the oral cavity. During the production of /f/, for example, the air is set into vibration by being forced to exit through the narrow passage between the upper teeth and lower lip.

The configuration (i.e., shape) of the cavities in the vocal tract at a particular moment determines which phoneme will be produced. Each phoneme has a unique configuration. During every second of conversational speech, as many as 14 phonemes are produced (Darley, Aronson, & Brown, 1975). This means the configuration of the vocal tract is continually in a state of transformation. Phonemes have been classified in a number of ways, depending on how they are produced. More detail on this classification system will be provided in Chapter 8.

When we produce speech, we do so with a moderate amount of what is called **fluency.** Of course, we all hesitate periodically while speaking. We also insert sounds, syllables, words, and even phrases in the course of a conversation. At times, we insert long pauses between words; prolong speech sounds; and stop to correct errors of pronunciation, syntax, and word usage. A certain amount of these pauses, insertions, and hesitations is considered to be a normal part of speaking. Indeed, unless we're listening to trained speakers or actors, we usually notice when someone's speech does not include any of these attributes.

Language
The code used for communicating ideas with others.

Speech
The production of phonemes by the vocal tract.

Phonemes
Speech sounds.

Vocal tract
The mechanism that molds the "buzz" generated by the vocal folds into speech sounds. It consists of the pharyngeal, oral, and nasal cavities.

Respiratory system
The organs that generate the raw material (i.e., air) for vibrating the vocal folds to produce voice.

Larynx
The structure that contains the vocal folds (i.e., the mechanism that produces voice). The larynx also functions as a valve which prevents food and liquids from getting into the lungs.

Pharyngeal cavity
The throat. Also referred to as the pharynx.

Oral cavity
The mouth.

Nasal cavity
The interior of the nose.

Fluency
Effortless and smooth production of speech.

| Figure 1.2 | **The Three Major Cavities of the Vocal Tract** |

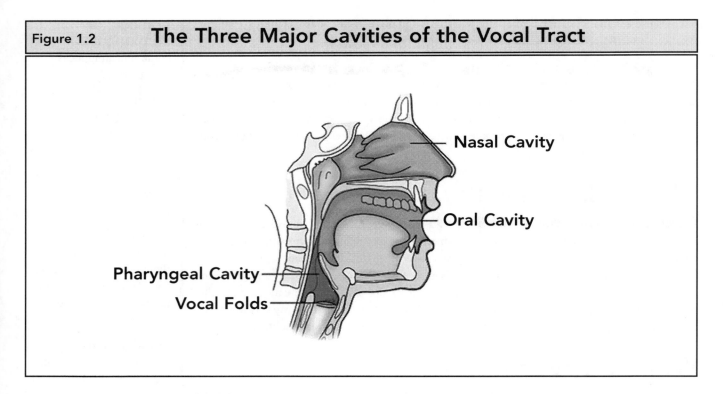

Nasal Cavity

Oral Cavity

Pharyngeal Cavity

Vocal Folds

Hearing
The perception of sound.

What Is Hearing?

The process of speaking involves the generation of speech sounds; the process of **hearing involves the perception of sound.** Within the context of communication, hearing means perceiving speech sounds. To understand hearing, you need some basic information about how sound is generated and transmitted—that is, the physics of sound. You'll also need to know a few basics about the anatomy and physiology of the ear. In Chapter 10 you will learn about (1) the physics of sound; (2) intensity; (3) the anatomy and physiology of the hearing mechanism; and (4) the inner ear, auditory nerve, and central auditory nervous system.

How Are Communication, Language, Speech, and Hearing Related?

In general, communication takes place through the processes of hearing and speaking, both of which rely on an understanding and command of the rules of the language being used to communicate. Of course, communication also takes place through modes other than speaking and hearing. However, almost all children first learn to communicate through speaking and hearing, and only later in their development are able to communicate through reading and writing.

Culture and Communication

Although communication is a universally shared human process, cultural groups vary significantly in how communication takes place within their culture, the various rule systems governing how people communicate within each culture, and how people in each culture view communication. Culture determines how we express (or suppress) emotions such as happiness, anger, joy, disapproval, and love. For instance, consider how your culture governs the expression of love in public settings. Is it acceptable to hold hands? Hug? Kiss?

Culture governs how we think about and communicate our ideas regarding etiquette, values, norms, rituals, and expectations, to name a few. Try the exercises in Study More 1.3 to think about your culture's communication patterns.

The important thing to remember is that every communicative act takes place within a cultural context, whether it's enjoying a conversation with a friend, participating in a political rally, listening to a lecture by a world leader, or writing a term paper. Every person exists within at least one cultural context; most of us live in more than one culture. Learning to communicate with people from other cultures is a necessary prerequisite for becoming a successful clinician.

Study More 1.3	Communication in Your Culture

1. Think about your culture's "rules" regarding personal space; patterns of touch; etiquette and ritual; and the expression of emotions.
    - How close is "too close" when talking to a good friend?
    - Can you touch a stranger on the arm during a conversation?
    - What is the etiquette for how you address your parents' friends (first name, last name)?
    - Does your family have any communication rituals? What are they?
    - How do you express anger or joy in your culture?
2. Think about your culture's ideas about food.
    - Is food viewed as a reward in your culture?
    - Is food viewed as something to enjoy?
    - Is food viewed as simply a necessity?
    - How do people talk about food in your culture?
3. Think about parent-child relationships in your culture.
    - How do children talk to their parents in your culture?
    - How do parents talk to their children?
    - How do nonfamily members speak to other people's children?
    - How do children address adults outside the family?
4. What are some ways of showing respect in your culture?
    - What are the most common polite forms you use? With whom? Under what circumstances?
    - Is it acceptable to show disrespect in your culture? How?
    - Are manners important in your culture? How do they show up?

Introduction to Communication Disorders and Communication Science Professions

Chapter 2

Learning Objectives

- Develop an awareness of how communication disorders affect people.

- Define and describe what constitutes a communication disorder.

- Explain how a communication disorder can impact personal relationships.

- Explain how culture plays a role in the diagnosis of a communication disorder.

- Describe the primary purposes and types of assessment used with communication disorders.

- Describe why it is necessary to track progress during the intervention process.

- Describe the professions in communication sciences and disorders.

- Name the work settings of professionals in communication sciences.

- Name the professional organizations in the area of communication sciences.

Introduction

Imagine that, when you woke up this morning, your tongue was paralyzed and you were completely unable to speak. You could understand speech and language just as well as ever, and your ability to think and reason was unimpaired. But when you tried to talk, your tongue wouldn't move—it was paralyzed on the floor of your mouth. A physician examined you and concluded that the paralysis was due to damage to the nerves that innervate the tongue musculature, and that your condition is unlikely to improve.

Or, imagine instead that you woke up unable to hear even the loudest sound. When your roommate talked to you, you could see his or her lips moving, but you couldn't understand anything because you could no longer hear. Your physician said you'd suffered sudden hearing loss, possibly due to two things: a series of upper respiratory infections you'd had over the past several months or prolonged exposure to loud noise in a music club where you listen to bands. It is possible that your hearing may not ever return to normal because of reduced blood flow to the inner ear.

Consider each scenario. What impact do you think your inability to talk or hear would have on your life? How would these two scenarios affect you differently? Similarly? Would you be able to remain a student with the same major? How would each of these scenarios affect your plans for the future? How would each affect your social life now, including dating? How would it affect how you feel about yourself as a person? Could either motivate you to succeed? For an example, see Temple Grandin's comments about her life in Study More 2.1 on page 16.

If you're like most people, you probably will have a difficult time answering these questions because you take talking and hearing for granted, just as you take for granted your ability to walk and use your hands. This is not particularly surprising because you have been able to do these things for as long as you can remember. Babies begin using their voices to communicate within a few minutes after being born. They communicate feeling uncomfortable by crying, and they cease crying to indicate they are feeling comfortable again. Only those who have had difficulty communicating, either temporarily or permanently, can fully appreciate the impact a communication disorder can have on a person.

One of the goals of this chapter is to increase your awareness of the importance of communication in everyday life, and, consequently, the effects a communication disorder can have on one's life. Although the field of communication sciences and disorders is based on scientific facts, professionals who interact with people with communication disorders must have tremendous insight into the impact a communication disorder can have on someone's life. This chapter includes excerpts from people who have communication disorders, in the hope that you can better understand how it feels to live with such a condition.

What Is a Communication Disorder?

The American Speech-Language-Hearing Association (ASHA; 1993) defines a communication disorder as:

> an impairment in the ability to receive, send, process, and comprehend concepts or verbal, nonverbal and graphic symbol systems. A communication disorder may be evident in the processes of hearing, language, and/or speech.

Study More 2.1	Living with Autism

I think in pictures. Words are like a second language to me. I translate both spoken and written words into full-color movies, complete with sound, which run like a VCR tape in my head. When somebody speaks to me, his words are instantly translated into pictures. Language-based thinkers often find this phenomenon difficult to understand, but in my job as an equipment designer for the livestock industry, visual thinking is a tremendous advantage.

Visual thinking has enabled me to build entire systems in my imagination. During my career I have designed all kinds of equipment, ranging from corrals for handling cattle on ranches to systems for handling cattle and hogs during veterinary procedures and slaughter. I have worked for many major livestock companies. In fact, one third of the cattle and hogs in the United States are handled in equipment I have designed. Some of the people I've worked for don't even know that their systems were designed by someone with autism. I value my ability to think visually, and I would never want to lose it.

One of the most profound mysteries of autism has been the remarkable ability of most autistic people to excel at visual spatial skills while performing so poorly at verbal skills. When I was a child and a teenager, I thought everybody thought in pictures. I had no idea that my thought processes were different. In fact, I did not realize the full extent of the differences until very recently. At meetings and at work I started asking other people detailed questions about how they accessed information from their memories. From their answers I learned that my visualization skills far exceeded those of most other people.

I credit my visualization abilities with helping me understand the animals I work with. Early in my career I used a camera to help give me the animals' perspective as they walked through a chute for their veterinary treatment. I would kneel down and take pictures through the chute from the cow's eye level. Using the photos, I was able to figure out which things scared the cattle, such as shadows and bright spots of sunlight. Back then I used black-and-white film, because twenty years ago scientists believed that cattle lacked color vision. Today, research has shown that cattle can see colors, but the photos provided the unique advantage of seeing the world through a cow's viewpoint. They helped me figure out why the animals refused to go in one chute but willingly walked through another.

Every design problem I've ever solved started with my ability to visualize and see the world in pictures. I started designing things as a child, when I was always experimenting with new kinds of kites and model airplanes. In elementary school I made a helicopter out of a broken balsa-wood airplane. When I wound up the propeller, the helicopter flew straight up about a hundred feet. I also made bird-shaped paper kites, which I flew behind my bike. The kites were cut out from a single sheet of heavy drawing paper and flown with thread. I experimented with different ways of bending the wings to increase flying performance. Bending the tips of the wings up made the kite fly higher. Thirty years later, this same design started appearing on commercial aircraft.

From *Thinking in Pictures: And Other Reports from My Life with Autism* (pp. 19–20), by T. Grandin, 1995, New York: Doubleday. © 1995 by Temple Grandin. Reprinted with permission of Doubleday, a division of Random House.

Speech-language pathologist (SLP)
An independent professional whose primary responsibility is helping persons who have speech and/or language disorders cope with them as impairments, disabilities, and handicaps.

Audiologist
An independent professional whose primary responsibility is helping persons who have a hearing disorder cope with it.

A communication disorder may range in severity from mild to profound. It may be developmental or acquired. Individuals may demonstrate one or any combination of communication disorders. A communication disorder may result in a primary disability or it may be secondary to other disabilities. (pp. 40–41)

Most professionals in communication sciences and disorders would add two conditions to the ASHA definition:

- There has to be something noticeably different about how the person talks or listens. If the person is not aware of the difference and most people would not detect it, he or she would not likely be looked upon as having a communication disorder. In this situation, the communication difference would not interfere with communication; call adverse attention to the person; or cause him or her to be self-conscious or maladjusted.

- The communicative deviation has to be regarded as "abnormal" by at least one person whose judgment is respected by the person who has it. This person can be a professional such as a **speech-language pathologist (SLP)** or **audiologist;** a family member; a friend; or the person himself or herself.

The ASHA definition and the two additional conditions are incorporated nicely into a conceptualization of communication disorders put forth by Charles Van Riper, one of the most respected and influential speech-language pathologists in the United States during the twentieth century.

Charles Van Riper's Definition of a Communication Disorder

Van Riper and Erickson's (1996) definition states that a communication disorder has three aspects: (1) a perception by others that the person's communication deviates enough from normal hearing, speech, or language that it interferes with communication; (2) the person's communication calls adverse attention to him or her; or (3) it causes the person to be self-conscious about it, or "maladjusted." The meanings of certain terms in this definition are addressed in the next sections. To learn more about Van Riper and how he conceptualized communication disorders, see Van Riper and Erickson.

Meaning of "Perceived Deviation from Normal" in the Definition

For a person to be regarded as having a communication disorder, some aspect of his or her speaking and/or listening behavior must be perceived as deviating from normal. A necessary first step for deciding whether a particular aspect of communication behavior is abnormal is defining *normal limits* for it. What is regarded as being normal is almost always a value judgment—an opinion. It depends on the percentage of the population that you are willing to classify as abnormal. Should it be regarded as abnormal, for example, for a two-and-a-half-year-old child not to be producing the /r/ sound correctly in words? For a speech-language pathologist to look upon it as such, he or she would have to be willing to classify more than 75 percent of two-and-a-half-year-olds as abnormal. On the other hand, should it be regarded as abnormal for an eight-year-old child not to be doing so? To view it in this way, an SLP would only have to be willing to classify fewer than 5 percent of eight-year-olds as abnormal. Therefore, two well-qualified SLPs could conceivably evaluate a five-year-old child and disagree about whether his or her failure to say words containing /r/ correctly is abnormal.

Meaning of "Hearing" in the Definition

Most disorders of hearing are caused by damage to the outer, middle, or inner ear (which are pictured in Figure 2.1 on page 18). Damage can be on one or both sides of the head or to some part of the **central auditory nervous system (CANS)**—the parts of the brain that process electrical signals from the ears. The location and extensiveness of damage will determine the amount of difficulty a person will experience in understanding speech.

Meaning of "Speech" in the Definition

Disorders of speech consist of perceived deviations from normal voice, articulation, fluency (or rhythm), and nasal resonance. These four types of speech disorders are briefly described next. They are discussed in depth in Chapters 6 through 9.

Voice disorders (disorders of **phonation**) result from a disturbance in the functioning of the **larynx**, particularly the part known as the **vocal folds**, or vocal cords. The most severe

---

Central auditory nervous system (CANS)
A group of sites within the central nervous system (brain) that process the electrical signals output by the auditory nerves. The CANS enables us to be aware of, and abstract information from, sounds in our environment.

Phonation
Voice produced by vibration of the vocal folds.

Vocal folds
Two mucous-covered muscles that stretch horizontally across the larynx; they vibrate to produce sound.

Figure 2.1	Anatomy of the Ear

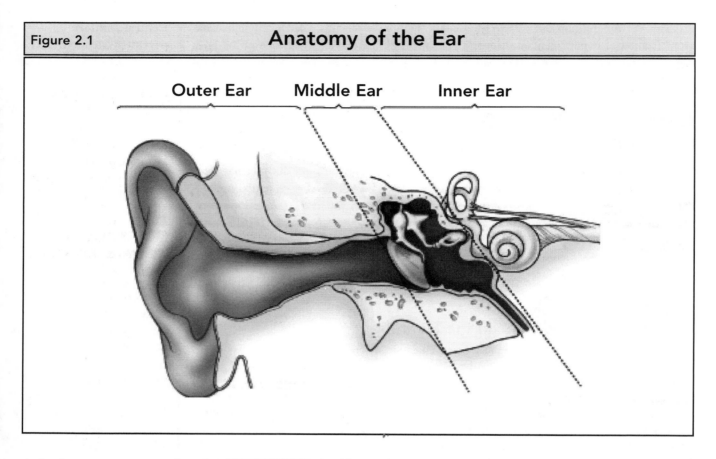

Outer Ear   Middle Ear   Inner Ear

Aphonia
The inability to phonate (i.e., produce voice).

voice disorder is **aphonia**. Since voice is the "raw material" from which speech sounds are formed, if you can't produce voice, you can't speak. Other disorders of voice are habitually speaking (1) too loudly or too softly; (2) at a pitch level that is too high or too low; and (3) with a breathy, hoarse, or other type of abnormal voice quality. You can listen to two people with voice disorders on Audio Clips 2.1 and 2.2. Voice disorders are discussed in more detail in Chapter 6.

Audio Clip 2.1	Organic Voice Tremor

◎ AUDIO	The voice of a woman with an organic voice tremor. The tremor isn't as obvious when she reads aloud as it is when she sustains a vowel at the end of the recording.

Audio Clip 2.2	Hoarse Voice

◎ AUDIO	Hoarse voice quality caused by pathology (e.g., a growth) on the vocal folds.

Articulation disorders are characterized by consistently making one or more errors in **phoneme** production. These errors can be of several types. One type of error is **sound substitution.** An English-speaking child, for example, might substitute /w/ for /r/ and say "wed wagon" rather than "red wagon." Another error type is **sound omission**. A child might omit the initial /s/ in a word when it is followed by another consonant, for example, and say "paghetti" instead of "spaghetti." A third type of error is **sound distortion**. A lateralized /s/ (an /s/ production in which the corners of the mouth retract and the air flows between the side teeth rather than the front ones) would be classified as a sound distortion in English because no words in this language contain such a sound. If there were such words, the error would be classified as a sound substitution. Audio Clip 2.3 provides an example of a sound substitution. Chapter 8 discusses articulation disorders in detail.

Audio Clip 2.3	**Sound Substitution**
AUDIO	A sound substitution on *vacuum*—substituting /r/ (as in *r*oom) for /j/ (as in *y*ellow)

Fluency disorders are characterized by disturbances in the normal flow (i.e., rhythm) of speech. Such disturbances include abnormally long pauses between words; frequent repetitions of speech sounds, syllables, words, or phrases; prolongations of speech sounds; and abnormal pauses between the syllables of words. **Stuttering** is the most frequently occurring disorder of this type. Audio Clip 2.4 provides an example of stuttering. Stuttering and other fluency disorders are discussed in detail in Chapter 9.

Audio Clip 2.4	**Stuttering**
AUDIO	A moment of disfluency (i.e., a break in speech fluency) containing a phrase repetition and an interjection

Nasal resonance disorders result from an abnormal amount of air flowing through the nose during speech. If too much air flows through it, the resulting speech is referred to as *hypernasal*. **Hypernasality** tends to be difficult to understand, and people who have it sound like they are "talking through their nose." **Hyponasality** (i.e., denasality) results if too little air flows through the nose. A person whose nose is "stuffed" as the result of a cold sounds hyponasal.

Meaning of "Language" in the Definition

People who have a language disorder do not understand and/or express themselves in their native language as well as most others their age, and their difficulty cannot be accounted for by a hearing loss or speech disorder. The disorder may have been present from early childhood or developed later in life after disease or injury to the brain.

Language disorders can affect any or all of a person's abilities to listen and understand, to speak, to read, and to write. If the disorder affects only the person's ability to understand speech

Sound substitution
An articulation error in which one phoneme that occurs in a language is substituted for another that occurs in that language.

Sound omission
An articulation error in which a phoneme is omitted from words.

Sound distortion
An articulation error in which a phoneme that does not occur in a language is substituted for one that does.

Stuttering
A fluency disorder that usually begins in early childhood.

Hypernasality
A disorder in which air flows through the nasal cavity while producing sounds for which it should not.

Hyponasality
A disorder in which air does not flow through the nasal cavity while producing sounds for which it should.

Receptive
Relating to the skills of listening and reading.

Expressive
Relating to the skills of speaking and writing.

or print, it is referred to as a **receptive** language disorder; if it affects only the person's ability to produce speech or to write, it is referred to as an **expressive** language disorder. Language development and disorders are discussed in Chapters 3 and 4.

Meaning of "Interferes with Communication" in the Definition

This is the first of three conditions that alone or in combination can transform a perceived deviation from normal speech, language, or hearing into a communication disorder. Deviations can be considerable and yet not interfere in any significant way with a person's ability to communicate. This is the case for some persons who speak with foreign dialects. Their pronunciations and arrangement of words may deviate considerably from what is acceptable in English, and yet after listening to them for a relatively short time, we become accustomed to these deviations and no longer have difficulty understanding what they are saying. This also is true for most persons who consistently substitute /w/ for /r/ or only occasionally stutter.

Meaning of "Calls Adverse Attention" in the Definition

A perceived deviation from normal hearing, speech, or language can call adverse attention to the person with the deviation. This can result in a person being classified as having a communication disorder even if it does not interfere with communication. While a /w/ for /r/ sound substitution is unlikely to impede an older child's or adult's ability to communicate, it is likely to cause him or her to be stereotyped in undesirable ways. Such stereotypes can keep individuals from achieving their highest potential of productivity, an outcome that our society regards as unacceptable. To learn more about how even a single sound substitution can cause a person to be stereotyped in undesirable ways, see Silverman and Flack (1992) and Silverman and Paulus (1989).

Meaning of "Self-Conscious or Maladjusted" in the Definition

How people react to their communication disorder and the reactions of others to it largely determines the degree to which it handicaps or benefits them. If they are self-conscious and embarrassed and attempt to conceal it, the disorder is likely to keep them from doing some things they want to do. A person's reaction to something abnormal about his or her speech, hearing, and/or language can be more handicapping than the deviation itself.

Merely having a communication disorder does not automatically cause a person to be handicapped. For example, the fact that Winston Churchill, the prime minister of England during World War II, stuttered did not keep him from doing what he wanted to do. The same was true for some other persons who had this disorder, including George Washington, Charles Darwin, Moses, Aesop, Virgil, Aristotle, Demosthenes, Mel Tillis, Carly Simon, Marilyn Monroe, Somerset Maugham, and John Updike (Silverman, 1996). To learn more about how it is possible to cope even while being almost completely paralyzed (i.e., having "locked-in" syndrome), see Bauby (1998).

Impact on Interpersonal Relationships

Van Riper and Erickson's (1996) definition of a communication disorder suggests that it can affect interpersonal relationships in the following ways:

1. It can interfere with communication between speaker and listener.

2. It can cause the listener to react negatively to the speaker.

3. It can cause the speaker to have a poor **self-image**.

These impacts and the reasons for them are explored further in the next paragraphs.

Interfering with Communication

A necessary condition for developing and maintaining interpersonal relationships is being able to transmit information to and receive information from (i.e., communicate with) other people. Anything that impedes our ability to communicate interferes with our ability to have a relationship with others.

A communication disorder can impede the transmission of information between speaker and listener in several ways. First, it can interfere with the listener's ability to receive information. For instance, if a listener can't hear much of what a speaker says, communication is adversely affected. Or a listener may not understand some spoken words because he or she cannot hear certain consonant sounds. If, for example, a listener were unable to hear /s/ at the end of nouns, he or she would have difficulty differentiating singular from plural forms. Furthermore, difficulty processing oral language can prevent a listener from understanding some of what a speaker says. A disorder of this type is particularly likely to interfere with communication when messages are relatively long.

A communication disorder also can impede the flow of information between a speaker and a listener by interfering with the speaker's ability to transmit information. This can happen in several ways. For example, when the speaker cannot remember some of the words that he or she needs in order to communicate messages, communication is impeded. Also, a communication disorder could prevent the speaker from fully controlling the musculature of the speech mechanism (e.g., the tongue), thereby reducing the **intelligibility** of what is said. Furthermore, a communication disorder could cause an individual to speak with abnormal hesitations and syllable repetitions. Such behaviors, if they occur frequently (as they do in the speech of some people with fluency disorders), can interfere with message transmission because the listener is distracted by the disfluencies.

Causing a Negative Reaction

Just as there are stereotypes for members of racial and religious groups, there are stereotypes for people who have certain communication disorders. These include stuttering, **lisping,** substituting /w/ for /r/, hearing loss, **dysarthria, spasmodic dysphonia,** and **aphasia.** If you expect a person to have certain personality characteristics or to behave in a certain way because he or she has a particular disorder, your expectation can cause you to perceive the person as having these characteristics and exhibiting these behaviors.

self-image
The manner in which a person views himself or herself.

Intelligibility
How understandable a speaker is to a listener.

Lisping
Either a substitution of the voiceless /θ/ sound for /s/ (e.g., *th*ip for *s*ip) or a distortion of /s/ in which the airstream is directed at the side rather than the front teeth. The former is referred to as a frontal lisp and the latter as a lateral lisp.

Dysarthria
A neuromuscular disorder that affects some or all of the vocal tract musculature.

Spasmodic dysphonia
A voice disorder in which the voice, at times, sounds tense or strained.

Aphasia
A language disorder resulting from damage to the brain in which the person loses some ability to understand speech, formulate speech, read, write, calculate, or some combination of these abilities.

Introduction to Communication Sciences and Disorders

Cultural sensitivity
Awareness that cultures differ in their views of the world; knowing there is no one "right way" to view things.

What characteristics do listeners ascribe to persons who have communication disorders? The characteristics that people are likely to ascribe to such a person will be determined by the following: (1) the type of disorder, (2) how the person reacts to it, (3) the listeners' previous experiences with persons who have the disorder, and (4) the listeners' cultural backgrounds.

The type of communication disorder determines to some extent the characteristics that listeners ascribe to a person. A man who has a frontal lisp (who substitutes /θ/ for /s/), for example, is more likely to be viewed as "feminine" than one who speaks with a whistling /s/.

How the person reacts to the disorder influences how listeners will react to it. If they sense that the person is embarrassed or ashamed about having the disorder, they are likely to ascribe more negative personality characteristics to him or her than they would otherwise (Silverman, 1988a; Silverman, Gazzolo, & Peterson, 1990).

A listener's previous experience with persons who have a particular disorder determines, to some extent, the characteristics he or she is likely to ascribe to those who have it. A listener who perceived those he or she met previously who had the disorder as having low intelligence may tend to perceive others who have the same disorder as not being very intelligent.

Finally, cultural background influences the characteristics a listener will ascribe to a child or adult who has a communication disorder (Bleile & Wallach, 1992). For example, an African American preschool-age child who has trouble speaking is likely to have some different characteristics ascribed to him or her by persons in an African American inner-city community than in a white middle-class community. And an African American preschool-age child who uses Black English vernacular at home is likely to have some different characteristics ascribed to him or her than if he or she uses it when speaking to a white middle-class preschool teacher—particularly one who lacks **cultural sensitivity** (Campbell, 1993). The characteristics ascribed will be determined, in part, by the beliefs in the person's culture about the causes and consequences of disabilities (Maestas & Erickson, 1992). To learn more about the influence of culture on how communication disorders are perceived, see Battle (1993).

Although the specific traits listeners tend to ascribe to people with communication disorders are not the same for all disorders and for all listeners, some are ascribed frequently, including the following:

1. *Relatively Low Intelligence.* One of the main factors people consider when judging a person's intelligence is how he or she speaks. They tend to regard people who express themselves well as being more intelligent than those who do not express themselves as well. Consequently, people who have a communication disorder are often perceived as being less intelligent than they really are. In Study More 2.2, two people with cerebral palsy describe their experiences with this perception. This thinking pattern, however, isn't universal. Some data, for example, suggest that few teachers tend to perceive students who stutter as less intelligent (Lass et al., 1992; Silverman, 1990).

2. *Immaturity.* A related characteristic often ascribed to adults who have a communication disorder is immaturity. People may treat someone with a communication disorder as they would a young child by doing one or more of the following:

   • Speaking loudly, at a rather slow rate, using relatively short sentences

   • Repeating a message several times

| Study More 2.2 | # If You Can't Talk, People Assume You're Deaf and Dumb |

If a person is perceived as having a communication impairment, certain assumptions will tend to be made about him or her, particularly about his or her intellect and personality. Such assumptions can have a more devastating impact on self-concept than the communicative disorder itself. Ricky Creech and James Viggiano, both of whom are unable to talk because they have cerebral palsy, communicate by means of electronic communication devices. The following comments were abstracted from a presentation they gave at the National Institutes of Health.

Ricky Creech

There is a great need for educating the public on how to treat physically limited people. People are still under the misconception that somehow the ability to speak, hear, see, feel, smell, and reason are tied together. That is, if a person loses one, he has lost the others.

The number one question people ask my parents is, "Can he hear?" When I reply that I can, they bend down where their lips are not two feet away from my eyes and say very loudly, "How—are—you? Do—you—like—that—talking—machine?" Now, I don't mind when that person is a pretty, young girl. But when it is an older or married woman, it is a little embarrassing. When the person is a man, I'm tempted to say something not very nice...

I would make a great spy. When I am around, people just keep talking—because I can't speak, they think I can't hear or understand what is being said. I have listened to more private conversations than there are on the Watergate tapes. It is a good thing that I am not a blackmailer. If people know that I hear and understand everything they say, some would die of embarrassment.

One of the results of this misconception is that people will ask my parents questions they should ask me. Since getting my HandiVoice [an electronic communication device that generates synthetic speech], I have had the hardest time training my parents not to answer those questions, but to let me answer. I can kid about people treating me as if I can't hear because I can see the humor in it. There is another conclusion which people make when first seeing me, which I don't kid about; I don't find it a bit humorous. That is that I am mentally retarded.

The idea that if a person can't speak something must be wrong with his mind is the prevalent belief in every class, among the educated as well as the not-so-educated. I have a very good friend who is a nuclear scientist, the most intelligent person I have ever known, but he admitted that when he first saw me his first conclusion was that I was mentally retarded. This was in spite of my parents' asseverations that I was not.

However, this man had a special quality, when he was wrong he could admit it with his mind and his heart, most people can't do both. There are people who know me who know with their minds that I am not mentally retarded but they treat me as a child because in their hearts they have not really accepted that I have the mentality of an adult. I am an adult and I want to be treated as an adult. I have a tremendous amount of respect for anyone who does.

James Viggiano

My biggest handicap isn't having cerebral palsy. It is people's ignorance about the nonspeaking person. The principal unmet need surrounds the basic right to live with dignity in such simple things as eating, toileting, and basic assistance in activities of daily living.

The most obvious problem occurred recently when I was in my room, in bed. I had pushed the call light for assistance. The staff, even though they knew I was nonspeaking, responded by querying me on the intercom five times before the light dawned on their marble heads. Finally, someone showed up and handed me a spelling board...

It is an honor to be addressing such brainy people who have degrees and credentials of an expert nature. Though with all your expertise, there is not a book which tells you how frustrating it is to be ignored when you have a life or death matter to communicate. For example, a so-called normal person just walked away before I could tell him that one of his psychotic patients is playing with matches while there were five other patients in the room who can't get out of the way. I just sat by the nurse's desk until a person finally paid attention and took away the matches. A good five minutes went by and six people could have burned. But, what the hell, I was in a hospital where patients aren't supposed to have constructive thoughts of their own. Or so they say.

Because society in general still does not understand how people who are nonvocal communicate, many times I have been exposed to the indignity of being treated as if I were retarded. Quite often even health care professionals pat me on the head and say, "Can you spell 'cat' Jimmy?" I am James, a 36 year old MAN, not a boy.

From "Consumers Speak Out on the Life of the Non-speaker," by R. Creech and J. Viggiano, 1981, *ASHA, 23,* pp. 550–552. © 1981 by the American Speech-Language-Hearing Association.

Culture
The ways of thinking, talking, understanding, and relating to others that are characteristic of groups of people with a shared history (Paul, 2001, p. 165).

- Being overly helpful (acting in a patronizing manner)

- Using the person's first name in situations in which it is customary to use a title (e.g., Mr., Doctor) and last name

Creating a Poor Self-Image

Having abnormal speech, language, or hearing can influence one's self-concept. It can make an individual dislike himself or herself, which can result in one or more of the following: unhappiness, depression, being overly sensitive, frustration, having suicidal thoughts and/or actions, embarrassment, pessimism, emotional instability, defensiveness, introversion, being frightened, or feeling tense.

Liking yourself is a necessary condition for developing and maintaining relationships with others that are both enjoyable and beneficial. Experiencing any of the emotions and feelings listed above can severely impact an individual's ability to form and maintain relationships.

A person who has a communication disorder may attempt to maintain a positive self-image by frequently employing one or both of the following strategies: (1) avoiding situations in which he or she would be expected to communicate or (2) entering them, but reducing speaking to an absolute minimum. Although doing either can reduce the number of times the person becomes embarrassed as a consequence of communicating abnormally, using these strategies can seriously impair interpersonal relationships. In fact, using them may contribute more to the person being handicapped than the communication disorder itself. Some of the responsibilities of SLPs and audiologists include encouraging people with communication disorders to communicate, teaching them ways to better communicate, and supporting their communication efforts.

The impact that a communication disorder has on a person's self-image is, in part, a function of how the person is reacted to by others in his or her culture (Anderson, 1992). Persons from different cultures may react differently to a child who has a particular communication disorder. To learn more about how a person's culture can affect the impact that a communication disorder has on his or her self-image, see Battle (1993), Hargrove and Katz (1992), and Terrell and Hale (1992).

Multicultural Issues and Concerns

People from different cultural groups may communicate differently from each other and hold different beliefs about what constitutes appropriate, and, therefore, disordered, communication. But what is culture, exactly? Rhea Paul (2001), an expert on language development and disorders, defines **culture** as "the ways of thinking, talking, understanding, and relating to others that are characteristic of groups of people with a shared history" (p. 165). People in a given cultural group share attitudes, values, goals, and practices over a period of time, passing them along to succeeding generations.

Differentiating between what constitutes a communication disorder and what is merely a cultural variation in communication style or custom requires knowledge of how different cultural groups communicate, what is considered "normal" in each cultural group, and what is considered "disordered." For instance, in virtually all cultures, severe language disruptions following a stroke constitute a language disorder, but dialectal variations in grammatical constructions do not. Similarly, in almost all cultures, a child who does not speak by age three would be at least evaluated for a language disorder, but a teenager with a hoarse voice might be sent for an evaluation in only some cultures.

People living in cultures that are heavily dependent on print (i.e., reading and writing) view difficulties learning to read and/or write as communication disorders, while people from cultures that rely more heavily on oral language may not. Similarly, people from cultures in which oral language is prized may view people who cannot tell complex, entertaining, and lengthy stories to be communicatively impaired, while those from cultures in which storytelling is not particularly valued may not.

A related issue concerns cultural perceptions of hearing loss and the use of sign languages. Most people with normal hearing view profound hearing loss and the inability to speak as a communication disorder, while most people with hearing impairment who use a sign language to communicate do not. Rather, people who sign argue that theirs is a separate culture from hearing culture and should be considered a cultural entity separate from any conceptualization of disorder imposed by the hearing community. One way to think about cultural groups is by examining the demographic characteristics of the United States.

Demographic Profile of the United States

Since the end of World War II, the cultural makeup of the United States has been changing at a steady pace. According to the 2000 census (United States Census Bureau, 2005), the total adult population in the United States was 281,421,906. Of those, approximately 98 percent identified themselves as being of one race. Of that 98 percent, approximately 77 percent identified themselves as White or Caucasian; approximately 14 percent as Hispanic; approximately 8 percent as Black or African American; not quite 3 percent as Asian; 1 percent as American Indian or Alaska Native; and less than 1 percent as Native Hawaiian or other Pacific Islander. (The numbers don't add up to 100 percent because of rounding.)

Of perhaps greater interest is the fact that the 2000 census identified 72.3 million children, an increase of 8.7 million since the 1990 census, and the largest number in the country's history (O'Hare, 2001). According to O'Hare, 98 percent of the growth in the number of children between 1990 and 2000 was in minority families; only 200,000 of the children were non-Hispanic White children. There are nearly 50.5 million individuals (18.3 percent) in the United States who speak a language other than English at home (American Community Survey, 2002). What this means for the field of communication disorders is that, as professionals, we must attend to the widening circles of diversity that make up our society in order to ensure that our clients can participate in it. Becoming familiar with multicultural issues and concerns affords us the opportunity to develop the necessary sensitivities and tools.

Defining Multicultural

Stockman, Boult, and Robinson (2004) write, "culture can be viewed broadly as the socially constructed and learned ways of believing and behaving that identify groups of people. Verbal and nonverbal communication behaviors readily identify cultural groups. By attaching the prefix *multi-* to the word *culture,* we can refer to more than one socially constructed and learned way of believing and behaving" (p. 6). These authors suggest that the term *multicultural* applies to everyone because everyone belongs to a multicultural group. Specifically, they say that people in every culture have "multiple and complex identities" (p. 6) that are created by their membership in various sorts of groups, including race, ethnicity, gender, social class, religious preference, geographical region, sexual orientation, and linguistic community.

Deciding whether a language variation is a disorder or a cultural difference is an important issue for today's professionals. This subject is discussed further on pages 77–80 in Chapter 4.

Assessment/Diagnosis and Management/Intervention

Two approaches to assessment and intervention are used in communication sciences and disorders: medical and developmental. The medical approach is used for conditions arising from a specific and known cause—a particular disease, injury, or condition—that has resulted in a communication disorder. Labeling the approach "medical" does not imply that the focus is strictly on medical aspects; rather, it means that the process of gathering data and diagnosing the disorder follows that used in the field of medicine, which is to identify and label the disorder and specify its cause. In the medical approach, management of the disorder arises directly from this identification, labeling, and specification of cause.

The developmental approach, on the other hand, focuses, not on diagnosis, but on deciding whether there is a significant problem in communication relative to what is known about normal development. Issues of cause are not of primary concern; rather, attention is given to describing the client's communication and determining what should happen next developmentally. Even when a potential cause can be identified and/or a developmental condition categorized, the focus remains on the developmental sequence of communication rather than on "treating" or managing the underlying cause.

Within the field of communication sciences and disorders, the medical approach is most often utilized when assessing and diagnosing voice disorders; dysarthria and dysphagia; hearing loss; adult neurogenic disorders; and fluency. The developmental approach is most often used when assessing children's language development and consequent disorders; intervention is designed to facilitate and enhance language development. A combination of medical and developmental approaches is used to assess children's articulation and phonological disorders.

Assessment/Diagnosis

The process of assessment leads to the diagnosis of the type and severity of communication disorder exhibited by the client. Here, the purposes, types, benefits, and limitations of assessment are described. Chapter 15 addresses the assessment process in considerably more detail.

Purposes of Assessing

Assessment in the medical approach focuses on three goals:

1. Identifying the underlying cause of the disorder

2. Diagnosing the disorder

3. Arranging for treatment

Assessment in the developmental approach focuses on four goals and methods (Paul, 2001):

1. Screening to find out whether there is a problem

2. Establishing the client's **baseline** function

3. Establishing goals for intervention consisting of appropriate targets and procedures

4. Measuring change across time in intervention to determine whether intervention goals have been met and when to dismiss the client from intervention

Types of Assessments

Professionals in communication sciences and disorders use several types of assessments. They range from informal conversations and interviews with family members, to standardized tests that are administered in quite specific ways, to measurements taken with sophisticated instrumentation such as an **audiometer.** There are five primary types of assessments used when evaluating communication systems. Each is briefly described as below.

Standardized Assessments

Standardized assessments, known as norm-referenced tests, are based on the data collected from a large number of people in statistical groupings based on chronological age. These groups are the norms against which an individual client's scores are compared (Polloway, Miller, & Smith, 2004). For instance, United States children between the ages of 5 and 12 could be a statistical grouping. Standardized tests are called "standardized" for two reasons: (1) they are administered, scored, and interpreted in a standard (i.e., specifically described) manner, and (2) because they are based on a set of norms (i.e., standards) collected from a representative population to which the client is then compared.

Nonstandardized Assessments

Nonstandardized assessments include criterion-referenced procedures, developmental scales, and dynamic assessment. Criterion-referenced procedures are methods that compare the client's performance to a performance standard (e.g., Which components of a story does the child include when telling a story?). Developmental scales provide what is known about a particular aspect of communication development. The clinician then compares the client's current developmental progress against the scale. Dynamic assessment is a method in which the clinician assesses the client's ability to learn a new skill or ability with graduated levels of support.

Interviews with Families and Caregivers

Families and caregivers represent a rich source of information about a client, more so when the client is unable to communicate fluently. The clinician can design an appropriate interview with family and/or caregivers depending on the communication disorder exhibited by the

Baseline
The reference point to which a client's current status is compared (e.g., the results of evaluation at the beginning of therapy) when measuring the degree of progress toward achieving a particular goal.

Audiometer
An instrument used to measure hearing acuity.

Standardized assessments
Tests that are based on the scores of a large number of people with the same characteristics as the person being tested.

Nonstandardized assessments
Instruments or procedures for which norms have not been collected and which may include procedures that are not standardized or specified completely.

Tympanometer
An instrument used to measure the mobility of the eardrum (i.e., tympanic membrane) at different levels of air pressure.

Calibrated
Precisely adjusted in order to measure a particular function.

Otolaryngologist
A physician who specializes in treatment of diseases of the ear, larynx, and upper respiratory tract.

Dysphagia
Difficulty, discomfort, or pain when swallowing.

client. For instance, when interviewing a family member of a child with a language disorder, the clinician will focus on the child's developmental history (including any medical and health issues or concerns); his or her understanding and use of language; and hearing acuity. When interviewing a family member of a client who has suffered a stroke, the clinician will want to obtain information about the client's health prior to the stroke; communicative ability and habits before the stroke; special interests and/or hobbies; personality characteristics; motivation level; current language ability; hearing acuity; and any medical or health problems beyond those associated with the stroke.

Observation of the Client in Familiar Environments

Although clinicians cannot always observe their clients at home, in school, or at work, the ideal scenario would be to make at least one visit to a place with which the client is familiar. Outside the clinic setting, the clinician will almost always be able to discover aspects about the client's communication abilities that were not apparent inside the clinic, hospital, health care facility, or rehabilitation center. Children, especially, are more noticeably comfortable in their own surroundings, and observing their play and routines offers invaluable information that can be utilized in both the assessment and intervention processes. Visiting a client with a voice disorder may reveal aspects of everyday life that impinge directly on the client's ability to progress during the management phase. Similarly, making a home visit to a client who has had a stroke and is back in a familiar environment may yield important clues about how to design subsequent intervention sessions that focus more directly on communication that will be functionally useful to the client in this setting.

Use of Calibrated Instrumentation

Audiologists rely to a large extent on calibrated instruments to measure various aspects of hearing acuity and function. To measure hearing acuity, they make use of audiometers of varying degrees of technological complexity. Assessing middle ear function is done with an instrument called a **tympanometer**. Central auditory function—how the hearing system functions once sound is translated from physical energy to neural energy in the inner ear—is measured with a variety of instruments including electrodes and audiometers. All of these instruments are **calibrated**.

Speech-language pathologists often use calibrated instruments when assessing voice function, particularly when evaluating respiratory and laryngeal function. Noninvasive instruments used include the spirometer (which measures respiratory volume) and strain gauges, magnetometers, and plethysmographs (which all measure respiratory movement). Invasive instruments, which are usually used by an **otolaryngologist** rather than an SLP, used to assess vocal fold condition and function include the endoscope and the stroboscope. The endoscope is a fiberoptic tube, often with a video camera attached (which makes it a videoendoscope), that is inserted into the nose or mouth to view the vocal folds. The stroboscope is a flashing light that is used to view the vocal folds during movement. (Topical anesthesia is required for both.) Speech-language pathologists working with clients with **dysphagia** often use a videofluoroscope. This instrument combines video and x-ray to provide a dynamic record of swallowing.

Benefits and Limitations of Assessment

The chief benefit of the assessment process is that it offers a way to collect information regarding a client's communication abilities, organize the resulting data, and generate relevant and meaningful goals for intervention. Without the assessment phase, developing intervention goals becomes virtually impossible. In addition, the assessment period allows the clinician to develop a relationship of trust with the client, who will be more likely to participate fully in the intervention process knowing the clinician is trustworthy and has his or her best interests at heart.

The assessment process also carries a serious limitation because it can only show limited "peeks" at the client's communication system. Assessment occurs at certain periods, in certain places, and for a limited period of time. In other words, assessment cannot be ongoing, nor can it be totally thorough by its very nature. For this reason, clinicians strive to make certain that the assessment procedures and instruments they use will yield representative samples of the client's communication abilities and not just snippets that may or may not be representative. Using **valid, reliable,** and efficient assessment methods and procedures in combination with an always-growing ability to make accurate clinical judgments, the clinician aims at gathering the most representative information possible during the assessment process. However, clinicians know that the collected information is always just a sample and not a complete picture of the client's communication abilities.

Management/Intervention

Managing communication disorders involves designing therapeutic intervention based on the outcomes of the assessment process described in the previous sections of this chapter. The purposes of intervention, the types of goals utilized in designing intervention, and how to measure progress are described next.

Purpose of Intervention

The intervention process is guided by the results of assessing and evaluating the communication disorder. The primary purpose of intervention is to assist the client in improving his or her communication abilities as much as possible given the nature and severity of the disorder; the client's desire and ability to make changes; and the existence of the resources necessary for making changes.

Types of Goals

Several types of goals are used in management and intervention. Generally, clinicians set both **long-term** and **short-term goals** (the latter are often called objectives). A long-term goal usually specifies the communication abilities and skills that will result from a course of management or intervention. For a client with an articulation disorder in which he substitutes /w/ for /r/, for instance, the long-term goal would be that he successfully produces /r/ in all positions in words 100 percent of the time. The clinician may want to establish a series of short-term objectives written for shorter time periods. For example, one of the first short-term objectives might be for the client to make a close approximation of an /r/ sound once every five tries. A later short-term goal might be for him to correctly produce an /r/ sound at the end of the words *clear, fire*, and *bear* 50 percent of the time he produces the words.

Clinicians working with students in school settings are sometimes required to write goals known as benchmarks or performance objectives. Benchmarks and performance standards are usually linked to abilities considered essential to school success and codified by each state in a set of learning standards to which all schools must adhere. For instance, a benchmark for a

Valid
Measures what it says it measures.

Reliable
Consistently gives the same result on successive trials.

Long-term goals
Statements that specify the measurable outcomes that the clinician is attempting to achieve through the intervention process.

Short-term goals
These are "stepping stones" to achieving long-term goals. They often have to be accomplished in a specific order. Also referred to as short-term objectives.

Efficacy of intervention
Demonstrating that changes in communication ability(ies) occurred that would not have occurred without intervention.

Speech-language pathology assistant (SLPA)
A paraprofessional who helps people who have speech and/or language disorders cope with them under the supervision of a speech-language pathologist.

Audiology assistant
A person working under the supervision of a licensed audiologist.

Phonetics
The study and classification of the sounds made in a spoken language.

Linguistics
The study of the structure and development of a particular language and its relationship to other languages.

child in early elementary school might be to "restate and carry out a variety of oral instructions." The clinician would then write a series of steps the client would need to carry out in order to reach that particular benchmark.

Measuring Progress

For intervention to be considered successful, the client must demonstrate measurable change directly related to the intervention process. To demonstrate the change, as well as to determine whether the intervention goals and/or methods need to be modified, the clinician collects data periodically and compares it with the information and data collected during the initial assessment. In this way, the clinician demonstrates **efficacy of intervention.**

Collecting data can range from a simple tally sheet to the administration of a standardized test. However, standardized testing is used more often at the beginning and end of the intervention process. Monitoring ongoing intervention progress usually involves designing some sort of data collection system that summarizes client progress. Table 2.1 shows an example of a data collection sheet designed for the client described earlier who substitutes /w/ for /r/.

The Professions of Communication Sciences and Disorders

The professionals who have the primary responsibility for helping people cope with their communication disorders are speech-language pathologists (SLPs), **speech-language pathology assistants** (SLPAs), audiologists, and **audiology assistants.** Another group of professionals, speech scientists, studies various aspects of **phonetics** and **linguistics,** including the physiologic, acoustic, and perceptual characteristics of speech.

Speech-language pathologists (also known as speech pathologists; speech therapists; speech clinicians; speech and hearing clinicians; and logopedists) have as their primary responsibility the promotion of the welfare of persons from birth (see Cirrin & Magnusson, 1992 and Rossetti, 2001) to more than 90 years of age who have speech and/or language disorders. Although important aspects of this responsibility include the evaluation, diagnosis, and treatment of these disorders, they are not the only roles of SLPs. SLPs also work with families,

Table 2.1 Data Collection Form (/w/ for /r/ Substitution)					
Initial /r/—Word Imitation	**Sessions**				
	1	**2**	**3**	**4**	**5**
Correct production					
Incorrect production					
Total attempts					
% correct					

teaching them how to communicate with the person with the disorder and how to strengthen their loved one's speech and language development. Many SLPs in school settings work closely with classroom teachers and other professionals in special education.

For people who would like to work with clients with speech and language disorders but are unable to pursue a master's degree in speech-language pathology, there are opportunities to work as a speech-language pathology assistant (SLPA) under the supervision of a speech-language pathologist. Many public schools and medical facilities employ SLPAs.

Audiologists have as their primary responsibility the promotion of the welfare of children and adults who have hearing losses or are at risk for developing them. As with SLPs, their responsibility to persons who have communication impairments is not restricted to the evaluation and treatment of the client's communication disorders. Audiologists engage in a variety of assessments of the integrity and acuity of the hearing mechanism, and they work to develop effective treatment programs for individuals with hearing impairments. In addition, they often fit and maintain hearing aids.

Audiology assistants work under the supervision of a licensed audiologist, performing selected tasks in patient assessment and working with hearing aids and other amplification systems. Their job includes testing the hearing ability of people by means of various hearing tests. Based on the results of the tests (and possibly supplementary examinations), audiology assistants establish where the hearing impairment is located: in the middle ear, the inner ear, the nerve pathways, or the brain. Audiology assistants can also adapt and adjust hearing aids in collaboration with a physician.

Work Settings

Speech-language pathologists, audiologists, and speech-language pathology assistants typically work either in health care (including private practice) or schools. Table 2.2 shows how professionals provide their services in these two settings. Audiology assistants usually work in either private practice or in corporate settings.

Table 2.2	Service Delivery Models	
Types of Service Deliveries	**Settings**	
	Health Care	**School**
Classroom based/Inclusive		X
Community based	X	X
Consultation	X	X
Home based	X	X
Individual "pull-out" intervention	X	X
Group "pull-out" intervention	X	X

American Speech-Language-Hearing Association (ASHA) The primary national professional and scientific organization in the United States that regulates the training and practice of audiologists, speech-language pathologists, and speech-language pathology assistants.

National Student Speech Language Hearing Association (NSSLHA) The preprofessional membership association for students interested in the study of communication sciences and disorders.

Professional Organizations

The primary national professional and scientific organization in the United States that regulates the training and practice of speech-language pathologists and audiologists is the **American Speech-Language-Hearing Association (ASHA).** It is to speech-language pathology and audiology what the American Medical Association is to medicine, the American Dental Association is to dentistry, and the American Psychological Association is to clinical psychology. Its current membership is more than 120,000.

Begun in 1925 as the American Academy of Speech Correction, the organization became the American Society of the Study of Disorders of Speech in 1927; the American Speech Correction Association in 1934; the American Speech and Hearing Association in 1947; and assumed its current name in 1978. Its activities include accrediting master's degree clinical training programs in speech-language pathology and audiology, certifying practitioners in these fields, and fostering improvement of clinical procedures for communication disorders. ASHA's activities include disseminating information through annual conventions in which juried programs are presented by members; publishing professional journals; and accrediting continuing education sponsors, as well as offering its own continuing education activities.

The **National Student Speech Language Hearing Association (NSSLHA),** an ASHA affiliate, is the preprofessional membership association for students who are interested in the study of communication sciences and disorders. Undergraduate, graduate, or doctoral students enrolled full- or part-time in a communication sciences program or related major can become members. For more information, visit their website (2004).

State associations of SLPs and audiologists exist in every state and in Washington, D.C. There is also an Overseas Association of Communication Sciences. Although the state associations are not directly affiliated with ASHA, they often work closely with ASHA on such activities as legislative efforts, professional licensure, and continuing education.

Part 2
Language Development and Disorders

The three chapters in this part of the book address language development and language disorders. Chapter 3 is an overview of typical child and adolescent language development. This chapter is important because understanding language disorders depends on a thorough understanding of how language develops.

In Chapter 4, language disorders are described within the context of the components of language form, content, and use. You will also learn about the language characteristics of children with specific etiologies and conditions, such as autism, language-learning disability, hearing loss, and others. There is also a section on differentiating between a language disorder and a language difference, emphasizing again the importance of taking a multicultural perspective in order to assess language disorders and design appropriate intervention programs for children exhibiting the various characteristics of language disorders.

Chapter 5 focuses on language disorders in adults arising from conditions, diseases, and traumatic events. It begins with a brief discussion of the causes of brain damage and then moves to a description of aphasia, how it is classified, and its symptomatology. Also included is a section on right hemisphere deficits that result from trauma and those that appear with dementia and Alzheimer's disease. The assessment and management sections focus on reducing the severity of the deficit and augmenting the client's remaining communication abilities.

Child and Adolescent Language Development

Chapter 3

Learning Objectives

- Identify the types of students with language disorders served by speech-language pathologists in schools.

- Describe language development from infancy through young adulthood.

- Describe metalinguistic development.

- Describe the relationship between oral language development and the development of writing.

- Describe factors contributing to students' literacy development.

Introduction

Understanding language disorders depends on a thorough understanding of how language develops. Knowledge of language development is the cornerstone for the decisions **speech-language pathologists (SLPs)** make regarding whether a client exhibits a language disorder, or whether that client's language is merely different from his or her age peers, perhaps because of cultural background. To help you better understand language disorders and their effects, the following sections explain the three categories of language **(form, content** and **use)**. The remainder of the chapter takes you through an overview of how language develops from infancy through young adulthood and describes the relationship among language development, literacy, and academic success.

Language Form

Language form refers to the structures we use to build words, phrases, and sentences. Languages are comprised of sets of rule systems that govern the arbitrary symbols used to make meaning at the word, phrase, and sentence level. The rule system governing how we combine sounds is called **phonology,** the rule system governing the markers we put on individual words to mark specific meaning is called **morphology,** the system governing how we combine words into phrases and sentences is called **syntax,** and the rule system governing how we combine phrases and sentences into larger units of meaning is called **discourse.**

Phonology

Phonology is the study of how sounds are used to make syllables and words. Out of the entire set of sounds humans can produce, individual languages each contain a set number of sounds, called **phonemes** that are considered pronounceable. Individual languages differ regarding which sounds are used and which are not. What this means is that, in each language, some speech sound differences matter, and some do not. For instance, in English, one can pronounce the /l/s in *little* with considerable variation without the listener mistaking the meaning of the word. Similarly, in English, *pure* can be pronounced with or without a puff of air on the /p/, but in some languages, a puff of air would change the meaning of the word.

Morphology

Morphology is the study of how people combine phonemes into syllables and syllables into words to convey meaning. **Morphemes** are the smallest grammatical units that carry meaning (phonemes can change meaning, but, individually, they don't carry meaning). An example of a morpheme is the word *cat,* which is considered a **free morpheme** because it can stand alone. Another example of a morpheme is the plural marker *-s,* which, when added to *cat,* results in *cats.* The *-s* plural marker is known as a **bound morpheme** because it cannot stand alone; it must attach to either a free morpheme (as in *cats)* or another bound morpheme that is already attached to a free morpheme. An example of a bound morpheme attaching to another bound morpheme that is already attached to a free morpheme is *-s* in the following: *calculate+tion+s* (calculations).

Language form
Phonology, syntax, and morphology.

Language content
Semantics.

Language use
Pragmatics.

Phonology
The rule system governing how we combine sounds.

Morphology
The rule system governing the smallest units of meaning in language.

Syntax
The rule system governing the use of the grammatical structures of language.

Discourse
The rule system governing how we combine phrases and sentences into larger units of meaning.

Morpheme
The smallest grammatical unit that carries meaning.

Free morpheme
A morpheme that has meaning on its own.

Bound morpheme
A morpheme that must be attached to a free morpheme or another bound morpheme.

Semantics
The rule system governing how words are used.

Each language has its own set of morphemic rules for marking meanings such as:

- plural (*-s* as in *dogs*)

- possessive (*-'s* as in *the girl's dress*)

- verb tenses (*-s* as in *He walks every day*, *-ed* as in *He walked there yesterday*, *-ing* as in *He is walking there now*)

- negation (*un-* as in *undesirable*, *dis-* as in *disinterested*, *im-* as in *impossible*).

Syntax

The rule system governing how people combine words into phrases and sentences is called syntax. Among other things, syntax explains:

- Word order

- When to use active or passive voice

- How to make declaratives, imperatives, or interrogatives

- How to form negatives

- How to make conditional statements

- How to combine sentences into compound and/or complex sentences

Some languages, such as English, rely more on word order (i.e., syntax) to convey meanings, while other languages, such as German, rely more on adding markers to words (i.e., morphology).

Discourse

Discourse refers to the various ways we combine words, phrases, and sentences into larger units to do things such as tell stories; explain how things work; relate experiences; describe events, actions, and ideas; or persuade others. Each type of discourse operates with its own rules, which vary from one language to another.

Language Content

Language content refers to the meaning we make when we string sounds together into syllables, words, phrases, and sentences. Language content is usually referred to as **semantics.** The primary component of semantic ability is vocabulary, although semantics also addresses the relations between specific words, such as homonyms (words that sound the same but have different meanings, such as *pare-pear-pair)*, synonyms (words that have similar or identical meanings, such as *couch-sofa)*, and antonyms (words that are considered to have opposite meanings, such as *top-bottom, big-little, sweet-sour, antonym-synonym)*, among others.

Language Use

Language use focuses on the functions of language. It is typically referred to as **pragmatics**—who says what to whom, how, and when, using the conversational code of conduct described in Chapter 1 on page 5. Pragmatics describes what people's intentions are in using language, how they use language to get what they want, and how they use language to get things done.

How people use language varies according to numerous factors, including:

- *The relative ages of the conversational partner(s).* We use different language when we talk to babies, familiars, and elders.

- *The power dynamic between conversational partners.* We usually use less formal language when the power relationship with a conversational partner is roughly equal, while we use more formal language if we perceive that our conversational partner has more social power. The person in the more powerful position can choose whether to use formal or informal language.

- *The gender of the conversational partners.* In most cultures, both men and women change how they use language depending on whether they're conversing with someone of the same, or different, gender.

- *The degree of respect we wish to convey.* Again, the specific ways in which people change their language to convey (or not convey) respect varies by culture, but in every culture, people make adjustments for this purpose. Interestingly, in some situations, using less formal language indicates a higher degree of respect, while other contexts call for using more formal language. For instance, fans addressing a well-liked athlete often use informal forms of address to show their respect, while these same people would most likely use much more formal language to address a member of the clergy in their faith.

- *The degree to which we know our conversational partners.* When speaking to someone we don't know, most of us use less slang, fewer idiomatic expressions, and more careful diction than when speaking to someone we know. When speaking to a stranger, we use vocabulary we assume the stranger will know, while when speaking with friends, we often use terms known only to our circle of friends.

Try the mind experiments in Study More 3.1 on page 40 to learn more about how you use language differently for different purposes.

Language Development

The arbitrariness of the symbols used in language allows for tremendous power in representing the ideas, feelings, thoughts, events, actions, experiences, possibilities, and wishes we want to communicate about. What does *arbitrary* mean in relation to language? Consider for a moment the word *apple* and the object to which it refers. There is nothing inherent in the actual apple that implies anything about which sounds are used to represent it, the order of those sounds, how they are pronounced, or how they look when written on the page. In short, the apple you see in your mind's eye is totally unrelated to the word *apple* except that it has

Pragmatics
The rule system governing how language is used.

Study More 3.1	**Pragmatics Mind Experiments**

In your mind…

1. Think about how you would ask your best friend if you can borrow some money until next month.

2. Think about how you would ask your parents if you can borrow some money until next month.

3. Imagine you are going to the credit union or the bank where you have a checking account. Think about how you would ask a loan officer to borrow some money until next month.

How did you change what you said and how you said it in each instance? Did you explain more in any of the situations? Was your language more or less formal? Did you use a different tone of voice? Different vocabulary? Did you use any softeners or qualifiers? When?

In your mind…

1. Tell your little brother or sister you are angry at him or her for ruining your favorite CD.

2. Tell your father or mother you are angry at him or her for giving away your favorite pair of jeans.

3. Tell your boss you are unhappy that the promotion you wanted was given to someone else.

Did you change your language in each situation? How? How did you change your vocabulary? Did you change your tone of voice? The length of your sentences? The formality of the language you used? Did you use any softeners or qualifiers? When?

Idioms

An expression with both a literal and nonliteral (i.e., figurative) meaning, the latter understood by a particular group of people to have its own unique meaning (e.g., *to kick the bucket* meaning *to die*).

become customary for a group of people to call it by that name because someone a long time ago called it that. There is nothing inherent in an apple to suggest that it be called an apple; hence, *apple* is an arbitrary symbol used to represent the object we're describing.

Language exists on more than one level. Think about this sentence: "Flying planes can be dangerous." On one level it means that flying planes can be dangerous to the people flying them, while on another it means that planes flying through the air can be dangerous. Or consider the **idiom,** "It's raining cats and dogs." On the literal level, it means cats and dogs are falling from the sky, but on the figurative level it means it's raining hard. To illustrate the idea of multiple levels of language, Study More 3.2 shows examples of double meanings.

What is important to remember is that children develop an awareness of the arbitrariness of language gradually. Similarly, when they are first developing language, they do not

Study More 3.2	**Examples of Double Meanings**

1. Read the sentence below and describe the two levels of meaning.

   Visiting relatives can be a nuisance.

2. Read the sentence below and describe its literal and the figurative meanings.

   He's been under the weather for a few days.

3. Read the words below and imagine how you would use each one to refer to something.

   hare-hair

   pare-pear-pair

   there-their-they're

   two-to-too

   Mary-merry-marry

understand that language has multiple levels; their development of the ability to understand the different levels of language occurs over time.

Children typically learn language in the social context of a family, although different cultures hold different views about how and when to talk to children, and some children grow up in different settings (e.g., foster homes, hospitals, group homes). Most children learn to speak well-formed sentences in spite of hearing the fragments and ill-formed scraps of conversations that are typical of normal communication. For this reason, most language researchers believe that children are born "hard-wired" to learn language, although they differ on the specifics of what constitutes the hardwiring. At the least, children must be in the presence of people using language in order to develop their own language system, whether it is oral or signed. At best, children engage in social interactions with people they trust and who attend to their emerging language skills with delight and pride.

If the child does not grow up hearing (or seeing, in the case of sign language) language, he or she will have a more difficult time learning anything beyond simple vocabulary words. In other words, there seems to be a critical period for developing the capacity to understand and use language; if the child has not learned a language system before puberty, he or she will likely not be able to acquire a complete language system afterward.

Although first spoken words do not appear in most children's communication before 9–12 months of age, children are actively engaged in learning important communication skills beginning in infancy. English language development from infancy through adolescence is described in the following sections.

Prelinguistic Language Development

The period between birth and the emergence of the child's first words is called the *prelinguistic* stage. Communication during this stage depends almost entirely on the efforts of the adults in the child's environment to interpret and react to the child's actions and reactions. Caring adults talk to their infants, respond to them as if they are communicating, and carry on conversations by taking both roles. This communication on the part of the adult, called **motherese,** emphasizes pitch, rate, loudness, stress, rhythm, and intonation rather than meaning or individual words (Polloway, Miller, & Smith, 2004).

Adults using motherese, regardless of gender or age, tend to repeat their utterances, use a singsong intonation pattern, and use exaggerated stress. Motherese focuses on things the infant can see, feel, and/or hear. The adult looks directly in the infant's eyes and smiles throughout the "conversation." If the infant vocalizes, the adult responds as if the baby were saying something and has taken a conversational turn. Adults continue using motherese until their babies reach approximately 6 months of age, after which the adults change their communication patterns to include the use of more informational language (Penman, Cross, Milgrom-Friedman, & Meares, 1983).

One of the most important prelinguistic developments during infancy is the infant's emerging skill in engaging in **joint attending** and **joint referencing** (Bruner, 1975). Both are necessary foundations for the acquisition of language. Joint attending is when the infant and adult both look at the same thing, first each other **(mutual attending),** and then at objects or one of the baby's limbs. Joint referencing emerges out of joint attending. As the baby develops, the

Motherese
The language used by adults communicating with infants in which they use altered pitch, loudness, and intonation patterns to talk about what is going on in the immediate environment.

Joint attending
An infant and adult attend to the same external object or process.

Joint referencing
An infant and adult jointly attend to an external object which the adult talks about.

Mutual attending
An infant and an adult attend to each other.

Babbling
The sounds produced by babies at approximately 6 months of age when they begin to experiment with sounds and before they produce real words.

adult tells the baby what things are called, naming them as they jointly attend to them. Gradually, the baby begins gesturing toward what the adult is talking about, to which the parent responds with enthusiasm. Soon, both adult and baby point to things to indicate joint reference. The baby develops the ability to refer to things through this process of jointly referring with an adult. As first words emerge, they replace pointing.

At around 6 months of age, babies begin producing consonant-vowel (CV) syllables called **babbling,** which seems to consist of experimenting with sounds, although no real words are produced. When babies begin babbling, their conversations with their parents change (Polloway, Miller, & Smith, 2004). They begin to imitate their parents and eventually to initiate conversations with them. During this period, babies develop considerable skill at communicating nonverbally to get what they want. As their mobility and motor abilities increase, they become adept at combining pointing, body gestures, and vocalizations to get adults to respond. They communicate their desires for more juice, a cookie, a visit to a grandparent's, or a hug. As most parents know well, babies in this period develop clear abilities to communicate interrogatives (i.e., questions) and negation.

Preschool Language Development

Preschool language development is usually described as occurring in two phases: the *emerging language* stage and the *developing language* stage. Preschool language development begins around 12 months and continues until about 46 months.

Emerging Language Stage

When children begin producing their first real words, they enter what is called the emerging language stage (Paul, 2001), which usually occurs sometime between 12 and 18 months of age. They rapidly learn a fairly large vocabulary of single words and use them to get a variety of things to happen. The most common communicative purposes for which children use words during the emerging language period are shown in Table 3.1.

When children are around 18 months of age, they begin producing two-word phrases, which marks a leap in the ability to communicate about relationships rather than being limited to referring to one thing at a time. They begin using early forms of syntax, their phonological abilities change considerably, and their pragmatic language shows increased complexity.

Syntax

Syntax in the emerging language stage remains relatively simple. Children's earliest syntactic structures are single words, accompanied by gestures, facial expressions, and intonation. At the end of this stage, they begin using two-word combinations, which are limited in the syntactic structure they can incorporate. The most typical kinds of syntactic constructions children demonstrate in their two-word phrases include:

- Agent + Action *(Car go)*
- Agent + Location *(Cup table)*
- Action + Location *(Go home)*
- Agent + Object *(Girl dress)*

Table 3.1	Emerging Language Stage Communicative Purposes
Communicative Purpose	**Possible Child Utterance**
Rejection	*no*
Nonexistence or disappearance	*all gone*
Cessation or prohibition of action	*stop*
Recurrence	*more*
Existence	*this*
Action on objects	*kiss*
Locative action	*up, fill, out*
Attribution	*big*
Naming, possession, commenting	*dog*
Social interaction	*hi*

During the emerging language stage, interrogatives (i.e., questions) and negations expand into two-word phrases. Negation is typically expressed by saying, "No," and naming whatever is to be negated (e.g., "No coat," meaning "I don't want to put my coat on!"). Questions are usually indicated through rising intonation, as in, "Go Nanny's?" meaning, "Can we go to grandmother's?"

Phonology

Children's phonological abilities develop well into elementary school age, and children in the emerging language stage exhibit wide variations in their phonological systems. Perhaps the most notable is that most children, unable to use adult phonological forms, choose forms that are obviously not adult forms, but they use them consistently so that their conversational partners recognize their meaning. For instance, when I was small, I was unable to say my name and called myself "Leelaw," which my family understood to mean "Lynda." Similarly, unable to say "Granddad," I called my grandfather "Lanlad" long enough that everyone in my family adopted it as his nickname.

Semantics

Children's vocabularies grow significantly during the emerging language stage. When they first start combining words, their vocabularies are somewhere around 20 words, but by the time they are two-years-old, they know approximately 200 words (Gillam & Bedore, 2000).

Pragmatics

Children in the emerging language stage communicate verbally with greater and greater frequency as they develop, engaging in conversations that increasingly take into consideration what the listener already knows or needs to know. Children become better able to ask for information in order to learn about the world, let the listener know his or her message was received, and respond appropriately to someone's request for information (Polloway, Miller, & Smith, 2004).

At the beginning of the emerging language stage, adults have to do most of the conversational work because children assume everyone else knows exactly what they know, what they are thinking, and what they mean in their communication. Even though children become better able to understand that others do not know what they know (and to adjust their communication accordingly), they still have difficulty providing enough information for listeners who do not know them well.

Turn taking, a crucial aspect of successful communication, has its foundation in the earliest give-and-take "conversations" mothers and fathers have with their babies. Joint attending and joint referencing provide early opportunities for babies to learn the rudiments of turn taking, and by the time they reach 18 months of age, most demonstrate basic turn-taking rules in their conversations (Bloom, Rocissano, & Hood, 1976). However, their turn-taking abilities continue to develop well into the elementary school years.

Developing Language Stage

The developing language stage in typically developing children begins at around 27 months and extends until about 46 months (Paul, 2001). During this period, children's language develops rapidly, elaborating on structures and competencies acquired during the emerging language stage. By the time children are around 4 years of age, they have acquired most of the basic structures of language, which they will refine and fine-tune as they enter the educational process and begin using their language abilities to learn in school.

Syntax and Morphology

Children in the developing language stage begin using morphological markers to refine word meanings, adding -s to *dog,* for example, to indicate more than one, or adding -*ing* to *eat,* to indicate present tense. As children learn the rules for morphological markers, they tend to overgeneralize them to those tricky irregular words, saying things like "eated," "drived," and "mouses." First they learn the rules; later they learn the exceptions, a process that lasts well into elementary school.

Phonology

During the developing language stage, children's use of phonology develops quickly. Between 3 and 5 years of age, children develop the ability to use almost all of the phonemes. However, as with syntax and morphology, some of the fine-tuning occurs after they enter school. The phonemes that are still emerging at the end of the developmental period are shown in Study More 3.3.

Semantics

Between ages 2 and 4, children's expressive vocabularies, the words they produce in their own conversations, expand from approximately 200 words to around 1,800 different words (Gillam & Bedore, 2000). Gillam and Bedore report that by age 4, children understand somewhere between 3,000 and 4,000 different words. The types of words they use also increase from nouns and verbs to prepositions (e.g., *in, on, up, down*), words related to time (e.g., *first, then*), adjectives (e.g., *little, big, happy*), and pronouns (e.g., *he, she, him, her*).

	Phonemes Still Emerging at the
Study More 3.3	**End of the Developing Language Stage**

Phoneme	Example
ʃ	<u>s</u>ure
θ	<u>th</u>rill
s	<u>s</u>ip
ð	<u>th</u>is
l	<u>l</u>ake
r	<u>r</u>un
z	<u>z</u>ip
ʒ	trea<u>s</u>ure

Source: Hulit and Howard (2006)

Pragmatics

During the developing language stage, children become much better at engaging in conversations, which means that their adult conversational partners have to do less work to keep the conversation going. By the end of this stage of development, children can take turns conversing over several turns, and they interrupt less. They also understand when their listener doesn't know what they're talking about and can make adjustments and provide more information. Their initial attempts at revising and/or repairing something for a listener may not actually result in a clarification the listener can use, but they become more adept at clarification toward the end of the period.

One of the most interesting aspects of children's pragmatics during this stage is their increasing ability to make indirect, as opposed to direct, requests. At the end of the emerging language stage, most children, when they want something, say something like, "Give me more milk." During the developing language stage, children learn to soften their requests by becoming less direct, saying things like "I need more milk" or "I want more juice, please." These less direct requests are correlated with what are considered polite forms; the indirect language social groups have developed for saying what one wants, thinks, believes, or desires. Without the ability to use polite forms, children may be regarded as rude, unintelligent, arrogant, and/or disrespectful.

Figurative Language

During the developing language stage, children discover other instances of nonliteral, or **figurative language,** including idioms. Idioms are sayings that, on the figurative level, mean something entirely different from what the actual words imply. For instance, *to kick the bucket* means *to die* in some areas of the English-speaking world, but *to die* is nowhere implicit—or explicit—in the words *kick* or *bucket.* Children in the developing language period learn, first, that there are such things as idioms (though they may not have any idea what these funny sayings are called), and, later, what some of them are. In fact, children may learn an idiom as a literal phrase, not knowing, for example, that *hang* in *hang out* has any meaning separate from the entire phrase.

Figurative language
Nonliteral language or language forms that say one thing and mean another (e.g., idioms, polite forms, metaphors, parables, satires, aphorisms, and axioms).

Introduction to Communication Sciences and Disorders

Basic episode
An early narrative form used by children; it consists of a problem, action taken by a character to solve the problem, and resolution of the problem.

Children's verbal humor begins to appear during the developmental language stage, although they do not become fully adept until they are between 8 and 10 years old. Among the first humorous forms to appear are knock-knock jokes and riddles, both of which first appear as unfunny routines that illustrate the child is engaged in learning the general format and only later develops the ability to juggle the demands of the format and the content. Study More 3.4 provides examples of children's developing abilities with knock-knock jokes and riddles.

Discourse

Stories and storytelling exist in all cultures and begin appearing in children's communication in the developing language stage. By the end of this period, children begin telling stories with fictional elements, and they begin retelling their own experiences using a narrative format. The earliest stories children tell usually take the form of a **basic episode**, which consists of an initiating event (some problem that begins the action), followed by an attempt by a character to solve the problem, and a consequence, or resolution of the problem. The ability to engage in narrative thinking and expression becomes especially important when children enter school and are expected to understand stories and to produce stories of their own. Table 3.2 summarizes the primary characteristics of preschool language development.

Study More 3.4	Example Child Joke Retelling

Four-year-old Sue Ann's knock-knock joke:

> Sue Ann: Knock, knock.
>
> Mom: Who's there?
>
> Sue Ann: Sue Ann! [laughs with glee]

Four-year-old Brian and five-year-old Sid are told the following riddle on Halloween:

> Adult: Why didn't the skeleton cross the road?
>
> Both boys: Why?
>
> Adult: Because he didn't have the guts. [Both boys laugh knowingly.]

Here's how each boy retold the riddle to their parents:

> Brian: Why didn't the skeleton cross the road?
>
> Parents: Why not?
>
> Brian: Because he fell down [laughs]

> Sid: Why didn't the skeleton cross the road?
>
> Parents: Why?
>
> Sid: He, he…[rubs his stomach]…he was afraid.

In this example, Brian clearly understood and could use the riddle format, and he may even have understood the double meaning of "guts." However, he was unable to tell the riddle using the double-meaning word. Sid, by rubbing his stomach, showed that he understood that "guts" can refer to stomach, and saying "he was afraid" indicates he knows that "guts" also refers to fear. He is developmentally closer to being able to manipulate both the riddle format and the double-meaning content.

Table 3.2	**Primary Characteristics of Preschool Language Development**	
	Emerging Language Stage: Birth–26 Months	**Developing Language Stage: 27–46 Months**
Syntax and Morphology	• Expands from first word to two-word combinations • Expands use of declaratives, interrogatives, imperatives, and negatives into two-word utterances	• Begins using morphological markers to indicate grammatical meanings (e.g, using -*s* to indicate plurality) • Learns most of the syntactic structures
Phonology	• Does not yet use adult forms, but is consistent in the forms used	• Develops almost all the phonemes in their language; fine-tuning still to come
Semantics	• Expands vocabulary knowledge and use significantly: uses approximately 20 words at the beginning of this stage to over 200 at the end	• Expands vocabulary comprehension and use significantly: uses approximately 200 words at the beginning of the stage to over 1,800 at the end; understands somewhere between 3,000 and 4,000 words at the end
Pragmatics	• Uses few (if any) indirect speech acts • Has little ability to take the listener's perspective • Has limited ability to respond appropriately to requests for clarification • Becomes increasingly adept at turn taking in conversations	• Extends turn taking over several turns during a conversation • Requires listeners to do less work to keep the conversation going • Begins using indirect speech acts (e.g., polite forms and softeners)
Figurative Language	• Does not understand figurative language forms	• Begins using nonliteral language forms such as idioms and colloquialisms • Begins to use verbal humor
Discourse	• Does not yet combine words into larger units to tell stories or explain/describe things	• Begins using basic story telling abilities, though most children in this stage cannot tell a complete story

School-Age Language Development

Between the time most children enter the formal schooling process in kindergarten or first grade and leave for middle school or junior high, their language continues to develop at a rapid pace. Their language expands and becomes more complicated and precise as they shift from learning language to using their language to learn in the classroom. Their burgeoning language skills shift from oral language to reading; writing; figurative language; and narrative and expository discourse. During this stage of development, children are expected to make what Westby (1991) calls the *oral-to-literate shift,* making the transition from using language primarily as a means to regulate social interactions and communicate in face-to-face conversations to using language as a vehicle for regulating thought; constructing abstract ideas; communicating over time and distance; and reflecting. Making this oral-to-literate shift depends on the oral language abilities children develop earlier in syntax, morphology, phonology, semantics, figurative language, pragmatics, and discourse.

Syntax

Because children have learned most of the syntactic structures of English in the developing language stage, their syntactic development once they enter school consists primarily of expanding on the forms they have already learned. In addition, they gradually acquire most of the more difficult forms. Polloway, Miller, and Smith (2004) describe several syntactic processes typical of children in the school-age language learning period.

1. *Expanding noun and verb phrases.* Children in this stage expand their noun and verb phrases through the addition of more adjectives and adverbs and through incorporating more prepositional phrases (e.g., "We went *into the mall* yesterday.") and subordinate clauses (e.g. "We went to the store *that has the cool shoes.*"). During this stage children also fine-tune their usage of irregular plural and tense markers (e.g., *deer, mice, cattle, sheep; ate, drove, swam),* and they include articles appropriately (e.g, "*The* big dog barked at me" when the listener knows which dog is being referred to; "*A* big dog barked at me" when the listener does *not* know the specific dog). Study More 3.5 tells the story of two 12-year-olds who experienced a "eureka" moment about verb tense markers, one example of the fine-tuning that continues throughout childhood and into adolescence.

2. *Decoding passive sentences.* Passive sentence constructions present special difficulties because the order of the words is opposite the order of the events being described, a cognitive mismatch that children at the beginning of this stage are unable to decipher. During this stage, children first figure out how to understand and use *nonreversible*

Study More 3.5   # Dennis Figures Out "Have Tooken"

I began my professional career as a junior high school English teacher in Westminster, Colorado, where I taught 7th and 8th grade English language arts and English literature. Dennis, a bright 7th grade student, had learned Spanish and English simultaneously in a family of migrant workers. He was adept at both languages and used a vernacular speech style in both.

At the end of Dennis's 6th grade school year, his family had moved into the area on a more permanent basis because his father had gotten a year-round job. When Dennis entered 7th grade, he discovered that he liked to read, an activity he hadn't had much opportunity to explore outside school.

I noticed that in his oral speech, Dennis (and several other students) would say things like "I've tooken the book to the library" or "My mom and dad have tooken the car to the garage." When we began studying past participles in English class, I had the students practice writing sentences using "have taken" to see if Dennis would figure out that the "standard" past participle of "take" was "have taken."

For a period of several weeks, none of the students remarked on "have taken" or "have tooken," and they con-

tinued using "have tooken" in their oral language. Then, one day when the students were reading during free time, Dennis came up to where I was sitting and excitedly pointed to a sentence in the book he was reading. "Miss Miller, guess what I just learned!" Thinking he'd read about an interesting event or idea, I asked him what it was. "You can't say 'have tooken!' This guy keeps saying stuff like, 'I've taken the kids to the store,' and 'He's taken the book to school.' Nobody says 'tooken!'"

When I asked him what had caught his attention about "have tooken," he said he didn't know and that it had just started to sound funny to him. When the students were sharing their new learnings after their free period, Dennis excitedly shared his new knowledge with his classmates. Mark, another student whose language included "have tooken," was taken aback because he, too, suddenly realized he had been using a form that didn't coincide with the standard usage. Both boys continued to point out examples of "have tooken" when they heard them, although not all their classmates were entirely happy having their language usage scrutinized.

The story illustrates how the finer points of language usage continue developing well into late childhood and into adolescence.

passives, which are sentences in which the meaning can only be expressed one way. For example, "The mouse was eaten by the cat" is nonreversible since it is extremely unlikely that a mouse could eat a cat, which would be the case if the sentence was "The cat was eaten by the mouse." Later in this period of development, children understand and use *reversible passives,* sentences in which the meaning can be expressed with either of two word orders. For instance, because either event: "The girl was chased by the dog" or "The dog was chased by the girl" is possible, the word order doesn't help children in their attempts to decode the sentence.

3. *Embedding.* Embedded phrases can encode a variety of complicated relationships. One of the first syntactic strategies children learn is to use word order as a primary cue for understanding sentences. To interpret a sentence, children assume that the order of words reflects the order of the events and/or relationships being described. Hence, they understand a sentence such as "The girl who won the election is my sister" as meaning something like "The girl won the election. That girl is my sister." Later in this stage of development, children begin to understand that some sentences cannot be relied on to provide clues to their meaning through word order alone. Children come to realize that a sentence such as "The girl the dog bit ran away" means that the girl ran home, not the dog.

4. *Conjoining.* Children at the beginning of the school-age language stage are able to manipulate straightforward conjoined sentences, most typically those with *and.* During this period, they develop proficiency with the other conjunctions as well. First, they develop the ability to express cause-effect conjunctions such as "We came inside *because* it was raining." Next, they begin using conjunctions that express a contrastive relationship such as "It was raining, *but* we didn't get wet." Later, as their cognitive understanding develops, they are able to use constructions using conditional conjunctions, such as "*If* I do all my chores, I can go to the movie."

Sentences that do not express things in a logical order are more difficult for children to grasp; thus, they develop in children's language later in this period. For instance, putting the effect in front of the cause, as in, "He was late *because* he missed the bus," does not follow the "logical" order of the cause, missing the bus, followed by the effect, being late. Facility with sentences that are "illogical" develops at the end of this stage, at around 10 or 11 years of age.

Morphology

Like syntax, morphology during the school-age language stage becomes a process of learning aspects of English morphology that elaborate on linguistic relationships to extend their meaning further. One example is learning how to produce *gerunds,* which are verbs turned into nouns by adding *-ing* (e.g., *build/building).* Another example of a morphological elaboration that occurs in the school-age language stage is learning to add *-er* to a verb in order to identify the person as the one engaged in the action of the verb (e.g., *paint/painter).* At the beginning of this period, children typically add the *-er* ending to every verb to produce this *agentive* effect (e.g., *type/typer,* or *draw/drawer).* By the end of this stage, children have learned which of these forms are correct in usage, and which are not. A third example of a morphological elaboration occurring in this stage of development is forming adverbs by adding *-ly* to adjectives, (e.g., *slow/slowly).* By the end of the stage, children have figured out the special cases in which adding *-ly* does not work, as in *fast.*

Phonological awareness
Understanding elements of words, such as syllables; initial, medial, and final sounds; sound sequencing; rhyming; and syllabication.

Graphophonemic awareness
The ability to associate letters of the alphabet with speech sounds.

Metalinguistic ability
The ability to think and talk about language.

Phonology and Phonological Awareness

Early in the school-age language development period, children's use of phonology is fine-tuned. Typically developing students can produce all phonemes correctly by approximately age 7. Once children enter school, **phonological awareness** skills becomes necessary in order to:

- Identify rhyming words

- Count syllables in words

- Segment words into syllables and sounds

- Match speech sounds to letters (i.e., **graphophonemic awareness**)

Most children acquire these phonological awareness skills by age 8, although some children require more time and may experience difficulty learning to read and write because both depend on these **metalinguistic abilities.**

Semantics

Vocabulary development, which occurred at a rapid pace during the developing language stage, continues during the school-age years. Vocabulary development is influenced considerably by children's developing knowledge of and interactions with print. Children during this period learn to use words they already know in new ways, to differentiate among words with similar meanings, to select among many words the one that is best suited for their purpose, and to use the same word to mean different things in different contexts (Polloway, Miller, & Smith, 2004). Vocabulary development at this age includes homonyms (words that sound the same but carry different meanings), antonyms (words with opposite meanings), and synonyms (different words with the same meaning). Much of this ability stems from their developing competency in reading as they encounter words used in ways that do not occur in oral language usage.

Two important semantic developments during this period are learning to classify words and learning the English pronoun system. Children first begin classifying words during the developmental language stage into categories such as "animals," "runny things," "people I know," "things I have experienced," and so on. At the end of that stage and into the beginning of the school-age language development period, children begin elaborating their categories to include, for instance, "wild animals," "animals likely to be at a zoo," "pets," and "extinct animals." These elaborations form hierarchical subcategories, which continue to develop into and through adulthood. Study More 3.6 contains an exercise that lets you explore how you think about and categorize words.

The pronoun system is one of the few holdovers from Old English (i.e., Anglo-Saxon) still in general use in English. Old English, like many other Teutonic languages, used a declension system to differentiate gender (masculine, feminine, neutral), person (1st, 2nd, and 3rd), position in the sentence (nominative, possessive, objective, or reflexive), and singular and plural. Table 3.3 on page 52 shows the modern English pronoun system, which children in the developing language stage begin to elaborate. Children vary widely in their pronoun usage, some becoming consistent in their use of pronouns referring to self and not so consistent with pronouns referring to others. Other children will demonstrate just the opposite, or they will develop consistency using first and second person pronouns but not third person. By the end of the developing language stage, typically developing children have mastered most of the

Study More 3.6	Categorizing Words		

1. List as many categories as you can to describe how you classify animals. Don't think about it before you start; just write down the categories that come to mind. Here are the categories I listed without any planning:

wild	free	beautiful animals	ugly animals
domesticated	nonmammals	slow	slimy
four-legged	insects	striped	whiskered
feline	arachnids	multicolored	spotted
canine	two-legged	smart	speedy
equine	slithery	mammals	vertebrates
feathered	graceful	reptilian	invertebrates

Notice that my list is simply an associative list rather than a hierarchically arranged system. Do your categories fit into a hierarchical system? What would be the main categories?

2. Now think about how you categorize words themselves. List as many categories of words as you can without any planning. Here are the categories I thought of without any planning:

nouns	verbs	pronouns	adverbs
adjectives	prepositions	gerunds	participles
articles	proper nouns	locatives	interrogatives
imperatives	indicatives	negatives	names
modifiers	antecedents	conjunctions	predicates
antonyms	synonyms	homonyms	contractions
interjections	collectives	abbreviations	portmanteaus

You can tell from my list that I've probably studied language and know the names of some types of words you've never heard of! Not to worry—look at your list and think how you could arrange the types of words into a hierarchical system. What would be the main categories?

pronouns, though not all, and their pronoun systems will generally reflect their unique approaches to figuring things out.

Figurative Language

Figurative language, which emerges in the developing language stage, becomes more frequent—as well as more fluent—in children's language during the school-age language development period. Children's interactions with print through both reading and writing provide encounters with various forms of figurative language, and afford opportunities for children to develop facility with figurative language that they might not develop otherwise.

Children's ability to manipulate idioms increases considerably during this period, especially after age 7 or 8, when their abilities to understand the multiple levels of language seem to spurt. They begin understanding that idiomatic expressions are best understood, not literally, but in a more abstract (i.e., figurative) manner. Where earlier a child might envision cats and dogs pouring down from the sky when someone said, "It's raining cats and dogs," now he or she understands that the phrase offers a humorous way to depict a particularly hard storm.

Table 3.3		English Pronouns					
		Singular			**Plural**		
		1st	**2nd**	**3rd**	**1st**	**2nd**	**3rd**
Subjective	**Female**	she	you			you	
	Male	he	you			you	
	Neutral	I*		it, one	we*		they
Possessive	**Female**	her, hers	your, yours			your	
	Male	his	your, yours			your	
	Neutral	my, mine*		its, one's	our*		their, theirs
Objective	**Female**	her	you			you	
	Male	him	you			you	
	Neutral	me*		it, one	us*		them
Reflexives	**Female**	herself	yourself			yourselves	
	Male	himself	yourself			yourselves	
	Neutral	myself*		itself, oneself	themselves*		themselves
		* Self-referring pronouns are assumed to carry the gender of the person using them.					

Metaphor
A figure of speech that involves an implicit comparison between two things (e.g., *He's a brick)*.

Simile
A figure of speech that involves an explicit comparison between two things with the use of *like* (e.g., *He's like a big cat)*.

Proverbs, adages, and maxims
Short, witty, popular sayings that impart wisdom.

During this period, children encounter **metaphors** and **similes,** and develop an understanding that each is a particular way of comparing two ideas, events, people, feelings, or experiences. Children also become more adept with **proverbs, adages,** and **maxims** such as "A stitch in time saves nine" or "A bird in the hand is worth two in the bush."

Children's humor continues to develop during this stage (and long after) as they become more proficient with juggling different levels of meaning to produce punchlines. By age 9 or so, children have developed the ability to utilize multiple meanings of words in order to tell jokes that are actually funny, as in this example from Hulit and Howard (1997, p. 230) which capitalizes on two meanings of *flies:*

"What's big and white, has four wheels and flies?"

"A garbage truck!"

Pragmatics

Children's conversational competence during the school-age years increases significantly. They become more proficient at taking turns during conversations with several other people, they learn how to interrupt appropriately, and they learn how to signal their readiness for taking and yielding turns. Their ability to clarify when their listeners don't understand also improves enough that they can use their listener's request for clarification as a guide for exactly how to repair (i.e., clarify) their previous sentences.

Indirect requests become much more frequent when children enter school, largely as a function of their discerning that they have a much better chance at getting what they want if they utilize less direct (i.e., polite) forms. After around age 8, most children have developed enough facility with indirect requests to know which ones to use with each listener.

Learning polite forms is tied to a child's development in understanding that language exists on several levels, and that what one says is not always exactly what one means. For instance, in many cultures, people greet each other by saying some version of "Hi, how are you?" The response is usually "Fine" or "Doing well," even though that may or may not be true. Consider your own behavior when you're greeting a casual acquaintance (we often suspend polite forms with close friends). How often have you wanted to say, "I feel horrid!" even as you respond in the appropriate, socially-sanctioned way? Another example of people saying one thing and meaning another is when an adult will ask a child a question, when what he or she really intends is to give a direction. For instance, the adult might say to the child, "Do you want to look at this book?" when what he or she really means is, "Look at this book." Children in this stage begin to understand these subtle social language skills.

During the school-age years, children also develop considerable **metapragmatic ability.** They become able to attend to their listeners' perspectives and prior knowledge (and consequent conversational needs), engage in different types of conversations (e.g., explanations, descriptions, reports, disagreements, arguments, persuasion, benign teasing), and engage successfully in classroom discourse. When they consciously think or talk about the behaviors and choices they make regarding how they are using language, they are demonstrating metapragmatic ability. They are reflecting on and talking about their use of language, which is more abstract than merely using language without reflection.

Becoming fluent with classroom pragmatics depends on metapragmatic ability, because classroom expectations vary from teacher to teacher and from grade to grade. Children must be able to "code switch," or use language differently in each setting. Sturm and Nelson (1997) also noted that to participate successfully in classroom discourse, students need to understand that:

- Teachers talk and students listen

- Teachers grant permission for students to talk

- Teachers tell students how to do things

- Teachers ask questions and expect specific responses

- Teachers give hints about how to answer

- Students give brief responses

- Students ask few questions, and those are expected to be short

- Students talk to teachers, not each other

- Students make few spontaneous comments

Metapragmatic ability
The ability to think and talk about how language is used.

53

Narrative discourse
Telling actions, feelings, or thoughts of fictional or nonfictional characters.

Expository discourse
Discourse types other than narratives.

Discourse

Not only are children in elementary school expected to make the shift from oral to literate language, they are also expected to develop fluency with new forms of classroom discourse. A sampling of these types are shown in Table 3.4.

Of particular interest during this stage of development are children's emerging facility with two types of discourse: **narrative discourse** and **expository discourse.** Stories take many different forms, some of which are more highly valued in one culture, others more highly valued in another culture. One familiar type of story begins with a protagonist (i.e., hero), set in a particular context, who encounters some sort of problem. The story unfolds through time as the hero takes action to solve the problem. After one or more episodes of trying to solve the problem, the hero reaches some sort of resolution, after which the story ends.

Discourse types other than narratives are called expository discourse and include:

- Descriptive
- Explanatory
- Persuasive/argumentative
- Compare-contrast
- Cause-effect
- Enumerative
- Sequential
- Problem-solution

Table 3.4	Examples of Discourse Types	
Expository Discourse	**Classroom Lectures and Directions**	• Teacher chooses the topic and takes most of the speaking turns • Language often used out of context—requires children to be able to think and talk about language
	Explanations and Descriptions	• Language decontextualized and usually organized hierarchically • Information is new to the student—requires thinking and talking about language
	Argumentative/Persuasive	• Statements or facts are put forth as "proof" • Logical sequence is followed • Others' perspectives taken • Thinking and talking about language are required
Narrative Discourse	**Personal**	• Children talk about own experiences • Usually told to a listener who was not part of the event • Sequence of events follows same pattern as the activities occurred
	Fictional	• Includes generation of own fictional story or retelling of a story • Logical sequence of events is followed • Starts with a problem that characters act to solve

Each of these types of expository discourse has a unique communicative intent and corresponding structure.

Writing

Writing during the school-age years develops almost directly from children's oral language skills and from their emerging reading abilities (Polloway, Miller, & Smith, 2004). When children first begin writing, their writing ability is considerably less well developed than their oral language abilities, but, as their reading becomes more fluent, their writing usually follows. Therefore, children who experience difficulties learning to read will likely experience similar difficulties in their writing.

Most writing in elementary school is done in response to teacher assignments or emerges from a particular child's enthusiasm for writing. Some time around fourth grade, children are expected to use their writing abilities to write for people other than themselves and their teachers. For instance, students may be asked to write to further a cause in their community, solicit information from a local business, or thank a visitor for coming to their classroom.

Children from homes in which writing and print are available and used as part of everyday life often arrive at school with the ability to write their own names and a few additional words, usually the names of others in their household. These children usually possess what is called graphophonemic awareness, the ability to associate letters of the alphabet with speech sounds. They know that print is speech written down and often play with "writing" squiggles, lines, and shapes along a line that suggests the linearity of print. As children explore and experiment with writing, they gradually gain mastery over their writing and begin trying new forms, such as poems, letters, or short essays. Table 3.5 on page 56 summarizes the primary characteristics of school-age language development.

Adolescent Language Development

Larson and McKinley (2003) have described adolescence as unfolding across three stages, each of which can be characterized according to the developmental tasks and stages that are unique to adolescence. Table 3.6 on page 57 shows their characterizations for the early, middle, and late stages of adolescence.

Language development during adolescence marks the transition from childhood to adulthood. The forms, contexts, and styles of language used by adolescents accompany a reduced reliance on family and the increasing importance of friends, music, popular culture, magazines, movies, and the Internet. According to Paul (2001), typically developing adolescents extend the language competencies they have already learned for use in:

- Peer social interactions, which are often intensive

- Literate contexts such as debate, presentations, and written discourse

- Critical thinking

Because language development after the childhood years is not as obvious as the development that occurs during the preschool and elementary school years, some people have concluded that not much development is actually taking place. However, those who study language

Table 3.5	**Primary Characteristics of School-Age Language Development: 4–11 Years**
Syntax and Morphology	• Expands syntactic structures already in use • Learns the most difficult syntactic forms, including passives, conjoining, and embedded phrases • Uses the most complex and least frequent morphological markers such as gerunds, agent -er, and adjectives
Phonology and Phonological Awareness	• Becomes able to use all phonemes appropriately • Develops phonological awareness skills such as rhyming, syllableness, and matching speech sounds to letters
Semantics	• Continues expansion of vocabulary, which is now influenced by rapidly improving reading skills • Elaborates classification of words • Masters most of the English pronouns
Pragmatics	• Becomes proficient in turn taking • Understands subtle social language rules • Interrupts appropriately • Develops metapragmatic ability • Uses conversational repair strategies • Follows classroom pragmatics • Uses indirect requests
Figurative Language	• Develops the ability to use more sophisticated figurative language forms (e.g., metaphors, similes, proverbs, adages, and maxims) • Becomes more proficient with different levels of meaning used in humor
Discourse	• Makes the oral-to-literate shift; from being primarily oral to being able to understand and use written language • Becomes aware of audience (both oral and written) and develops the ability to speak and/or write from that perspective • Becomes able to tell complete stories • Develops the ability to understand and use various forms of expository discourse, though this continues to develop throughout adolescence and young adulthood
Writing	• Uses writing skills that reflect the development of reading skills (i.e., the better the student reads, the better he or she will write) • Becomes able to write complete stories, poems, letters

Metacognitive ability
The ability to think and talk about thinking.

development in older children and adolescents have shown that two crucial aspects of language development occur during this period: (1) the development of meta-awareness about one's own thinking, speaking, listening, and writing, and (2) the development of skills in written language. Adolescent development is characterized by growth in their metalinguistic, **metacognitive,** and metapragmatic abilities. The metalinguistic skills adolescents need include being able to analyze, reorganize, synthesize, and talk about both oral and printed language. Writing puts a particularly heavy demand on adolescents' metalinguistic skills because it cannot be done effectively without reflecting on and manipulating various aspects of language and language levels.

Table 3.6	Characteristics of Tasks and Stages of Typical Adolescence		
Developmental Task	***Stage of Typical Adolescence***		
	Early (10–13 females; 12–14 males)	**Middle (13–16)**	**Late (16–20)**
Acceptance of the Physical Changes of Puberty	• Physical changes occur rapidly but with wide range of person to person variability • Self-consciousness, insecurity, and worry about being different from peers	• Pubertal changes almost complete for girls; boys still undergoing physical changes • Girls more confident; boys more awkward	• Adult appearance, comfortable with physical changes • Physical strength continues to increase, especially for males
Attainment of Independence	• Changes of puberty distinguish early adolescents from children, but do not provide independence • Ambivalence (childhood dependency unattractive, but unprepared for the independence of adulthood) leads to vacillation between parents and peers for support	• Ability to work, drive, date; appearance of more maturity; dependency lessens and peer bonds increase • Conflict with authority, limit testing, experimental and risk-taking behaviors at a maximum	• Independence a realistic social expectation • Continuing education, becoming employed, getting married—all possibilities that often lead to ambivalence about independence
Emergence of a Stable Identity	• Am I OK? Am I normal? • How do I fit into my peer group? • Paradoxical loss of identity in becoming a member of a peer group	• Who am I? • How am I different from other people? • What makes me special or unique?	• Who am I in relation to other people? • What is my role with respect to education, work, sexuality, community, religion, and family?
Development of Cognitive Patterns	• Concrete operational thought: present more real than future; concrete more real than abstract • Egocentrism • Personal fable • Imaginary audience	• Emerging formal operations: abstractions, hypotheses, and thinking about future; personal interests and identity emerging	• Formal operations: thinking about the future, things as they should be, and options; consequences can be considered

From *Communication Solutions for Older Students* (p. 36), by V. L. Larson and N. L. McKinley, 2003, Eau Claire, WI: Thinking Publications. © 2003 by Thinking Publications. Reprinted with permission.

Adolescents must develop metacognitive skills in order to understand and comprehend information; organize information and materials; reflect on their own learning processes and skills; and monitor themselves as they progress through the curriculum. To develop facility with written discourse, for instance, adolescents need to develop competence in outlining logical hierarchies; devising numerical schemes to illustrate ordinate and subordinate relationships; and construct diagrams to represent how information and/or ideas are related.

Larson and McKinley's (2003) summary of the contrasts, general trends, and specific trends between early and later language learning, shown in Table 3.7, describes some of the most salient characteristics of language development during this stage. The specific aspects of language development during adolescence are described in the following sections.

Syntax and Writing

Adolescents typically produce longer, more complicated sentences than they used in the previous stage of development, and they become adept at using specific sentence structures for each type of discourse (e.g., descriptive, explanatory, argumentative). Their sentences contain more

Table 3.7	Contrasts, General Trends, and Specific Trends between Early and Later Language Learning
Contrasts	The major language goal for young children is to acquire spoken language. The major language goal for school-age students is to acquire written communication skills.
	The primary source of language stimulation for young children is spoken communication. For preadolescents and adolescents, both spoken and written communication forms are significant sources of language stimulation.
	Young children learn language in nondirected, informal settings. Older children and adolescents learn a great amount of language through formal instruction.
	Language development in younger children does not require metalinguistic competency. Metalinguistic competency is required for language development in older children and adolescents, especially as they learn to read and write.
	Young children are literal in their interpretations of language. Older children demonstrate increasing ability to appreciate figurative meanings.
	Young children's language and reasoning are concrete. Preadolescents and adolescents are learning language and acquiring reasoning processes that are abstract.
	Young children do not always take the perspective of others when communicating. Preadolescents and adolescents are more aware of listeners' and readers' needs and adjust their spoken and written messages accordingly.
General Trends	In adolescence, it is difficult to state in detail by age level the specific thinking, language, and communication developmental milestones because individuals become increasingly individualistic in their thinking and language abilities.
	During early childhood (birth to age 5), language is acquired rapidly, and the changes that occur from year to year are highly visible. During preadolescence and adolescence, these changes are more subtle, which has probably reinforced the concept that not much happens in language development after age 5.
	Analyzing written communication is as critical as oral communication after about the fourth grade. Written communication may influence oral communication and vice versa during the preadolescent years and beyond.
	During preadolescence and adolescence, the student develops meta-awareness (i.e., the ability to think about one's own thinking, listening, and speaking performance) and thus is capable of revising communication performance based on evaluative feedback.

Table 3.7—*Continued*	

Specific Trends	The child's lexicon (word development), especially word usage, improves greatly during the adolescent years. Quantitatively, upon graduating from high school, the average adolescent has learned the meaning of at least 80,000 different words. Qualitatively, old words take on new and subtle meanings, and it becomes easier to organize and reflect on the content of the word meanings.
	Syntactic structure is greatly affected by the context in which the utterances occur (i.e., setting [school or home]; channel [spoken or written]; and discourse genre [narrative or expository]). The more structured the setting, channel (written), and discourse genre, the more formal, complex, and complete the syntactical utterance.
	At about the age of 9, an important transition occurs in the literacy acquisition process. Children who have thus far been exposed primarily to narrative structures (stories) must begin to comprehend textbooks that are written in expository prose. Around the third grade, the student must read to learn instead of learn to read.
	Thinking becomes more abstract around age 11 years and older. At this time, the adolescent can think about thinking and operate on ideas, not just tangible objects and events.
	Figurative language includes metaphors, similes, idioms, and proverbs. It has been suggested that growth in figurative language production follows a U-shaped curve (i.e., novel, imaginative expressions are frequently produced by preschoolers; then decrease during the elementary years; and then increase during the adolescent years).
	Linguistic ambiguity can be in various forms, such as in isolated sentences, humor, and advertisements. Humor continues to develop during adolescence, and ambiguity alone is viewed as too simplistic by most adolescents. They like humor that is cognitively challenging with abstract themes, such as irony or witty remarks and spontaneous anecdotes.
	Narratives or story-telling ability occurs around 7 years of age; at 7 to 11 years of age, students are producing stories with multiple, embedded narrative structures. Between 13 and 15 years of age, students are capable of analyzing stories. From 16 through adulthood, individuals are capable of more sophisticated analysis (i.e., can generalize about story meaning, formulate abstract statements about the message or theme of the story, and focus on their reaction to the story.

From *Communication Solutions for Older Students* (p. 53–54), by V. L. Larson and N. L. McKinley, 2003, Eau Claire, WI: Thinking Publications. © 2003 by Thinking Publications. Adapted with permission.

interrogatives, negatives, and verb tense markers than younger children's, and they use more literate forms in their writing. Adolescent writing begins to reflect a knowledge of the intended audience, how much information the reader already has (or does not have) regarding the topic, and an organizational framework appropriate for the type of writing.

Semantics

Vocabulary development during adolescence reflects the ever-increasing importance of the literate language forms used in writing. Paul (2001) described adolescent vocabulary development in the following categories:

- Advanced adverbial conjuncts (e.g., *moreover, similarly, consequently, nonetheless*)

- Adverbs of likelihood (e.g., *possibly, probably, definitely, likely*) and adverbs of magnitude (e.g., *considerably, significantly, greatly*)

- Terms related to specific curriculum content (e.g., *photon, obtuse, quadrangle, axis*)

- Specific verb types, such as presuppositional (e.g., *regret*), metalinguistic (e.g., *predict, infer*), and metacognitive (e.g., *hypothesize, conclude*)

- Multiple-meaning words (e.g., *sore, pitch*)

- Multiple-function words (e.g., *soft face, soft water, soft blanket*)

Adolescents also come to understand how words are related through:

- Derivation (e.g., *music-musician; phonetics-phonetician*)

- Meaning (e.g., antonyms such as *pleased-disappointed*, synonyms such as *mesa-butte*, sound such as *pear-pare-pair)*

Pragmatics

Though some parents would disagree, most adolescents are fluent conversational partners. That is, they usually understand what they need to say so listeners will understand what is being said; they know how to take turns appropriately during the conversation; they know how to repair a conversational breakdown; they can interrupt appropriately in various social contexts; and they know how to ask for clarification if they don't understand something that is being said. Of course, one of the characteristics of adolescents is that they don't always see the need to demonstrate their knowledge of appropriate pragmatic language use, especially with their parents.

Metapragmatic ability is required in order to engage in virtually all literate discourse, because one must know the purpose of each type of writing; who one's audience is and what they already know; which discourse genre best matches the purpose and the audience; and how to build one's sentences for the particular discourse genre and audience (Polloway, Miller, & Smith, 2004).

Figurative Language and Slang

Adolescents develop considerable fluency with figurative language of various sorts. Much of adolescent humor depends on multiple meanings and levels of language, especially idioms. Adolescent slang requires a sophisticated metalinguistic ability and plays a major role in how adolescents are perceived and accepted by their peers. The ability to use the slang characteristic of one's peer group may be the single most important language development to occur during adolescence.

Discourse

Adolescents also develop considerable expertise with the multiple types of discourse they encounter in school, both through different teaching styles manifested by multiple teachers, and through the diverse expository texts they are required to read and comprehend. After children leave elementary school, they are expected to be relatively fluent with more extensive forms of expository and narrative discourse in both oral and written form. Table 3.8 summarizes the primary characteristics of adolescent language development.

Young Adult Language Development (Ages 20+)

Language development continues throughout adulthood; however, language development in adulthood has not been studied as thoroughly as language development at younger ages. According to Owens (2001), although language continues to grow in all areas during adulthood, the most prevalent changes occur in the semantic and pragmatic areas. Semantic development continues throughout adulthood as people continue to add new words to their lexicon. Young adults enrolled in higher education typically add significantly to their lexicons as they take

Table 3.8	Primary Characteristics of Adolescent Language Development: Ages 12–19
Syntax and Writing	• Produces longer, more complicated sentences • Uses specific sentence structures for each type of discourse • Uses more literate forms in writing • Begins to reflect a knowledge of the intended audience in writing
Semantics	• Vocabulary development reflects literate language forms used in writing • Comes to understand how words are related through derivation and meaning
Pragmatics	• Becomes fluent conversational partners • Increases metapragmatic ability
Figurative Language	• Bases humor on multiple meaning words • Use of slang plays a major role in peer perception
Discourse	• Develops expertise with multiple types of discourse types in school • Becomes relatively fluent with more extensive forms of argumentative and persuasive discourse

courses replete with terms specific to particular fields of study. Too, their reading assignments introduce them to words they would not encounter in oral language. Young adults continue to expand their abilities to understand relationships among words, particularly if they study foreign languages, many of which have contributed substantially to the English vocabulary.

A recent examination of persuasive writing in children, adolescents, and adults found that the syntactic, semantic, and pragmatic language used improved steadily from childhood to adulthood (Nippold, Ward-Lonergan, & Fanning, 2005). The changes included a "gradual increases in essay length; mean length of utterance; relative clause production; and the use of literate words, including adverbial conjuncts (e.g., *typically, however, finally),* abstract nouns (e.g., *longevity, respect, kindness),* and metalinguistic and metacognitive verbs (e.g., *reflect, argue, disagree)"* (p. 125).

Pragmatic development in young adults reflects their continuing cognitive growth, especially their ability to take the perspective of others and to communicate on an abstract level about topics with many dimensions and perspectives (Owens, 2001). As young adults gain competency in understanding other people's viewpoints, they gain greater control of language structure in their efforts to take their audience into account. As they shift perspective from one person to another, their language reflects the shifts through choice of vocabulary, sentence structure, and style of discourse. Young adults typically belong to more than one social group, each of which uses its own style of language. In addition, workplace environments use different styles of language; young adults may find themselves using a variety of language styles within one workplace, as, for instance, in talking on the phone; writing reports; sending e-mail messages; talking to superiors or subordinates; and presenting information to colleagues.

Communicating on an abstract level about topics with different dimensions and perspectives requires the young adult to use language that can describe coordinated, multiattributional descriptions of objects, events, and ideas (Owens, 2001). This sort of language use is a distinct change from the more personal, one-dimensional descriptions used by younger children and adolescents. As pointed out above, young adults' lives take place in more than

Conjunct
A device used to signal a logical relationship between sentences (e.g., *still, to conclude*).

Dysjunct
A device used to indicate the speaker's attitude toward the content of a sentence (e.g., *frankly, honestly*).

one communication context, including those requiring the use of more formal, literate language. Young adults frequently find themselves in situations in which they must make a bridge between one topic and another in order to change the subject of conversation, which necessitates using a sentence or two to segue from one topic to another, perhaps unrelated, topic. Young adults also become more adept with what are called **conjuncts** and **dysjuncts**. The primary characteristics of young adult language development are shown in Table 3.9.

Relationships among Language Development, Literacy, and Academic Success

Previous sections have referred to the oral-to-literate shift children undergo as they make the transition from primarily using oral language to using print language for learning and communication. Although social, cognitive, and motor skills are involved in moving from orality to literacy, language development remains the most important and necessary component of the shift.

Factors Contributing to Becoming Literate

Several factors contribute to children becoming literate. Among the earliest influences is the literacy level of the child's family. Children from families in which literate language is a part of everyday life arrive at school with many of the preliteracy skills necessary for making the shift into literate language. For instance, these children already know that:

- Print generally represents speech (though what print represents changes as children become more adept at using print)

Table 3.9	Primary Characteristics of Young Adult Language Development: Ages 20⁺	
Syntax and Writing	• Develops skills in tandem with educational achievement • Increases essay length • Increases mean length of utterance • Produces relative clauses
Semantics	• Uses literate words • Continues to add new words to lexicon • Adds terms specific to a field of study in higher education
Pragmatics	• Takes the perspective of people whose experiences are not shared • Takes greater command of language structures to speak and write for a particular audience • Uses more formal language • Uses the discourse style of various groups • Learns the pragmatics of the work setting • Segues from one topic to another

- Words have smaller components

- You can talk about language and about talking

- Letters correspond to sounds

- Stories involve a problem, characters who try to solve the problem, and a solution to the problem

- Print is read left to right, and book pages turn from right to left

- Pencils, pens, markers, and crayons can be used to write

- Signs (e.g., road signs, billboards, advertisements) contain messages

A second factor contributing to children's emerging literacy is their own language ability. Children whose language development is atypical may experience difficulty acquiring the literacy skills necessary for school success, particularly if they have a language disorder associated with cognitive disabilities, severe hearing loss, behavior disorders, or moderate to severe autism. Even children with mild or moderate language disorders not associated with other disabilities may struggle to acquire the literacy skills they need.

A third factor affecting literacy development is **bilingualism.** Children learning English as a second language sometimes exert such energy to learning the basic content, forms, and uses of English that they fall behind their English-speaking age peers in developing literacy skills. In their native language, these children may possess the language abilities that underlie becoming literate, but their development of English may not be sufficient to make the transition.

Language Bases for Academic Success

As children progress in school through the early elementary grades, literacy and academic success become more entwined. By the time children exit elementary school, they are expected to use their language abilities to understand and produce a variety of literate language forms, both oral and print. These language abilities include:

- Applying phonological awareness skills (e.g., segmenting words into smaller units, synthesizing sounds and syllables into words)

- Using an extensive vocabulary

- Defining words

- Applying metalinguistic, metapragmatic, and metacognitive skills

- Understanding and producing compound, complex, and compound-complex sentences

- Understanding and using advanced morphological markers (e.g., exceptions to general rules and markers for infrequent grammatical constructions)

- Understanding their audience and their purpose in speaking or writing

- Using appropriate organizational and stylistic conventions for each discourse genre

Bilingual
Proficiency in (or developing proficiency in) two languages.

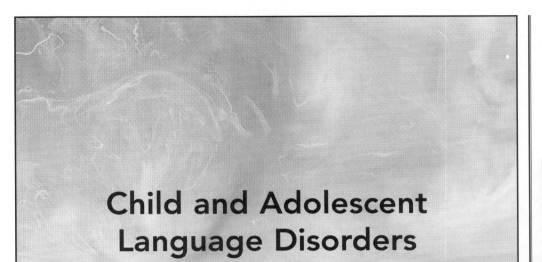

Child and Adolescent Language Disorders

Chapter 4

Learning Objectives

- Describe disorders of language form, content, and use.

- Describe the language characteristics of children and adolescents with various etiologies.

- Differentiate between language disorder and language difference.

- Explain how to design assessment and intervention for multicultural clients.

- Describe the primary types of language intervention used with children and adolescents.

Introduction

According to the National Institute on Deafness and Other Communication Disorders (NIDCD; 2002b), there are approximately six to eight million people in the United States with a language disorder; approximately 6 percent of children in preschool and early school years have a **specific language impairment (SLI).** In addition to children with SLI, children with related disorders, such as **cognitive disabilities** and learning disabilities, may have language disorders related to their primary disorder. **Speech-language pathologists (SLPs)** provide language services to all these populations of children and adolescents.

The majority of SLPs providing services to children with language disorders work in school settings. According to a survey conducted by the American Speech-Language-Hearing Association (ASHA) in 2003, 71 percent of SLPs employed full time indicated that they provide services in a school setting (ASHA, 2004a). Table 4.1 shows the percentage of SLPs in schools who serve children with SLI and other impairments that have accompanying language disorders. As this shows, SLPs in school settings spend considerable time providing services to children and adolescents with language disorders.

A child or adolescent with a language disorder may have difficulty with any or all areas of language—phonology, morphology, syntax, semantics, or pragmatics. Roseberry-McKibbin and Hegde (2000) believe that children and adolescents who have a disruption within their language systems are unable to "interact, within their families, communities, or cultures, in a manner consistent with that of their peers or with societal expectations" (p. 178). The main symptom of a childhood or adolescent language disorder is the lack of ability to understand

Specific language impairment (SLI)
Difficulty with language (i.e., communication) in the absence of another problem such as cognitive disability, hearing loss, or emotional disorders (NIDCD, 2005e). Also referred to as language-learning disability (LLD).

Cognitive disability
A condition characterized by significantly below average intelligence and limitations in daily life functions; appears before the age of 18.

Table 4.1	Types of Students Served by SLPs in Schools
Disorder	**Percentage of SLPs Who Serve Students with This Disorder**
Articulation/Phonological disorders	93.4
AD/HD	70.5
Auditory processing disorder	66.9
Autism/Pervasive developmental delay (PDD)	80.2
Learning disabilities	74.5
Mental retardation/Developmental disabilities (MR/DD)	73.6
Nonverbal, augmentative/alternative communication (AAC)	48.9
Pragmatics/Social communication	76.2
Reading & writing/literacy	39.7
Specific language impairment (SLI)	57.0
Traumatic brain injury (TBI)	19.3

Source: American Speech-Language-Hearing Association (2004a)

Phonological disorder
A language disorder in which sound substitutions and omissions result from a lack of awareness of the phonemes that words contain, rather than errors programming the articulators to produce desired phonemes (as is the case with an articulation disorder).

Syntactic disorder
Difficulties understanding sentence structures and/or combining words into phrases and sentences.

Morphological disorder
Difficulties understanding and/or producing morphemes, the smallest units of meaning.

and/or formulate language as well as other children the same age. With older children, adolescents, or young adults who have a language disorder, the deficit may be relatively subtle. For example, they may have poorer comprehension of humor or **figurative language** than peers, or they may have difficulty writing.

It is important for you to have read Chapter 3 carefully in order for the material in this chapter to make sense. The information on language development will help you understand the discussions of how language disorders are described, identified, and remediated.

Disorders of Language Form, Content, and Use

Children and adolescents can exhibit language disorders in form, content, use, or any combination of these three aspects of language. Disorders in **language form** include difficulties with **phonology** (i.e., speech sound system), **syntax** (i.e., use of grammatical structures), and/or **morphology** (i.e., use of markers). Disorders in **language content** typically appear as problems with vocabulary development and word meaning (i.e., **semantics**). Disorders of **language use** appear as difficulties adjusting language form and content to match varying social settings and conditions (i.e., **pragmatics**).

Disorders of Language Form

The American Speech-Language-Hearing Association (ASHA) describes a **phonological disorder** as "an impaired comprehension of the sound system of a language and the rules that govern the sound combinations" (ASHA Ad Hoc Committee on Service Delivery in the Schools, 1993). The committee indicated that, compared with their age peers, children with phonological disorders have difficulty producing the speech sounds of their language and that, for the majority of these children (80 percent), the disorder is severe enough to require treatment by a speech-language pathologist (SLP).

Many (50–70 percent) of children who are identified as having a phonological disorder at a young age experience subsequent difficulties with reading, writing, spelling, and mathematics (ASHA Ad Hoc Committee on Service Delivery in the Schools, 1993). In a 2004 survey, over 93 percent of school-based SLPs indicated that they provided services to children with phonological or articulation disorders (ASHA, 2004a). ASHA estimates that phonological disorders affect approximately 10 percent of children in the first grade (2005n).

Children and adolescents with **syntactic** and **morphological disorders** may demonstrate reduced ability to understand and/or produce longer or more complex sentences. They frequently use short, simple syntactic structures. Their syntax and morphology is slow to develop and often remains at a relatively unelaborated level. They rely on the most common morphological markers and may have difficulty learning exceptions to morphological and/or syntactic rules. In addition, children with syntactic and morphological disorders produce a limited variety of syntactic structures; their sentences may exhibit persistent errors; and they have difficulty using connectives (e.g., *because, but)* and words indicating relationships, such as *moreover* and *therefore.*

Disorders of Language Content

Children and adolescents who experience difficulty with language content are usually identified as having **semantic disorders.** They may have problems with word-retrieval in conversational speech, which can result in various disfluencies (e.g., repeating, starting over, or revising). In addition, they may have difficulty defining words and they may not be able to elaborate on word meanings beyond simple, basic statements. Another characteristic of the language of children and adolescents with semantic disorders is difficulty in using specific referents that actually name what they are referring to. Instead, they use words such as *stuff, thing, this, that,* or they use nonverbal cues to indicate what they are referring to.

Students with semantic disorders also have difficulty understanding word relationships such as derivatives (e.g., *science-scientist),* antonyms (e.g., *graceful-clumsy),* synonyms (e.g., *couch-sofa),* and sound (e.g., *two-to-too).* They may be unable to form adverbs (e.g., *happily, slowly, gracefully)* or use adverbial conjunctives (e.g., *therefore, nonetheless).*

Disorders of Language Use

Children and adolescents who struggle with language use are described as having a **pragmatic disorder.** These students often are unable to participate effectively in conversations because they are unable to take the perspective of their listeners, they may not know how to take turns appropriately, and they may be unable to provide clarification if a listener asks for it. These students also have difficulty participating in the various discourses they encounter in school because they are unable to shift the form and content of their language to fit individual settings and contexts.

Students with pragmatic language disorders often experience difficulty with figurative language and **metapragmatics.** As a result they struggle with humor; idioms; slang; using language to learn; and reflecting on their own language use and learning strategies. They may ask questions in class that seem irrelevant or disrespectful, interrupt at inopportune times, and use non sequiturs. Because of their difficulty with metalinguistic processes, students with pragmatic language disorders continue to use direct rather than indirect language, which often results in others thinking them impolite or rude. In addition, they have difficulty discerning the difference between facts, opinions, arguments, and hypotheses.

Language Disorders with Specific Etiologies

Language disorders arise from a variety of etiologies or conditions. Roseberry-McKibbin and Hegde (2000) organize language disorders into three categories:

- Specific language impairment (SLI), also called language-learning disabilities (LLD)

- Language problems associated with physical and sensory disabilities

- Language difficulties subsequent to a combination of physical and social-environmental factors (e.g., poverty; neglect or abuse; alcohol or drug exposure in utero; and **attention-deficit/hyperactivity disorder)**

Semantic disorder
Difficulty understanding and/or assigning meaning to words.

Pragmatic disorder
Difficulties understanding how to use language in different ways for a variety of intentions, situations, and listeners.

Attention-deficit/hyperactivity disorder (AD/HD)
A neurobiological condition affecting an individual's ability to maintain attention.

Dyslexia
Learning disabilities associated with reading.

Word-finding problems
Difficulty retrieving specific words accompanied by pauses, repetitions, starting over, and use of generic terms such as *thing,* or *stuff.* Also referred to as word-retrieval problems.

Unintelligible
Speech with so many errors it is difficult or impossible to understand.

The following sections discuss language characteristics of children and adolescents with some specific etiologies.

Language-Learning Disabilities (LLD)

The terms language-learning disabilities and specific language impairments are often used interchangeably. However, some speech-language pathologists use SLI to refer to children prior to their entering elementary school and LLD to refer to children once they have entered elementary school. The relationship between language and learning disabilities, although not linear, certainly seems to suggest that early language problems often reappear in the school years as a learning disability sometimes called **dyslexia.** ASHA explains that language-based learning disabilities interfere with reading, writing, and spelling (2005h), while dyslexia refers to learning disabilities with reading only. The term LLD is used in this textbook because the term highlights the importance of language to learning and the relationship between language disorders and learning disabilities. However, because states use their own terminology to define disorders related to language and learning disabilities, you may encounter different terminology in your own state.

Children are identified as having a language-learning disability when their difficulties are specific to language and not secondary to some other disability. The cause of LLD is not known, nor do these children exhibit associated conditions such as cognitive disabilities, neurological impairment, or sensorimotor problems. Approximately 60 percent of SLPs in school settings indicate that they provide services to students with SLI (ASHA, 2003a).

Children with LLD frequently begin talking later than their peers, acquire words relatively slowly, and have **word-finding** (i.e., word-retrieval) **problems.** Although children with LLD have delayed language skills, their language development usually follows the same sequence of their typically developing peers in spite of their difficulties with specific components of language.

Many children with LLD have problems with articulation and phonology. These children are often difficult to understand (i.e., their speech is relatively **unintelligible),** and their phonological development proceeds at a considerably slower rate than their typically developing peers. Children with LLD commonly have problems with **phonological awareness.** They often struggle to learn the alphabet and to understand the relationship between print and speech. They have difficulty sequencing the sounds in a word, particularly if the word is more than one syllable in length.

Children with LLD often have difficulty with syntax and morphology. Their utterances are frequently short and simple, retaining essential meaning but omitting smaller grammatical units such as *the, a,* and *an.* Their syntax is usually simple and contains few compound, complex, and/or compound-complex sentences. In addition, they may have difficulty comprehending directions, questions, or complex sentences. Children with LLD may show errors in singular and plural forms of words (e.g., "That a cats" for "That is a cat"), possessives (e.g., "There is the dog bed" for "There is the dog's bed"), the present progressive –*ing* (e.g., "Dog eat" for "The dog is eating"), third-person singular noun form (e.g., "He go outside" for "He goes outside"), is verb forms (e.g., "Dog eating" for "The dog is eating"), past tense markers (e.g., "He walk" for "He walked"), and pronoun forms (e.g., "Him is at the movie" for "He is at the movie").

The pragmatic abilities of children with LLD are often affected. Some children with LLD are relatively passive conversationalists, expressing and responding little to their conversational partners. Others may be expressive yet unresponsive to their partners. These children experience difficulties with turn taking; introducing and maintaining topics appropriately; interrupting appropriately; maintaining coherence throughout a story or explanation; and repairing conversations that have suffered a breakdown. They seem relatively unable to take the perspective of their listeners and have little concept of varying audiences.

Children with LLD often do not understand how stories are constructed and organized, nor can they tell stories using the usual story structures that include a problem, a character attempting to solve the problem, and a resolution of the problem. They also find expository discourse difficult to comprehend and may not be able to see the organizational frameworks of the various types of expository discourse (e.g., descriptive, explanatory, cause-effect, compare-contrast, argumentative/persuasive).

Cognitive Disabilities

A cognitive disability, is characterized by significantly below average intelligence and limitations in daily life functions. Cognitive disabilities may arise any time before age 18. Approximately 1 percent of children age 3–10 in the United States have a cognitive disability (National Center on Birth Defects and Developmental Disabilities, Centers for Disease Control and Prevention, 2002).

Because they can arise from a wide range of conditions, cognitive disabilities constitute a diverse group of individuals. It can be caused by injury, disease, or brain abnormality. The most common known causes are Down syndrome, fragile X syndrome, and fetal alcohol syndrome (National Center on Birth Defects, 2002). Some cognitive disabilities are mild, while others are severe. The more severe the disability, the greater the consequences to communication and language development.

The language development of individuals with mild cognitive disabilities usually follows the same sequence as typically developing children, albeit at a slower pace. Thus, their language abilities often resemble those of younger children. However, if the disability is severe, the individual may exhibit language that is **idiosyncratic** and unlike younger children.

Children with even a mild cognitive disability may show difficulties with all aspects of language form, content, and use. Their articulation and phonological skills are often delayed, making it difficult to understand their speech. Their semantic abilities are compromised by their relatively small receptive and expressive vocabularies and difficulties in understanding relationships between words. Their syntax is more typical of younger children; that is, they understand and use short, simple utterances and have difficulties comprehending and expressing longer, more complex syntactic structures. The morphological abilities of children with cognitive disabilities are often more compromised than their syntactic abilities, primarily because of the abstract nature of morphological markers (Roseberry-McKibbin & Hegde, 2000). Lastly, their pragmatic abilities suffer. They have difficulty understanding the nature of less direct language forms; the nature of turn taking; taking others' perspectives; and organizing and telling a story.

Idiosyncratic
Unique, one-of-a-kind, or distinctive.

Autism
A neurologically based developmental disability with social, developmental, and physical symptoms. Usually described in terms of autism spectrum disorder.

Pervasive developmental disorder (PDD)
A set of five syndromes including autistic disorder, Asperger syndrome, childhood disintegrative disorder, Rett's syndrome, and pervasive developmental disorder (not otherwise specified).

Executive functions
The many skills required to prepare for and execute complex behavior (e.g., plan, organize, multitask, use feedback).

Autism Spectrum Disorders

Autism is a neurologically-based developmental disability with social, developmental, and physical symptoms (ASHA, 2006). The symptoms of autism, which continue throughout the lifespan, typically appear sometime in the first three years of life and are four times more prevalent in males than females. The three primary symptoms of autism are (1) difficulties with social interaction, (2) problems with verbal and nonverbal communication, and (3) repetitive behaviors or narrow, obsessive interests (National Institute on Neurological Disorders and Stroke, 2003). Each of these symptoms can range from mild to severe. Over 80 percent of school-based SLPs report that their caseloads include students with autism spectrum disorders (ASHA, 2004a).

Although many people refer to the disorder as autism, the American Psychiatric Association (APA; 2000) lists the disorder as **pervasive developmental disorder (PDD)** with five diagnoses along the spectrum:

- *Autistic disorder,* which begins in childhood, is characterized by significantly abnormal and/or impaired development in social interaction and communication, along with significantly restricted range of activities and interests. How the disorder manifests depends on the chronological and developmental age of the individual affected (ASHA, 2006).

- *Asperger syndrome,* which is characterized by challenges in social competence, (e.g., friendship/relationship development, perspective taking, social skills, nonverbal communication) and the academic areas of **executive functions,** self-management, reading to learn, writing, sensory perception, and motor control (Kaufman & Larson, 2005).

- *Childhood disintegrative disorder,* a rare disorder associated with severe cognitive impairment, is characterized by at least two years of normal development, followed by significantly severe and prolonged regression in multiple areas, such as language, social skills, adaptive behavior, play, motor skills, or bowel/bladder control. Children with childhood disintegrative disorder show qualitative impairment in social interaction, communication, and play, as well as idiosyncratic repetitive and stereotyped behavior patterns (ASHA, 2006).

- *Rett's syndrome,* which is believed to be the result of a chromosomal mutation on the X chromosome, is a progressive neurological disorder beginning with a period of normal development. Between 1 and 4 years of age, previously acquired skills are lost and muscle tone is reduced. Purposeful hand movements are replaced with repetitive hand movements such as washing, licking, clapping, and/or wringing. The syndrome occurs almost exclusively in girls and is accompanied by a reduced ability to express feelings; reduced eye contact; abnormalities in gait; seizures; and delayed head and brain development (ASHA, 2006).

- *Pervasive developmental disorder–not otherwise specified (PDD–NOS),* is used to describe children who show marked impairments in social interaction and communication and/or stereotypic behavior patterns or interests, but who do not exhibit all the features of any of the other categories of pervasive developmental disorder. Usually, social skills are less impaired than in classic autism (APA, 2000).

Roseberry-McKibbin and Hegde (2000) describe the general characteristics of children with any of the diagnoses under PDD as:

> a lack of responsiveness to and awareness of other people; a preference for solitude and objects rather than people; a lack of interest in nonverbal and verbal communication; stereotypic body movements such as rocking; a dislike of being touched or held; self-injurious behaviors such as head banging (in some children); unusual talent in some areas such as arithmetic. (p. 184)

Children with diagnoses under PDD exhibit a variety of communication and language problems. Their communication problems include a lack of interest in communicative interaction; a lack of **joint attending** and **joint referencing,** and a general lack of interest in the human voice. Language problems include:

- A slow developmental rate overall

- Pragmatic difficulties, including knowing how to maintain eye contact; take turns; interrupt; introduce and maintain a topic; use indirect language; and take the listener's perspective

- Greater ease of learning words associated with objects than words associated with emotions or feelings

- **Perseveration** on certain words or phrases

- Inability to generalize word meanings and to understand relationships between words

- Frequent pronoun reversals (e.g., *you* for *I*) and referring to self in the third person (i.e., *she* for *I*)

- Use of short, simple syntactic structures

- Frequent use of **echolalia**

Attention-Deficit/Hyperactivity Disorder

According to the American Psychiatric Association (2000), attention-deficit/hyperactivity disorder (AD/HD) is the most common mental health disorder in children, affecting 3–5 percent of school-age children. Children with AD/HD frequently have language problems, which means that SLPs provide services to a relatively high proportion of children with AD/HD. In a 2004 ASHA survey, almost 71 percent of SLPs in school settings indicated they worked with students with AD/HD (ASHA, 2004a).

Although AD/HD is seen most often in school-age children, it continues to affect people throughout their lives. AD/HD is treatable, but it is a permanent condition that extends into multiple contexts and environments. AD/HD may exist alone or be associated with other **comorbid** conditions such as learning disabilities, psychiatric disorders, or other **developmental disabilities** (Geffner, 2005). According to ASHA, the two primary symptoms of AD/HD are inattention and hyperactivity-impulsivity (2005b).

Inattention seems to stem from difficulty concentrating; sensory stimuli and one's own thoughts impede focusing and attending. Consequently, students with AD/HD appear as if they

Perseveration
Continuing to repeat a behavior to an exceptional degree (e.g., saying a word or phrase over and over).

Echolalia
Repeating what others say without communicative intent.

Comorbid
The presence of coexisting or additional diseases with reference to an initial diagnosis.

Developmental disability
A diverse group of physical, cognitive, psychological, sensory, and speech-language impairments that arise any time before age 18.

are not listening. Inattention seems to vary according to the interest of the person affected. This means that a child may be able to attend to and concentrate on some activities for extended periods but be unable to plan, organize, or complete other tasks of less interest. In addition, students with AD/HD may not be able to monitor their own behavior in some situations and contexts.

Hyperactivity and impulsivity often appear together, though they are somewhat different. Hyperactivity means difficulty sitting still—fidgeting, squirming, moving about, tapping pencils, wiggling, and touching things. Students with hyperactivity often switch quickly from task to task without completing any of them. Students exhibiting impulsivity appear to have problems thinking before they act. For instance, these students may barge into a game, interrupt speakers, or hit someone when they are frustrated.

Students with AD/HD often have difficulties with various aspects of communication, language, and speech. Pragmatic language is often affected because of the impulsivity, hyperactivity, and inattention associated with AD/HD. Students with AD/HD frequently have problems modifying their language to fit specific settings and conversational partners, which often appears to others as being rude or impolite. Students with AD/HD frequently barge into conversations without knowing the topic, without acknowledging that someone else (e.g., a teacher) is speaking, and without any apparent knowledge of likely consequences. In addition, these students do not seem to consider their listener's background and knowledge, resulting in statements that cannot be understood by their listeners. Pragmatic language in students with AD/HD is also affected by their relative inability to switch from the informal language of home and the playground to the more formal and literate forms required for participation throughout school. These students may talk to authority figures using the same casual language they use with their friends, again resulting in being thought rude and/or disrespectful.

Discourse in students with AD/HD is often disorganized. They frequently have difficulties telling stories because they cannot put together all the necessary components and because they cannot sustain attention throughout the entire story. In addition, they may experience considerable difficulty following what is being said in stories and in other discourse forms, particularly those with relatively abstract organizational schemes such as argumentative/persuasive, explanatory, compare-contrast, and descriptive.

Hearing Impairments

Normal hearing is essential to acquiring spoken language, but individuals without normal hearing may learn other communication systems. Hearing allows an infant to become aware of environmental and speech sounds and to understand and use spoken language, which includes monitoring one's own voice, speech, and language production (Roseberry-McKibbin & Hegde, 2000). Roseberry-McKibbin and Hegde reported that the degree to which a hearing impairment affects speech, language, and voice depends on both the age of onset and the degree of the hearing loss. Children who experience **prelingual deafness** are more likely to have difficulties with language acquisition than those who experience **postlingual deafness** (Roseberry-McKibbin & Hegde). In addition, the more severe the hearing loss, the more severe its impact is likely to be on the child's communication development. However, people respond in different ways to hearing impairments. Some individuals with relatively severe hearing loss use language well, while others with the same onset and degree of loss struggle to acquire language.

Many individuals with prelingual deafness find it difficult to communicate orally, preferring instead to use signs, gestures, and/or other types of **manual communication systems.** Children exposed to a fully developed sign language are usually able to acquire the language without difficulty and use sign language as their primary mode of communication. However, even though they may be fluent with sign language, spoken and written English may not be easily accessible. Depending on their educational experiences, they may also learn to read and write in English, with the result that they become **bilingual.**

When prelingually deaf children are exposed only or primarily to oral language, they frequently exhibit specific characteristics, including:

- Limited oral communication

- Reduced understanding of oral communication

- Difficulties with pragmatic language, especially providing background information and maintaining topic

- Reduced understanding and use of compound and complex syntactic structures

- Difficulties using various morphemes such as tense markers, possessives, present progressive *-ing,* conjunctions, articles, prepositions, and indefinite pronouns (Roseberry-McKibbin & Hegde, 2000)

- Low reading comprehension

- Poor writing skills

Cultural Deprivation

Cultural deprivation refers to a variety of situations and conditions that are correlated with language disorders, including low socioeconomic status (i.e., low income), low educational levels of family members, and limited access to adequate health care. However, you should note that these factors do not cause language disorders, nor do they always result in language disorders. In fact, the factor most closely related to language development is the mother's educational level (Battle & Anderson, 1998).

Many children who grow up in families with low income and limited access to health care develop excellent language skills. Among families in which educational level is low and there is a history of low literacy levels, children's language development suffers. Language development is adversely affected by inadequate oral stimulation from adults; few (if any) opportunities to engage in the preliteracy activities known to enhance language development (e.g., being read aloud to, seeing print used as an integral part of everyday life, hearing adults talk about language); few opportunities to be exposed to enriching activities that stimulate language development (e.g., going to a children's museum, an art fair, or a zoo); and limited access to toys and books that stimulate language development (Roseberry-McKibbin & Hegde, 2000).

The language of children with limited access to language-enriching experiences and activities includes these characteristics (McKibbin & Hegde, 2000):

- Limited oral vocabulary

- Limited oral expression

Manual communication system A communication system that uses gestures, body language, and facial expressions in place of the voice to mediate a message.

Prenatal
An event occurring prior to birth.

Perinatal
An event occurring during the birth process.

Postnatal
An event occurring just after birth.

Traumatic brain injury (TBI)
Injury to the brain that results from an accident (e.g., a traffic accident involving a motorcycle). TBI is the most common cause of brain damage in children and young adults.

Cerebral palsy (CP)
A neuromuscular disorder resulting from damage to the brain occurring prior to, during, or shortly after birth.

Congenital
Present at birth.

Degenerative
Causing a gradual decline in quality, value, or strength.

- Problems using language to sequence events and experiences

- Inability to use the language of school (e.g., reciting the alphabet, reading books, rhyming)

- Slow development of syntax and morphology

- Difficulties in reading and writing

Brain Injury

Two types of brain injury in children result in language disorders: (1) **prenatal, perinatal,** or **postnatal** brain injury; and (2) **traumatic brain injury (TBI)** that occurs some time after the birth process. Examples of prenatal brain injury are maternal rubella (i.e., measles), mumps, or accidents; examples of perinatal injuries are problems during the birth process (e.g., breech delivery or prolonged labor); examples of postnatal injuries are reduced oxygen to the brain, infection, diseases (e.g., meningitis), or accidents (Roseberry-McKibbin & Hegde, 2000).

Brain injuries occurring pre-, peri-, or postnatally result in **cerebral palsy (CP),** which is characterized by various neuromuscular problems. The language disorders resulting from cerebral palsy depend on which parts of the brain are damaged and whether there are other problems such as cognitive disabilities. Some children have severe impairments; others do not.

Traumatic brain injury (TBI) is caused by an external physical force rather than **congenital, degenerative,** or birth-related injuries to the brain. It can be either an open head injury or a closed head injury. TBI can result in total or partial disability in any of several areas of functioning, including language (Individuals with Disabilities Education Improvement Act, 2004). According to Roseberry-McKibbin & Hegde (2000), the most common causes of TBI in children are car accidents, sports-related accidents, falls, physical abuse, assaults, and gunshot wounds.

The language disorders resulting from TBI may be temporary or long-term, or a combination of both, depending on the nature and severity of the injury. Children who have suffered a TBI often have difficulty understanding what is being said, struggle to find words, are slow to process information, and have difficulty remembering things. They tend to struggle with attending, often losing focus easily. Their abilities to reason and organize may be affected, including the ability to organize long, complex sentences. Often their pragmatic abilities are affected, particularly knowing how to take turns in conversations, maintain a topic of conversation over multiple turns, and provide appropriate background information to listeners. They may have problems with figurative language, which affects their ability to understand and produce humor, idioms, and metaphors.

Adolescent Language Disorders

An adolescent with one of the disorders discussed above will most likely have been diagnosed earlier, except in the case of TBI, which can occur at any time throughout the life span. For most adolescents, language disorders are related specifically to problems with reading, writing, and academic achievement. The secondary curriculum makes considerable demands on students' reading and writing. For students with weak language systems, the academic challenges can be profound. In addition, the social intricacies of adolescence require considerable language facility in order to fit in and interact successfully with peers.

Adolescents with language disorders often exhibit difficulties with the varied language styles used by different teachers; the increased amount of work in secondary school; the increased reliance on writing as a way to learn and think; longer class sessions covering one or more topics; a wider variety of test formats to negotiate; the increased decontextualization of the information being taught (i.e., the information is more abstract and removed from the here and now); and the introduction of new symbol systems used to encode information (especially in mathematics and the sciences). Adolescents encounter many more instances of figurative language across all content areas, which may present particular difficulties for students with language disorders. Also, students in secondary school are expected to reflect on their own thinking, learning, and language use—another situation that presents problems for students with language disorders. These students may need additional help in learning how to use resources; learn; study; and use language to evaluate and present information in a variety of discourses.

Larson and McKinley (2003) have categorized the language disorders of adolescents into eight categories:

- *Cognitive deficits,* which surface as difficulty learning concepts

- *Metalinguistic deficits,* which can impede their ability to reflect on language

- *Linguistic feature deficits,* which affect their ability to comprehend spoken and written language

- *Discourse deficits,* which limit their ability to participate easily with peers, in the various discourses used in the classroom, and in conversations with teachers and other adults

- *Nonverbal communication difficulties,* which impede their ability to understand and use the nonverbal markers that are essential to communication

- *Reading deficits,* which limit their ability to make the oral-to-literate shift into reading to learn, as well as limiting their continued development of the more complex forms of oral language

- *Writing deficits,* which can interfere with their production of coherent and logical writing

- *Spelling deficits,* which can occur even if they have no difficulties with reading and/or writing, and which can reduce the clarity of their writing

Language Disorders versus Language Differences

Language usage varies across cultural groups. What is acceptable, or even preferred, in one cultural group may not be in another. For this reason, SLPs need to differentiate between what constitutes a language disorder and what constitutes a language difference related to cultural usage.

Introduction to Communication Sciences and Disorders

Language disorder
Impaired comprehension and/or expression of language form, content, and/or use.

Language difference
Variation of language used by a group of individuals with shared regional, social, or cultural/ethnic factors.

Code switching
Switching from one style of language usage to another, depending on context and the social situation.

A **language disorder** is impaired comprehension and/or expression of language content, form, and/or use. ASHA defines a **language difference** as "a variation of a symbol system used by a group of individuals that reflects and is determined by shared regional, social, or cultural/ethnic factors" (2004b ¶1).

In recent years, increasing numbers of people from a large number of countries have immigrated into the United States, each group speaking its own language and/or dialect. The Clover Park School District in Lakewood, Washington, reports that students there speak 36 different languages (2005), the Community Unit School District in Wheaton, Illinois, reports over 60 different languages spoken by their students (2004), and the Dallas Independent School District reports approximately 70 languages are spoken there (2003).

Each of the students in these districts is likely to be developing competence in English at a different rate and in a relatively unique fashion, though students from the same cultural backgrounds probably share some of the same patterns of English language development. Factors that influence children's learning English as a second language include how long they have been in the United States; the level of education of family members; English fluency of family members; age of the child; previous exposure to English; how long the child has been learning English; and family attitudes toward school and academic success.

Bilingual children who are learning English as a second language, or who speak a dialect other than Standard American English, frequently exhibit language characteristics that might be mistaken for a language disorder unless careful consideration is given to each child's situation. Children learning two languages, whether simultaneously or sequentially, often demonstrate growth bursts in one language, while development in the other language seems to plateau for a period of time. These growth bursts can continue throughout the course of acquiring the languages, seesawing between the two. If viewed in isolation, the child's development in the language that is on a plateau compared to the one that is showing a growth burst may appear to be delayed, or even disordered in comparison.

In addition, children learning two languages, especially in the early stages, often engage in what is called **code switching.** Code switching, while it may call attention to itself, is not considered a communication disorder because it is a normal progression in the acquisition of a second language. What is important is the child's overall language system that includes both languages. If this overall language system contains the forms, content, and usages that are customary and appropriate in the child's environment and culture, a communication disorder cannot be said to be present.

People in different geographic regions of the United States also speak different dialects of English. Each dialect uses its own unique semantics and syntax. Texans, for instance, are recognized by their use of "y'all" (you all), "fixin' to" (preparing), and "fur piece" (far away). New Englanders agree by saying, "Ayup," get a drink from a "bubbla" (drinking fountain), and eat a "grindah" (sub sandwich or hoagie) for lunch. Dialects also follow their own syntactical rules. African American English (AAE), for example, repeats the noun subject with a pronoun (e.g., "My father, he work there.") and uses the same form for singular and plural nouns (e.g., *one girl, five girl).* Dialectical differences such as these, must be seen as language differences, not disorders.

The dialects spoken by the greatest number of people in the United States are AAE, Spanish-influenced English, and Asian English (Owens, 2001). Within these dialects, there is considerable variation related to country of origin (e.g., Puerto Rico, Mexico, Spain; Vietnam, Indonesia, or Thailand), geographic region in the United States (e.g., West coast Spanish-influenced English, or Texas Spanish-influenced English), and socioeconomic characteristics (e.g., "upper class" dialects, and "lower class" dialects).

People from different cultures view communication in different ways, often using different means to accomplish the same end, such as having a request met. For instance, people who live in cultures oriented toward the individual tend to use direct language that can easily be understood outside the immediate context of the conversation, which is called *low-context* language (e.g., if someone writes, "I bought a shirt yesterday," you understand all the referents without having to be present in the immediate context). In these cultures, being too indirect can be seen as a sign of weakness or a lack of self-assuredness, or as a sign of a feminine way of communicating. On the other hand, people from cultures oriented more toward the collective, or larger social group, tend to use language that is more indirect and tied to the immediate context. Language with these characteristics is called *high-context* because it is not so easily understood outside the context of the immediate conversation (e.g., "I bought one, too" isn't immediately understandable unless you are present to know what *one* refers to). In these cultures, people use language to promote group cohesion, and being too direct can be seen as bringing too much attention to the individual.

Different cultures also have different ideas about how status and connection influence communication. Tannen (1992) reports that in some Asian cultures such as Japanese, Chinese, and Javanese, people in close relationship (e.g., parents and their children) tend to communicate in a more hierarchical manner, while those in less close relationship (e.g., business associates) tend to communicate in a more egalitarian way. In contrast, people in Western European cultures who are in close relationship communicate in a more egalitarian manner, while those in less close relationship communicate in a more hierarchical manner.

Cultural variations also exist regarding appropriate distance between conversational partners. Edward T. Hall (1966), an anthropologist who studied spatial relationships in communication, found that in the United States people engaged in conversation stand between four to seven inches apart—just close enough to touch. In many countries, the expected social distance is roughly half that. In Arab countries, for example, friends are expected to stand close enough to smell each other's breath because "to deny the smell of your breath to a friend is considered an insult in most Arab cultures" (Gudykunst, 1998, p. 101).

Other cultural variations in communication include:

- In Japan, a collective culture, people are viewed as more truthful the less they speak (i.e., silence is seen as directly connected with truthfulness). In individualistic cultures (e.g., American), silences are seen as awkward and in need of filling.

- In Arab cultures, the use of assertion and exaggeration is the norm, while in Western and most Asian cultures these characteristics are often viewed as offensive.

- French and Italian cultures use a more animated style of communicating, using a far wider range of intonation, volume, and body gestures than people in many other cultures.

- In many cultures, not making eye contact is a nonverbal sign of respect for someone in authority, rather than the dishonesty or avoidance associated with it in other cultures.

It would be impossible for any individual SLP to know all the characteristics of the languages and dialects spoken by school children today. However, SLPs can become attuned to multicultural issues and develop a set of resources for making certain that children receive appropriate assessments and intervention when warranted. ASHA recommends that SLPs develop an understanding of the following (2003b, ¶3):

- Cultural differences in verbal and nonverbal communication

- Cultural differences in communicative discourse and narrative style

- Cultural norms for greeting and addressing individuals

- Culturally based learning style preferences

- Cultural differences in rules for adult-child discourse

- Cultural differences in the conversational roles of children

- The impact of cultural communication and learning style differences on the educational and/or clinical process

Management of Language Disorders

Management of language disorders is influenced by a number of factors, including:

- The age of the person with a language disorder—child, adolescent, or adult

- The cause of the disorder, if known

- The developmental level of the client's language

- The severity of the disorder

- The age at which the disorder was first diagnosed and what has been done to ameliorate it since

- The family's and client's attitudes toward intervention

- The setting in which the assessment and intervention will take place (e.g., school, clinic, hospital)

- Whether English is the native language of the client

- If the client speaks a dialect of English

Management typically consists of three phases: (1) assessment; (2) intervention and ongoing data collection; and (3) reassessment. The assessment process determines what the intervention will be and how it will be provided, although other factors, such as where intervention will take place (e.g., school or clinic), also contribute to the design of intervention. For instance, language intervention that will occur in a clinic may not include classroom collaboration between the SLP and the child's teacher, while school-based intervention may take place entirely in the child's classroom, necessitating ongoing collaboration.

Purposes of Intervention

Olswang and Bain (1991) believe there are three purposes for language intervention with students: (1) changing or eliminating the problem causing the disorder; (2) changing the language disorder itself; and (3) teaching compensatory strategies. Changing or eliminating the problem causing a language disorder is difficult or impossible in most cases, because the underlying cause is either unknown or unchangeable. Changing the language disorder involves teaching the client specific language components, which is the approach that the majority of SLPs use. Teaching compensatory strategies is also used, although it may require the client to use metalinguistic, metacognitive, and/or metapragmatic abilities, which makes it a more suitable approach for upper elementary students, adolescents, and young adults.

Paul (2001) believes that identifying the purpose of intervention is a critical first step in designing the exact nature of the intervention processes and activities. Which purpose is selected depends on the nature and severity of the language disorder, the age of the client, previous intervention successes and/or failures, and the child's communication needs in everyday life.

Larson and McKinley (2003) point out that, although younger children may not always know the purpose of the intervention they are receiving for a language disorder, adolescents not only must know the purpose, they must also be full partners in planning their goals and objectives. That is not to say the clinician does not provide guidance; however, adolescents are more highly motivated to engage in the intervention process if they have formulated their own language goals.

Types of Intervention

All language intervention is not alike. As you might imagine, the type of intervention selected for any particular client with a language disorder will be affected by the same factors that influence the choice of purpose for the intervention, including age, severity of the disorder, degree of support from family, previous intervention successes and/or failures, and the child's specific communication needs in everyday life. Intervention can be family-based; individual- or group-based; or classroom-based.

Family-Based Intervention Programs

Often young children and clients with severe language disorders receive intervention through a family-based program. In family-based intervention, the SLP works directly with the family members closest to the child, teaching them how to interact with the child (or adolescent or young adult, in the case of a severe disorder) to promote the child's acquisition of specific communication and language skills. For children just learning to use words, for example, the SLP demonstrates to family members how to draw the child's attention to an object; name the object; offer it to the child; and play with the child and the object, all the while emphasizing the name of the object throughout the interaction. The SLP provides the family with a list of the words to emphasize in their interactions with the child and specific behaviors to look for in the child to indicate comprehension of the words on the list. The SLP also teaches the family members how to generally interact with the child in such a way to facilitate language development, both comprehension and expression, perhaps through reading aloud to the child, singing songs, or reciting rhymes.

Family-based intervention for an older child who has suffered a TBI might involve providing family members with a list of language behaviors characteristic of the particular injury suffered by the child, along with information on how to respond to emotional outbursts and frustration. Immediately following the TBI, the SLP may function more as a resource for parents rather than providing face-to-face intervention for the child. As the child regains brain function, the SLP may take a more direct role in the intervention process.

Individual and Group Therapy

Clients in hospital and clinical settings receive intervention in individual sessions, group sessions, or both. Students in schools also receive language intervention individually or in small groups; they can also receive intervention in their classrooms. Whether to provide intervention in individual or group sessions is not only determined by the type of intervention needed to address the disorder, but sometimes by the SLP's scheduling constraints. Some children benefit greatly from interacting with their peers throughout the intervention process, while others respond much more favorably when they receive one-to-one intervention. The primary factor in deciding whether to see individuals alone or in groups is determining which would be most beneficial to each client.

Classroom-Based Intervention

SLPs who work in schools increasingly provide language intervention in classrooms, working with classroom teachers to design and deliver the intervention. Some SLPs design an intervention plan and consult with the classroom teacher about how it can most effectively be implemented by the teacher. Other times, the SLP and the teacher collaborate in the design of intervention and then co-teach the plan in the classroom. In this situation, the SLP and the teacher jointly plan the intervention and then take turns teaching the plan, acting as the lead teacher and teaching consultant during the lesson, or using flexible groupings to each work with a group of students. In these situations, the language targets are embedded into the lesson and taught to all students. A third situation involves the SLP coming into the classroom to teach a small group of students with language disorders using a plan designed by the SLP. Although students without language disorders may be part of the group, the primary focus of the intervention is on specific language skills and processes.

Intervention with Adolescents

Language intervention with adolescents requires a somewhat different approach from that used with younger children because of their developmental needs. Larson and McKinley (2003) describe some general guidelines to use with adolescents at three different stages. For preteens and youth in early adolescence, they advocate developing the language students will need in order to be successful academically and to be accepted by their peers. For students in middle adolescence, language goals include academic growth, interacting successfully with peers, and beginning to think about vocational considerations. For students in late adolescence, language goals shift away from the academic to focus more on the language students will need for vocational success and for establishing and maintaining one-to-one personal relationships.

Larson and McKinley (2003) emphasize that one of the SLP's most important roles is to assist adolescents to take responsibility for their communication disorder and the behaviors necessary to change it. They offer these specific suggestions for SLPs:

- Take time to sit down with the student to listen and to talk.

- Ask the student questions about his or her communication and organization problems.

- Suggest ways the student could address his or her communication and organization problems.

- Stick to what the student wants to talk about.

- Assist the student in knowing his or her legal rights and becoming a self-advocate.

In addition to their suggestions regarding how SLPs can best support adolescents in learning to take responsibility for their communication disorder and how to manage it, Larson and McKinley (2003) also offer a list of things SLPs should avoid when communicating with an adolescent:

- Jump to conclusions before the student finishes talking

- Ignore the topic the student raises

- Hurry the student

- Avoid talking with the student about her or his concerns

- Show a flat affect

- Ignore the student as he or she is talking (e.g., working on something else)

Language intervention with adolescents requires that clinicians be flexible; be willing to counsel when necessary; listen attentively and thoroughly; and offer guidance grounded in their professional knowledge and experience.

Intervention with Multicultural Populations

Cultural perceptions of health, disease, communication, and authority all play significant roles in the intervention process. ASHA (1996) has identified four primary factors to consider when planning intervention with multicultural (bilingual and nonstandard English-speaking) populations:

1. Determine the most appropriate language of intervention.

2. Identify the cultural factors that might influence the intervention process.

3. Implement a culturally appropriate intervention program.

4. Select culturally sensitive materials and activities.

Appropriate Language for Children and Adults

Planning any sort of communication intervention with any client involves knowing his or her primary language and any secondary languages. Choosing which language to use during the intervention process differs depending on the age of the client (child versus adult), the desires of family members, and, particularly in the case of bilingual children, the political climate regarding bilingual education.

Choosing which language to use during the intervention process will depend on the nature of the communication disorder and the family's wishes regarding their child's fluency in their first or subsequent languages. For instance, parents of one bilingual child with a voice disorder may wish for intervention in his or her native language, while the parents of another bilingual child with the same disorder may wish the intervention to proceed in the child's second language. In the first case, a clinician who speaks the child's native language would be preferable. In the second case, the clinician must determine whether the child's second language is sufficiently developed for the intervention to proceed in an effective and efficient manner. If not, the clinician will need to counsel the parents about the need to conduct intervention in the child's native language.

Adult clients who cannot speak for themselves because of disease or injury to the brain will most often have family members who will be able to describe to the clinician the client's language abilities prior to intervention. In most cases, it will be obvious which language will be most effective and efficient to use during intervention. In those rare instances when a client has been equally fluent in more than one language, initial diagnostic testing will focus on determining which language faculties, if any, have been retained and are thus available to the intervention process. Ideally, the clinician will be fluent in whichever language appears during diagnostic testing to be most intact.

The political climate regarding bilingual education in the United States often dictates what language may be used in educational settings or how long a child's native language may be used in instruction. Language researcher Judith Johnston (2006) has pointed out that these policies are rarely based on objective research data.

Service Delivery with Multicultural Populations

Communication sciences and disorders professionals address the needs of linguistically diverse clients in a number of areas, including accent training for adults who wish to modify their accents for occupational and/or social reasons; diagnosis and intervention for children who have speech, language and/or hearing disorders; and diagnosis and intervention for adults who have communication disorders following injury or disease. According to Roseberry-McKibbin (1997), service delivery with multicultural populations is based on a foundation of understanding and knowledge about:

- The culture's beliefs and practices, including general beliefs, as well as beliefs and practices regarding religion; family life; health and disabilities; and education

- Linguistic considerations, including the culture's communication styles and linguistic characteristics and patterns

The American Speech-Language-Hearing Association (2005d, 2005o) recommends the following guidelines for those working with clients from different cultures.

1. Obtain a thorough case history to determine:

   - How long has the family resided in the United States?

   - When was English introduced?

   - In what settings is English spoken?

   - What language is used at home, work, and/or school?

   - What language does the family use?

- How does the client's language compare to that of peers who have been exposed to two languages?

- What are the dialectal variations typical of the accent or dialect?

- Who is responsible for health care and the overall wellness of the client?

- What forms of medicine or health care service delivery are used?

2. Conduct a preliminary assessment.

   - Determine whether there is a communication difference or a language disorder.

   - Obtain a language sample.

   - Determine whether one language is dominant.

   - Translate all written documents into the family's native language.

   - Use culturally and linguistically appropriate test materials.

   - If further speech and language assessment is necessary, conduct the assessment in the client's dominant language (if there is one). If necessary, work with an interpreter to complete the assessment.

3. Provide intervention for a speech-language disorder.

   - When designing intervention, consider how the client's native language or dialect may have influenced performance during assessment.

   - Distinguish between a language difference (e.g., dialectal variations) and a language disorder.

   - Provide intervention services to clients with communication disorders after counseling with the family. Be aware of the family's attitudes and beliefs regarding communication disorders.

   - Provide accent modification for clients who elect such service.

4. Provide intervention for clients with hearing disorders.

   - Use oral or sign language interpreters during aural rehabilitation.

   - Consider the client's culture when discussing treatment options and anticipated treatment outcomes.

ASHA has also designed a set of self-assessment checklists for cultural competency that is available online (2005l). The checklists offer an opportunity for you to gauge your beliefs and attitudes toward other cultures, and the degree to which an agency or clinic attends to the needs of linguistically and culturally different populations.

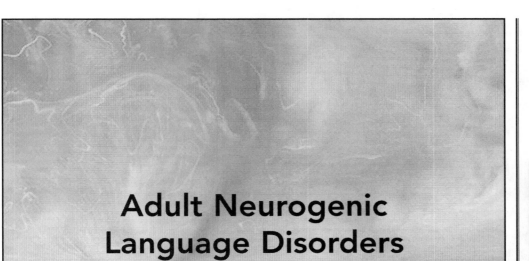

Adult Neurogenic Language Disorders

Chapter 5

Learning Objectives

- Describe the neurology of aphasia.

- Identify the primary causes of brain injury and resulting aphasia.

- Describe the primary types of aphasia and their language characteristics.

- Describe the most common nonlanguage characteristics of people with aphasia.

- Describe right hemisphere deficits and language characteristics.

- Describe dementia and associated language characteristics.

- Discuss the primary types of intervention used with aphasia, right hemisphere deficits, and dementia.

Chapter

5

Introduction

Adults, like children, can be impaired in their ability to comprehend and/or use language. Most adults who have such impairments were able to comprehend and use language normally when they were younger but lost their language abilities because of damage to their brain, usually somewhere in the **left cerebral hemisphere** (see Figure 5.1).

The adult language disorder that speech-language pathologists (SLPs) have been concerned with primarily is **aphasia,** which is the main focus of this chapter. Right hemisphere deficits can also produce symptoms requiring the services of an SLP. The two discussed in this chapter are **dementia** and **traumatic brain injury (TBI).**

People who have aphasia—mostly adults over 40—have lost some ability to understand and/or formulate language because of damage to the brain—specifically, to the **cerebral cortex.** Language abilities that may be impaired include understanding speech, speaking, reading, writing, and calculating (e.g., doing simple addition, subtraction, multiplication, and division). Although it is possible for only one or two of these language abilities to be impaired, in most cases all are impaired. The degree of impairment, however, varies across abilities and between people. One person who has aphasia, for example, may be more impaired in his or her ability to speak than to understand speech while the opposite may be true for another person. Part of these differences depend on the exact nature and extent of the damage to the brain.

Left cerebral hemisphere
The left half of the brain. Damage may impair the ability to comprehend and/or use language.

Dementia
A progressive disorder resulting from damage to the brain that impairs memory and cognitive functioning.

Cerebral cortex
The thin layer of nerve cells on the surface of the brain.

Figure 5.1 **The Lateral Surface of the Left Cerebral Hemisphere**

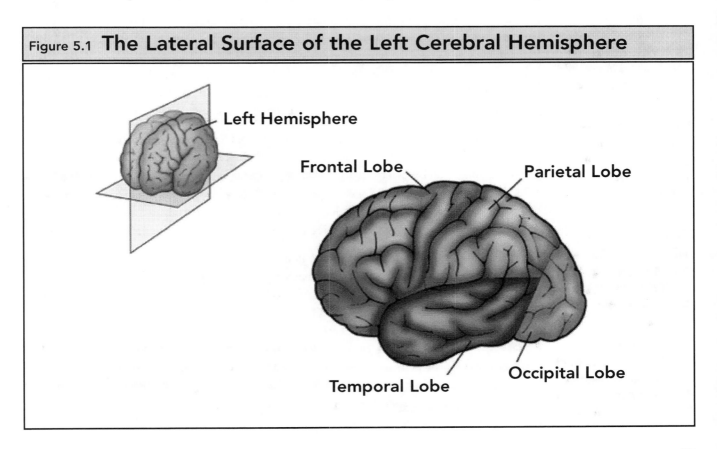

Left Hemisphere

Frontal Lobe   Parietal Lobe

Temporal Lobe   Occipital Lobe

Global aphasia
Aphasia that causes severe impairment in all language areas.

Corpus callosum
The structure that connects the right and left cerebral hemispheres.

Frontal lobe
One of the four lobes of the cerebral cortex. The left frontal lobe facilitates cognitive functioning and motor speech.

Temporal lobe
One of the four lobes of the cerebral cortex. The left temporal lobe facilitates speech comprehension.

Parietal lobe
One of the four lobes of the cerebral cortex. The left parietal lobe facilitates one's ability to repeat.

Occipital lobe
One of the four lobes of the cerebral cortex. The left occipital lobe facilitates visual functioning.

Cerebral localization of function
Dedication of nerve cells at specific locations in the cerebral cortex to performing specific functions.

Right hemiplegia
Weakness or paralysis of the right side of the body due to damage to the left cerebral hemisphere.

Furthermore, the degree of impairment of a particular language ability can range from minimal to profound. Impairment of the ability to comprehend speech, for example, can range from an inability to understand highly abstract words to not being able to understand any words. Fortunately, the impairment is more likely to be mild or moderate than it is to be profound. If the degree of impairment in all language abilities is profound, the person is referred to as having **global aphasia.**

Neurology of Aphasia

A structure known as the **corpus callosum** unites the left and right hemispheres of the brain. Because the left hemisphere is more important than the right one for mediating language functions, damage to the left hemisphere produces more severe and long-lasting language disturbances than does comparable damage to the right hemisphere.

Each hemisphere of the cerebral cortex is divided into four lobes: **frontal, temporal, parietal,** and **occipital.** The location of each lobe is illustrated in Figure 5.1 on page 89. Just as the two hemispheres of the cerebral cortex are important for mediating different functions, so too are the lobes and specific locations within each lobe. This specialization of the nerve cells in the cerebral cortex is referred to as **cerebral localization of function.**

The cerebral cortex mediates all motor, sensory, and "intellectual" (including language) functions. Which disturbance(s) will result from damage to specific nerve cells is determined by the function(s) they mediate. One of the ways neurophysiologists initially identified these functions was to note the types of disturbances shown by patients who had lesions (i.e., damage) at specific sites in the cerebral cortex. If a number of patients had a lesion at a specific site and exhibited a particular type of disturbance, neurophysiologists hypothesized that the nerve cells located there were responsible for mediating the function that was disturbed.

Aphasic-type language disturbances can result from lesions at specific sites (i.e., to specific nerve cells) in all the lobes of the left hemisphere of the cerebral cortex: the occipital, temporal, parietal, and frontal. Impairment of the ability to read is caused by lesions in the occipital lobe. Impairment of the ability to understand speech is caused by lesions in the temporal lobe. An impairment in the parietal lobe results in the inability to repeat. And, an impairment of the abilities to formulate speech and to write is caused by lesions in the frontal lobe.

Conditions that damage nerve cells important for mediating language functions usually also damage cells that are important for mediating other functions. Damage to the cerebral cortex is rarely limited just to a small group of cells. Therefore, people with aphasia are also likely to have certain other impairments, usually resulting from damage to nerve cells that are in close proximity to the damaged cells that produce aphasia. One of the most common of these impairments is a **right hemiplegia.** Nerve cells within the left hemisphere of the cerebral cortex control muscle contractions on the right side of the body. Consequently, since the lesion that produces aphasia is usually on the left side of the cerebral cortex, the hemiplegia would usually be on the right side of the body. Some other impairments that people with aphasia may exhibit are described on pages 96–97.

Aphasic impairments often decrease in severity during the first six months posttrauma, a phenomenon known as **spontaneous recovery.** When there is trauma to the brain, some brain cells are destroyed, while others are only damaged. At least some of the damaged cells are likely to begin functioning again during the first six months posttrauma. However, few damaged cells are likely to begin functioning after six months. Consequently, the prognosis for improving a client's ability to comprehend speech, formulate speech, read, and/or write a year or more posttrauma is usually poor. However, this is not the same as saying that the prognosis for a client learning to communicate better is not very good. It often is possible to improve a client's ability to communicate through the use of what are known as **augmentative/alternative communication (AAC)** strategies, which are discussed on pages 99–101. To learn more about the neurology of aphasia, see Bhatnagar (2002).

Causes of Brain Damage and Resulting Aphasia

The cortical lesions that produce aphasia can be caused by a number of conditions, the most common being **strokes.** Tumors and traumatic brain injuries (TBIs) can also cause aphasia depending on the site of the damage. If the area damaged is important for language functioning, the person is likely to become aphasic.

Three conditions can stop the flow of blood through a cerebral artery and thereby cause a stroke. In the first—which results in what is known as a **thrombotic stroke**—a blood clot forms in a cerebral artery and blocks blood flow. In the second—which results in what is known as a **thromboembolic stroke**—a clot forms in an artery outside the brain, a piece (i.e., **embolus**) breaks off, and the embolus is carried to a cerebral artery and blocks it. Note that the only difference between these two is where the clot originated. The third condition that can cause a stroke differs from the first two in that it does not result in a blockage. What happens is that a cerebral artery bursts and **hemorrhages.** Because there is now an opening in the artery, blood no longer flows through it to the areas of the brain it nourishes. Also, the blood that is released through the opening rips into the brain tissue, causing intense inflammation and swelling. Such strokes are called **hemorrhagic strokes.**

Another cause of aphasia is **neoplasms.** Some are malignant (i.e., cancerous) and some are benign (i.e., noncancerous). Both types can impede the functioning of adjacent tissue by pressing against it or by obstructing blood circulation to it. In addition, malignant tumors can impair tissue function by invading and destroying it.

Aphasia can also result from TBIs. TBI is the most common cause of brain damage in children and young adults. As with strokes and tumors, the site and the amount of damage will determine the severity of the language or other disorders.

Language Characteristics of Aphasia

Although the language of individuals with aphasia varies according to which area of the brain has been damaged, these are some of the language processes that are commonly affected:

Spontaneous recovery
The tendency for aphasic impairments to decrease in severity during the first six months posttrauma.

Augmentative/ alternative communication (AAC)
Communication strategies and devices used to supplement or replace speech.

Stroke
Occurs when a cerebral artery is blocked and the area of the brain it nourishes is damaged or destroyed. Also referred to as cerebrovascular accident or CVA.

Thrombotic stroke
Occurs when a blood clot forms in and blocks a cerebral artery.

Thromboembolic stroke
Occurs when a piece breaks off a blood clot that formed outside the brain, and the clot is carried to a cerebral artery and blocks it.

Embolus
A blood clot that moves from its site of origin.

Hemorrhage
A loss of a large amount of blood in a short time.

Hemorrhagic stroke
When a cerebral artery bursts and blood can no longer flow through it to the areas of the brain it nourishes.

Neoplasms
Tumors (i.e., abnormal masses of tissue) either malignant or benign.

Wernicke's aphasia
A disorder of the central auditory nervous system in which the person loses some ability to relate heard words to units of experience. It is also referred to as receptive aphasia and fluent aphasia.

First temporal convolution
A location in the temporal lobe of the left cerebral hemisphere that is referred to as Wernicke's area. A lesion in this area produces Wernicke's aphasia.

- The ability to name objects, pictures, events, experiences
- Language fluency
- Conversational speech
- Expository speech
- Auditory comprehension
- The ability to form speech sounds
- The ability to repeat what has just been said
- Reading
- Writing

Study More 5.1 lists some informative aphasia websites.

Study More 5.1	**Aphasia Websites**

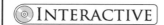	Informative aphasia websites are available on the CD-ROM

Classification of Aphasia

Wernicke's Aphasia (Receptive Aphasia, Fluent Aphasia)

Wernicke's aphasia is a disturbance in the ability to comprehend speech. It usually is caused by a lesion on the part of the temporal lobe known as the **first temporal convolution.** This location is also referred to as Wernicke's area. Carl Wernicke, a nineteenth-century German neurologist, is thought to be the first to attribute receptive aphasia to a lesion in this area.

What would it be like to have difficulty deriving meaning from the words you hear? If your comprehension problem was severe, what you would experience would be similar to listening to someone speak in a language you had never studied. You would hear the words, but they would have no meaning for you. If your comprehension problem was not severe, the experience would be similar to taking a year or two of a foreign language and visiting a country where it is spoken. You would understand some of what you heard, but not all.

Because adults with Wernicke's aphasia have difficulty in deriving meaning from words, they also have difficulty choosing appropriate words to use in their own speech. Without realizing it, they use inappropriate words. In severe cases, almost all of their nouns and verbs are inappropriate. Their speech sounds like a foreign language or jargon. A reading of the poem "Jabberwocky," reprinted in Study More 5.2, will give you an idea of what their speech is like.

Study More 5.2	Jabberwocky

What might the language of people with relatively severe receptive aphasia look like? The poem "Jabberwocky" from Lewis Carroll's book, *Through the Looking Glass,* is close to that which they tend to produce—language that is grammatically correct but for the most part meaningless.

'Twas brillig and the slithy toves
Did gyre and gimble in the wabe;
All mimsy were the borogoves
And the mome raths outgrabe.

"Beware the Jabberwock, my son!
The jaws that bite, the claws that catch!
Beware the Jubjub bird, and shun
The frumious Bandersnatch!"

He took his vorpal sword in hand:
Long time the manxome foe he sought–
So rested he by the Tumtum tree,
and stood awhile in thought.

And as in the uffish thought he stood,
The Jabberwock, with eyes of flame,
Came whiffling through the tulgey wood,
And burbled as it came!

One, two! One, two! And through and through
The vorpal blade went snicker-snack!
He left it dead and with its head
He went galumphing back.

"And has thou slain the Jabberwock?
Come to my arms, my beamish boy!
O frabjous day! Callooh, Callay!"
He chortled in his joy.

'Twas brillig and the slithy toves
Did gyre and gimble in the wabe;
All mimsy were the borogoves
And the mome raths outgrabe.

Source: Carroll (2001, p.17)

People who have this type of aphasia tend to be quite fluent because they are not aware of their errors and, consequently, don't revise them. For this reason, Wernicke's aphasia is sometimes referred to as fluent aphasia. Can you recall a time in a high school or college foreign language class when you volunteered to translate an English sentence because you thought you knew how to do it but were wrong? Since you were not aware of your error(s) while translating it, you probably were quite fluent—like someone with receptive aphasia. To learn more about Wernicke's aphasia, see Davis (1993) and Sarno (1998).

Broca's Aphasia (Motor Aphasia, Expressive Aphasia, Verbal Apraxia, Disfluent Aphasia)

Broca's aphasia is an impairment in the ability to produce speech voluntarily. It usually is caused by a lesion in the part of the left frontal lobe referred to as the **third frontal convolution.** This portion of the frontal lobe is known as Broca's area. Broca, a nineteenth-century neurologist, is credited with being the first to demonstrate a relationship between a lesion in this area and an impairment in motor programming for speech.

Broca's aphasia
An impairment in the ability to produce speech voluntarily (i.e., moving the articulators in the manner required to produce words). Also known as motor aphasia, expressive aphasia, verbal apraxia, or disfluent aphasia.

Third frontal convolution
A location in the frontal lobe of the left cerebral hemisphere that is referred to as Broca's area.

Articulators
The structures within the oral cavity that move to change the configuration of the vocal tract (e.g., the tongue and velum).

Delayed auditory feedback (DAF)
A procedure where you speak into a microphone and hear your voice through earphones, delayed by a fraction of a second.

Anomic aphasia
A disturbance in word finding. Persons with this problem have difficulty remembering the names of things. Also referred to as dysnomia.

Persons with this condition have difficulty moving their **articulators** in the manner required to produce the words they want to say when they want to say them. They know the words they want to say, but cannot say them. In severe cases they may be unable to say any words voluntarily. In mild cases they will be able to say most words voluntarily, but not necessarily fluently. Their speech tends to be slow, labored, and lacking normal inflection. For this reason, Broca's aphasia is sometimes referred to as disfluent aphasia.

Persons with Broca's aphasia tend to be more impaired in their ability to produce purposeful "intellectual" speech than in their ability to produce "emotional" speech. If they are upset, they may swear. Persons with Broca's aphasia convey meaning by the manner in which they use their words (i.e., through the pragmatics of their words). If they are angry, for example, the tone of their voice may communicate this. Furthermore, they are more impaired in their ability to produce voluntary speech than they are in their ability to produce rote speech. They may be able to count from one to ten consecutively but not be able to begin with three and count to ten or repeat a number when asked to do so.

What would it be like to have difficulty programming your articulators to say what you want to say? It would be somewhat similar to what you would experience if you tried to say a tongue twister rapidly. Try the examples in Study More 5.3

Another way you can experience not being able to program your articulators is speaking under the condition of **delayed auditory feedback (DAF).** The speech of some people using DAF tends to be relatively slow, and vowels and some consonants tend to be prolonged. The frustration you experience if you try to speak normally under this condition is somewhat similar to that experienced by people with Broca's aphasia. Audio Clip 5.1 is an example of the speech of someone with Broca's aphasia. To learn more about Broca's aphasia, see Davis (1993) and Sarno (1998).

Anomic Aphasia

Anomic aphasia is a disturbance in word finding, most likely caused by a posterior lesion in the temporal-parietal region. People with this problem have difficulty remembering the names of things even though they recognize the objects. Although most persons who have

Study More 5.3	Tongue Twisters

"Peter Piper picked a peck of pickled peppers."

"Twin-screw steel cruiser."

"Shall he sell sea shells?"

"She sells sea shells by the seashore."

Repeat each rapidly! Does it make you upset to have difficulty doing so? Do you feel compelled to keep working at it? If your answers to these questions are yes, you have experienced in a relatively mild form what people with Broca's aphasia experience.

Audio Clip 5.1	**Broca's Aphasia**

 An audio recording of a person with Broca's aphasia

this condition are senior citizens, it can have its onset during childhood. (See Casby, 1992, for a case study of an 11-year-old boy who developed anomic aphasia.)

We have all had the experience of being unable to remember the names of people we know well. We recognize them and are able to remember many things about them, but no matter how hard we try, we cannot think of their names. We say that their names are "on the tip of our tongue." We usually remember them a short time later after we have stopped trying consciously to do so. This is similar to what people with dysnomia experience. The main differences are that they are likely to have difficulty finding at least a few words every time they speak, and their problem isn't limited to people's names. If people with anomia are told a word they cannot remember and then are asked to repeat it, they are usually able to do so. However, they may forget it again in a few minutes.

Although the word-finding problems of people with anomia are caused by damage to the brain, the condition can have a **psychological overlay.** The harder they struggle to think of words and the more upset they become about having difficulty doing so, the more severe the disorder is likely to become. Consequently, it is often possible to reduce their word-finding difficulties at least a little by getting them to accept the fact that the difficulty will occur and to get on with their life—that is, by getting them to reach the final stage in the grieving process. To learn more about the word-finding problems exhibited by people with anomic aphasia, see Davis (1993) and Sarno (1998).

Conduction Aphasia

Conduction aphasia, which occurs in less than 10 percent of people with aphasia, results when there is damage to the group of fibers that connects Broca's area to Wernicke's area and the **supramarginal gyrus.** It can also occur when there is damage to the parietal lobe. The spontaneous speech of individuals with conduction aphasia is usually fluent, but their ability to repeat what they hear is more impaired.

The primary speech difficulty with conduction aphasia is in **phoneme** sequencing. People with conduction aphasia may distort words by adding syllables or sounds to words or they may transpose sounds in a word (i.e., **paraphasia).** People with conduction aphasia produce more paraphasias when they are trying to repeat. Although they can repeat some short utterances, they are unable to repeat multisyllabic words or syntactically complex utterances. These patients often try to correct their errors by saying a word over and over.

Transcortical Aphasia

Transcortical aphasia is caused by damage to the cerebral cortex surrounding Broca's area or Wernicke's area. Transcortical aphasias usually occur in older people because they result from

Psychological overlay
When psychological factors influence the severity of an organic impairment.

Supramarginal gyrus
A brain structure above Wernicke's area that carries out some language functions.

Paraphasia
Producing unintended syllables, words, or phrases during speech.

Petit mal seizures
Seizures characterized by frequent, momentary loss of contact with the environment.

Grand mal seizures
Seizures characterized by loss of consciousness.

Visual field disturbance
Blindness in a portion of the visual field.

Hemianopia
A visual field disturbance in which there is a loss of vision in either the right or left halves of the visual field in each eye.

a gradual deterioration of the blood supply to arteries. Two types occur, depending on where the lesion is located:

1. *Transcortical sensory aphasia* is characterized by comprehension difficulties. Both reading and writing are affected. Verbal output is relatively fluent (although it may include jargon), and repetition is relatively good.

2. *Transcortical motor aphasia* is characterized by expressive language difficulties. Comprehension and repetition may be very good, but there is little spontaneous speech output. The patient can read but not write.

Global Aphasia

Global aphasia occurs when the damage to the left hemisphere is extensive, covering a wide area of the cortex involved in language functioning. Because such a wide area of cortex has been affected, there is no discernible speech or language pattern that characterizes this type of aphasia. In the most severe forms of global aphasia, patients may be unable to utter more than one or two words (if any at all) in response to any kind of communication. They may also use gestures that are unrelated to their communicative intent.

Other Characteristics of Left Hemisphere Damage

Extreme Fatigue

Individuals with aphasia often experience periods of extreme fatigue. This fatigue can occur at any time and can cause an individual to have a poor memory. Fatigue can also make it difficult for individuals with aphasia to concentrate. Because of this, therapy sessions for some individuals with aphasia are relatively short. To learn more about the extreme fatigue experienced by people with aphasia, see Davis (1993) and Sarno (1998).

Seizures

Another disturbance people with aphasia may experience is epileptic seizures. They may experience **petit mal** or **grand mal seizures.** The medications clients take to control their seizures can add to their fatigue level. To learn more about seizures, see Eisenberg, Glueckauf, and Zaretsky (1999).

Visual Field Disturbances

Individuals with aphasia may also have a **visual field disturbance.** People with this impairment are partially blind. If, for example, they look straight ahead, they may be able to see objects to the left of their bodies but not to the right. Loss of vision in either the right or left halves of the visual field in each eye is called **hemianopia.** To learn more about visual field disturbances in people with aphasia, see Davis (1993) and Sarno (1998).

Perseveration

The inability to stop doing something is known as **perseveration.** An individual with aphasia who shows perseveration may repeat the same word over and over regardless of whether or not doing it is appropriate. For example, if a person who has this condition is shown a comb and says "comb," he or she may also respond "comb" if shown a pencil or some other object. To learn more about perseveration and aphasia, see Davis (1993) and Sarno (1998).

Abstract-Concrete Imbalance

People with aphasia who have an **abstract-concrete imbalance** have less than normal ability to categorize. For example, they may remember only some of the attributes that cause an object to be categorized as an animal and therefore, may categorize dogs, but not cats or pigs, as animals. Their lack of normal ability to categorize can contribute significantly to the severity of their speech comprehension; speech formulation; and reading and writing problems. It can also contribute significantly to their problems with mathematics. To learn more about abstract-concrete imbalance, see Goldstein (1948).

Catastrophic Reaction

If too many demands are made on a person who has severe aphasia, he or she may have a **catastrophic reaction**. For example, being asked by a spouse to say "thank you" for a meal tray after it is delivered may cause an expressive aphasic to throw it. This type of reaction can be looked upon as a form of nonverbal communication. Viewed in this way, it should be possible to eliminate it by providing the person with aphasia with a more socially acceptable way to communicate anger or frustration, perhaps by pointing to line drawings on a communication board that convey these feelings. To learn more about such challenging behaviors and their management see Durand (1993).

Despondency

It should not be particularly surprising that many people with aphasia experience depression. Some are suicidal and/or cry frequently for no apparent reason. While depression is a normal aspect of the grieving process that occurs following a loss, it can impede rehabilitation if it persists for too long. Depression may persist if individuals feel life no longer has meaning because they can no longer do what they used to be able to do. Unless they can find new meaning for their lives, their despondency is likely to persist. To learn more about the despondency in individuals with aphasia when they grieve for their loss of the ability to communicate normally, see LaFond, Joanette, Ponzio, Degiovani, and Sarno (1993) and Tanner (1980).

Altered Relationships

Because people with aphasia have lost the ability to communicate normally, their relationships with family members, friends, and co-workers are likely to change in highly undesirable ways. These changes can be more disabling to them than their language deficits. To learn more about the impacts that the communication impairments of people with aphasia can have on their families, see LaFond et al. (1993), Luterman (1995), and Zraick and Boone (1991).

Abstract-concrete imbalance
Having less than normal ability to categorize.

Catastrophic reaction
A reaction in which the person loses control and does something violent (e.g., throws something) when too many demands are made on him or her. Also referred to as challenging behavior.

Anosognosia
Denial of illness, demonstrated by some persons who have damage to the right cerebral hemisphere.

Left neglect
Lack of attention to environmental stimuli on the left. Also referred to as hemi-attention.

Prosopagnosia
Failure to recognize familiar faces, such as that of one's spouse.

Dressing apraxia
A deficit in which individuals may put on their clothes in a disorganized manner. For example, they might put their shirt on backwards.

Amusica
A disturbance in the recognition and processing of music, demonstrated by some persons who have damage to the right cerebral hemisphere.

Neglect dyslexia
A tendency to frequently misread the beginnings of words. It is demonstrated by some persons who have damage to the right cerebral hemisphere.

Alzheimer's disease
A brain disorder that often results in dementia.

Right Hemisphere Deficits

Damage to the right half of the cerebral cortex results in right hemisphere deficits. There are several types of right hemisphere deficits, including those associated with loss of visuospatial and musical skills. These disorders of perception and orientation can underlie language problems. As a result, clients who have them are often referred to SLPs for assessment and treatment.

The types of disorders of perception and orientation that people with right hemisphere damage exhibit include the following:

- *Anosognosia.* William O. Douglas, an Associate Justice of the United States Supreme Court had **anosognosia.** Following a stroke that damaged his right hemisphere and weakened his left arm, he insisted that his arm was injured in a fall.

- *Left neglect.* One woman with right hemisphere damage who exhibited **left neglect** "appeared in public only half made up, the left side of her face void of lipstick and rouge" (Sacks, 1985, p. 74).

- *Deficits in the recognition of objects and/or faces.* People who have this deficit may have difficulty identifying objects visually. They may, for example, put cigarette ashes in a sugar bowl (Shallice, 1987). They may also experience **prosopagnosia.** Furthermore, they may see faces where there are none or vice versa. One patient who had such a deficit looked around for his hat and tugged his wife's head, thinking it was his hat (Sacks, 1985).

- *Deficits in the recognition of spatial relationships between objects.* Persons with such a deficit may experience **dressing apraxia.** Or they may have difficulty finding their way around (e.g., reading maps, remembering familiar routes or learning new ones [Meyers, 1999]).

- *Auditory dysfunctions.* These are usually related to the recognition and processing of music. Such dysfunctions are sometimes labeled **amusica.**

Deficits in perception and orientation, such as those described above, can adversely affect a person's language functioning. Here are two examples. Some people with left neglect frequently misread the beginnings (i.e., left side) of words—for example, they may read *rose* as *nose* (Patterson & Wilson, 1990). This condition is referred to as **neglect dyslexia.** Also, some people who have recognition deficits have difficulty interpreting emotion in faces, scenes, and the tone of utterances. This can cause them to misunderstand what is being communicated.

Causes of Right Hemisphere Deficits

Dementia

Approximately 15 percent of people over the age of 85 suffer from some form of dementia, an acquired persistent compromise in intellectual function with impairments in at least three of the following spheres of mental activity: language, memory, visuospatial skills, personality, and cognition (e.g., abstraction, judgment, mathematics). About 65 percent of dementia is of the Alzheimer's type. While **Alzheimer's disease** is more prevalent in older adults, it does strike in middle age and on rare occasions can affect people below the age of 25. This progressive, degenerative disease usually begins with forgetfulness and disorientation and, over a period of

6 to 12 years, progresses to severe memory impairment (e.g., family not recognized), lack of responsiveness to speech, and mutism.

People who have Alzheimer's disease and other types of dementia tend to exhibit disturbances in language functioning. One of the most frequently mentioned is difficulty naming objects. However, the reason for their difficulty does not appear to be the same as for people with aphasia. Whereas the person with aphasia recognizes the object but cannot remember what it is called, the person with dementia fails to recognize the object in the first place.

All dementia results from brain damage. The specific type of damage is a function of the condition that is responsible for the dementia. In Alzheimer's disease, for example, the impairment seems to result from abnormalities known as **neurofibrillary tangles** that develop in nerve cells. Other conditions that can damage the brain to produce dementia include viruses and multiple strokes.

Traumatic Brain Injury

Brain trauma can occur whenever the head sustains a blow or wound that causes the brain to twist; turn; stop or start suddenly (as in a car accident); or be pushed against the skull. Brain injuries can affect many different parts of the brain, regardless of which part sustains the blow or wound. For instance, when the head strikes a hard object in a car accident, the skull hits the brain on the side of the impact, which forces the brain to bounce off the other side of the skull. The result is damage to both sides of the brain. In addition, hemorrhages that arise as a result of the injury can form a **hematoma,** which puts pressure on the brain.

The severity of the head wound or injury depends on the force of the impact and how much brain tissue is affected. The weaker the force and the less tissue that is damaged, the more likely the resulting effects on motor, cognitive, and communication functions will be mild. Greater force and more brain tissue involvement makes it more likely the resulting effects on these functions will be severe.

Management

Aphasia

The primary goal of the SLP is to maximize effective use of communication and participation in life for adults with aphasia in their natural settings. That is, the goal is to enable them to communicate more effectively in everyday conversational exchanges and to minimize the extent to which their condition limits their activities.

Two general approaches are used for improving the ability of people with aphasia to communicate. One is to reduce the severity of their impairment in understanding speech, formulating speech, reading, writing, and calculating. The other is to augment their residual communication abilities through the use of gestures, communication boards, and/or electronic devices. An example of a basic-needs communication board can be seen in Figure 5.2.

The first approach, to decrease deficits in affected language abilities, is most likely to be successful during the first six months posttrauma, while spontaneous recovery is still occurring.

Neurofibrillary tangles
Brain abnormality in persons who have Alzheimer's disease.

Hematoma
Blood that has formed as a result of a broken blood vessel.

The clinician attempts to manipulate the environment to maximize spontaneous recovery. One way that he or she does this is to arrange for the person to have frequent opportunities to stimulate language abilities that are impaired. The clinician may do some stimulation in the therapy room, and some may be done by encouraging the person to interact frequently with other people. This may involve encouraging him or her to participate in a therapy group, a stroke support group, and/or in a "golden age" club. Usually, the more practice the person with aphasia gets in communicating (i.e., the more his or her impaired language abilities are stimulated), the more he or she is likely to improve during the spontaneous recovery period.

The second approach, to augment the client's residual communication abilities, is used both during and after the spontaneous recovery period. The goal is to augment the client's existing communication abilities to be adequate for meeting his or her communication needs. These could range in complexity from being able to communicate feelings to family and friends; describe physical needs to doctors and nurses during a period of hospitalization; or use professional language necessary to return to his or her job.

Although the prognosis for improving communication using the first approach tends to be poor beyond the period of spontaneous recovery, this is not necessarily true with the second

Figure 5.2	**A Basic Needs Communication Board**

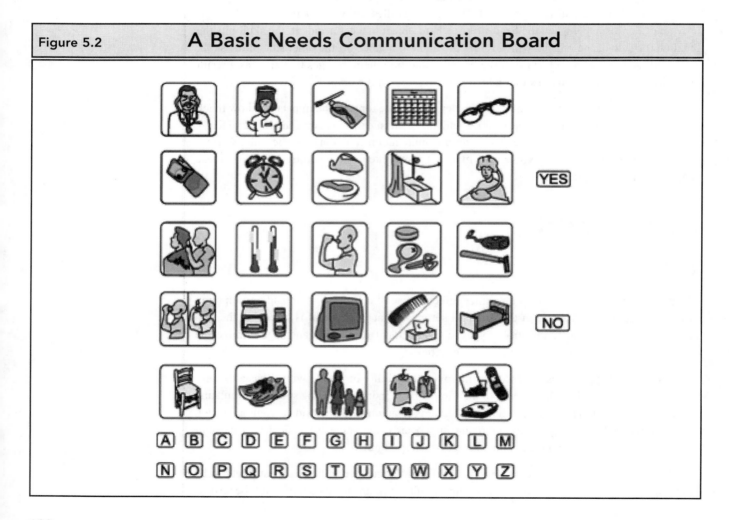

approach. For example, although it may not be possible to improve the speech of a client who has severe Broca's aphasia, it may be possible to improve the client's ability to communicate by teaching him or her to use a portable computer that can generate speech.

It may also be possible to teach strategies for coping with communication difficulties to those who frequently communicate with the person who has aphasia (e.g., family members and friends). To learn more about the management of aphasia, see Chapey (2001), Nadeau, Gonzales-Rothi, and Crosson (2000), and Wallace (1996).

Right Hemisphere Disorders

Speech-language pathologists often can be helpful to people who have right hemisphere deficits if the clients are adequately motivated. Many such clients, however, either are not aware of or deny their deficits; consequently, they are not highly motivated to work on reducing (or compensating for) them. This is unfortunate because some symptoms (e.g., neglect dyslexia) can be treated successfully. To learn more about the impairments resulting from right hemisphere dysfunction and their management, see Davis (1993), Halper, Cherney, and Burns (1996), and Meyers (1999).

Currently there is no specific drug available that can stop or reverse Alzheimer's disease. Although the majority of persons with this condition are not suitable candidates for traditional speech-language therapy programs, they and their families can often be helped by SLPs. The goal is to help the patient to maintain his or her ability to communicate with family members and others for as long as possible.

One way to help clients continue to communicate is to teach the family to minimize the client's specific communication deficits and, consequently, maximize his or her ability to communicate with them. One device that the family could learn to design and encourage the patient to use is a **memory wallet** (see Bourgeois, 1992, for additional information). To learn more about dementia and its management, see Bellenir (2003), Glickstein and Neustadt (1993), Lubinski (1995), Mace and Rabins (1999), and Wilcock, Bucks, and Rockwood (1999).

Memory wallet
A small loose-leaf binder containing photographs and words on index cards (e.g., names and photographs of family members and friends) that a person with Alzheimer's disease or dementia has difficulty remembering

Part 3
Speech Disorders

This section contains four chapters that deal with speech disorders. Chapter 6 begins with an overview of voice production. This overview is followed by a discussion of voice disorders and their management.

Chapter 7 discusses difficulties associated with dysarthria. Dysarthria in children and acquired dysarthria are both discussed. Speech disorders and difficulties with swallowing related to dysarthria are both described.

Chapter 8 describes the production of speech sounds. You will learn about how speech sounds are classified. Articulation and phonological disorders are discussed, and a distinction between the two disorders is explained.

Chapter 9 discusses fluency disorders. You will learn the difference between normal and abnormal speech fluency. This chapter focuses on the disorder of stuttering, since it is the most common fluency disorder.

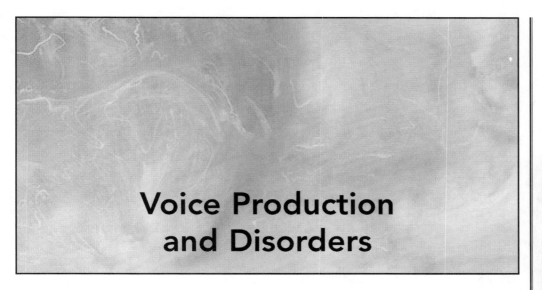

Voice Production and Disorders

Chapter 6

Learning Objectives

- Describe the respiratory system and its function in voice production.

- Describe the motor system and its role in voice production.

- Describe the anatomy and function of the larynx in voice production.

- Describe the five major types of voice disorders and their characteristics.

- Describe laryngectomy and consequent voice production.

Chapter 6

Introduction

This chapter begins with an overview of the anatomy and physiology of the entire speech mechanism, including the **respiratory system, larynx,** and **vocal tract.** The major speech functions of these mechanisms, as illustrated in Figure 6.1, are described below. This section also includes an explanation of how the vocal tract is controlled by the **motor system.** This overview is followed by a more detailed discussion of voice production. This chapter concludes with a description of voice disorders and their management.

Overview of the Speech Mechanism

Respiratory System

The respiratory system produces the raw material—air under pressure—from which speech is generated. The main component of the respiratory system is the **lungs.** Air from the environment is drawn into the lungs through **inhalation.** Air is stored in the lungs for a short time, during which oxygen is extracted and waste products are added. The air is then expelled from the lungs under pressure through **exhalation.** To learn more about the anatomy and physiology of the respiratory system, see Deem and Miller (2000).

Larynx

During exhalation, air under pressure is sent from the lungs to the larynx, which is illustrated in Figure 6.2. on page 108. The function of the larynx (particularly the **vocal folds**) is to set the molecules of this breath stream into vibration. For sound to be produced, these molecules have to vibrate at a rate that falls within a particular range, resulting in **phonation.** Voice production is described in more detail on pages 110–113. To learn more about the anatomy and physiology of the larynx, see Deem and Miller (2000).

Motor system
The parts of the peripheral and central nervous systems that regulate the contraction of muscle fibers.

Lungs
The two lungs are the main component of the respiratory system. They are the source of the air for vibrating the vocal folds to produce voice.

Inhalation
The process by which air from the environment is drawn into the lungs.

Exhalation
The process by which air is expelled from the lungs under pressure.

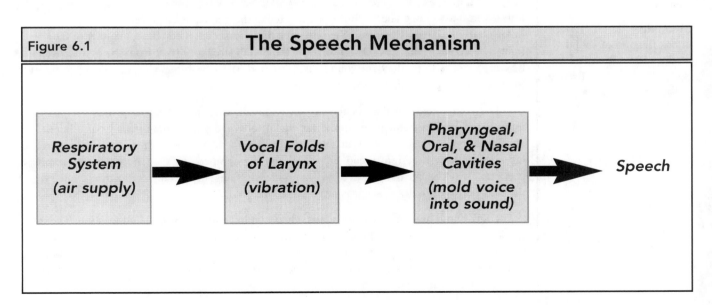

Figure 6.1	The Speech Mechanism

Respiratory System (air supply) → Vocal Folds of Larynx (vibration) → Pharyngeal, Oral, & Nasal Cavities (mold voice into sound) → Speech

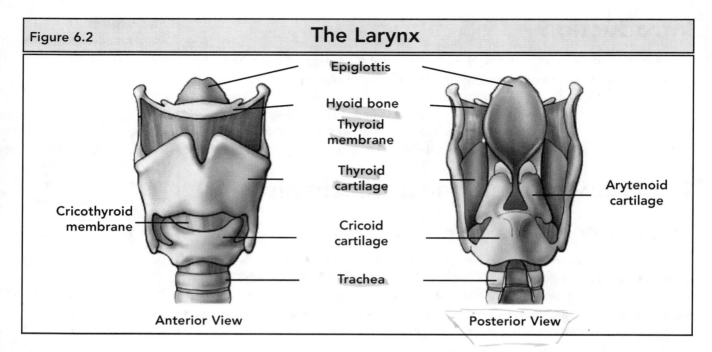

Figure 6.2 — The Larynx

Epiglottis
Hyoid bone
Thyroid membrane
Thyroid cartilage
Cricothyroid membrane
Cricoid cartilage
Trachea
Arytenoid cartilage

Anterior View | Posterior View

Laryngeal tone
The buzzing sound produced by phonation.

Mandible
Lower jaw.

Velum
The posterior portion of the roof of the mouth. Also referred to as soft palate.

Resonate
Intensification of sound produced by vibrations interacting with the tissues of the vocal tract.

Vocal Tract and Resonance

The vibration pattern of molecules produced by phonation is complex. It contains a wide range of frequencies and has a buzzing sound. This sound, called the **laryngeal tone,** is molded into phonemes by the vocal tract.

The vocal tract can be imagined as a box containing three major cavities that mold voice into speech sounds. The vocal tract consists of the **pharyngeal cavity** (i.e., pharynx), **oral cavity,** and **nasal cavity** as illustrated in Figure 1.2 on page 10. The configuration (i.e., shape) of the vocal tract at a particular moment determines which speech sound will be produced. This configuration can be changed by the movement of several structures within it: the tongue, lips, **mandible,** and **velum.** The first three are located in the oral cavity. The velum, which is located in the pharyngeal cavity, controls the influence of the nasal cavity on the remainder of the vocal tract. The velum either stays down to allow the breath stream to flow from the oral cavity into the nasal cavity (to produce the sounds /m/, /n/, and /ŋ/), or it lifts up to close the opening into the nasal cavity. In the latter, the oral cavity alone shapes the speech sound.

The components of the vocal tract act as resonators; in this capacity they increase the intensity of certain frequencies in the laryngeal tone and reduce the intensity of others. The configuration of these cavities at any given moment determines which frequencies in the laryngeal tone will be reinforced and which will be damped. That is, the voice **resonates** in particular ways because it passes through, bounces off, and echoes inside the throat (pharynx), the oral cavity (mouth), and the nose (nasal cavity).

Think about how your voice sounds when you have a cold or nasal congestion. The congestion changes the resonating qualities of the nasal cavities, rendering your voice less nasal (i.e., hyponasal). Each person's voice quality results in part from their own unique resonating characteristics of the vocal tract. To learn more about the anatomy and physiology of the vocal tract, see Deem and Miller (2000).

Motor System

Movement of the parts of the vocal tract is controlled by the motor system. These movements change the configuration of the vocal tract, which changes the resonance of the laryngeal tone.

The tongue plays a significant role in changing the vocal tract configuration. The tongue contains muscle fibers which contract to change its shape, thereby changing the configuration of the vocal tract. For example, the contraction of certain muscle fibers within the tongue raises its tip, thus changing the shape of the oral cavity. The contraction of muscle fibers is controlled directly by the peripheral nervous system (PNS) and the central nervous system (CNS), and indirectly by the autonomic nervous system (ANS). The motor system is diagrammed in Figure 6.3 and described in the following paragraphs.

The **pyramidal system,** which includes the **upper motor neurons** and **lower motor neurons,** determines which muscles will contract. To elevate the tongue tip, for example, certain muscle fibers in the tongue have to contract. For this to happen, the upper motor neurons send messages to their lower motor neurons, which cause the lower motor neurons to send electrical signals to the muscle fibers that innervate in the tongue, causing those muscles to contract. The pyramidal system is also involved with the inhibition of certain reflexes that can interfere with voluntary movement. If the pyramidal system is not functioning properly, there is both reduced ability to make voluntary movements and hyperactive (i.e., increased) reflexes. Both of these conditions can interfere with the functioning of the speech mechanism.

Pyramidal system
The system responsible for controlling voluntary motor movements.

Upper motor neurons
Motor neurons in the central nervous system that control the lower motor neurons in the peripheral nervous system.

Lower motor neurons
The structures within the motor system that come into most direct contact with muscle fibers. They conduct electrical signals to muscles.

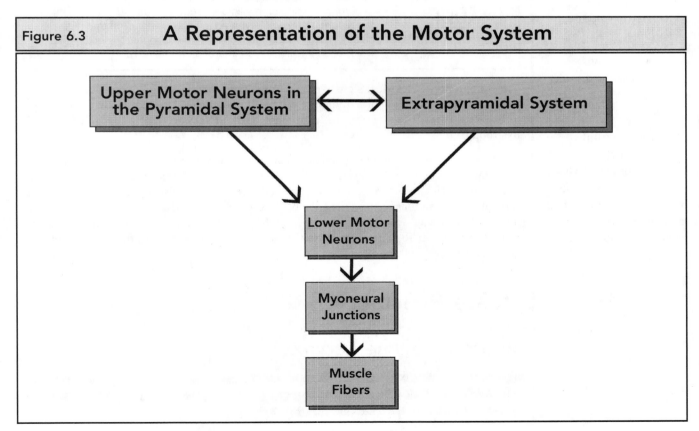

Figure 6.3   A Representation of the Motor System

Extrapyramidal system
Groups of neurons within the central nervous system that are responsible for the refinement of movement patterns.

Parkinson's disease
A neuromuscular disorder resulting from abnormal functioning of the extrapyramidal system.

Cerebellar ataxia
A neuromuscular disorder resulting from abnormal functioning of a part of the extrapyramidal system know as the cerebellum.

Myoneural junctions
The space between the tips of lower motor neurons and muscle fibers that contain a chemical for conducting electrical signals.

Myasthenia gravis
A neuromuscular disorder characterized by muscle weakness.

Muscular dystrophy
A neuromuscular disorder of genetic origin in which muscle weakness results from muscle abnormality, rather than myoneural junction or nerve abnormality.

Trachea
A hollow tubelike structure below the larynx through which air flows to the lungs.

The **extrapyramidal system** is concerned with the refinement of movement patterns. It allows movements to be made smoothly and accurately at a rapid rate. If the extrapyramidal system is not functioning properly, it may be possible to make movements only at a very slow rate; it may be possible to make rapid movements, but not accurately; or movement patterns may be accompanied by involuntary movements, such as tremors. People with **Parkinson's disease** or **cerebellar ataxia** have an abnormality in the functioning of the extrapyramidal system. People with Parkinson's disease are unable to make movements rapidly, and they make involuntary movements (i.e., tremors). Those with cerebellar ataxia cannot make rapid movements accurately and may appear intoxicated. Either of these conditions obviously can disturb the functioning of the speech mechanism. To learn more about Parkinson's disease, visit the National Institute on Neurological Disorders and Stroke (NINDS; 2005d) webpage.

Lower motor neurons conduct electrical signals to muscle fibers through **myoneural** (i.e., muscle-nerve) **junctions.** Lower motor neurons and muscle fibers do not come into direct contact; rather, there is a thin layer of chemical between them at the myoneural junction. If particular myoneural junctions do not function properly, electrical signals will not reach certain muscle fibers, and the muscles will not contract. This occurs with the partial paralysis that accompanies **myasthenia gravis,** which is caused by an abnormality in the chemical makeup of the myoneural junctions. Audio Clip 6.1 illustrates how myasthenia gravis sounds. To learn more, visit the NINDS (2005c) webpage on myasthenia gravis.

Audio Clip 6.1	Myasthenia Gravis
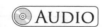	This man's myasthenia gravis causes him to have severe hypernasality and unintelligible speech. About 40 seconds into the recording he was given an injection of tensilon that sufficiently improved the functioning of his myoneural junctions for his speech intelligibility to improve dramatically.

If appropriate electrical signals pass through their myoneural junctions but some of the fibers in a muscle are abnormal, the muscle will not contract. One disease with this characteristic is **muscular dystrophy.** To learn more, visit NINDS (2005b) webpage on muscular dystrophy.

Emotional states, particularly anxiety, can influence motor functioning through the activity of the autonomic nervous system (ANS). The activity of this system affects the functioning of the pyramidal and extrapyramidal systems. The speech mechanism appears to be particularly susceptible to disturbance by anxiety. People tend to repeat sounds and syllables when they are highly anxious (e.g., when experiencing stage fright). And some authorities think anxiety is a cause of stuttering. To learn more about the anatomy and physiology of the motor system, see Deem and Miller (2000).

Voice Production

Anatomy of the Larynx

The production of voice (i.e., phonation) is the responsibility of the respiratory system and larynx. A key component of the larynx is the vocal folds, illustrated in Figure 6.4. The larynx is located on top of the **trachea** and below the pharyngeal cavity.

Figure 6.4 — Laryngoscopic Views of the Vocal Folds

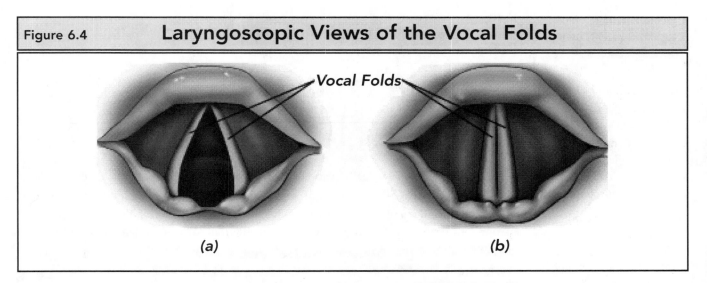

Vocal Folds

(a)   (b)

The location of the vocal folds in the larynx is at the level of the right and left **arytenoid cartilages.** The posterior ends of the vocal folds (which are at the bottom in Figure 6.4) are attached to these cartilages, whose movement **abducts** and **adducts** the vocal folds. The anterior (i.e., front) ends of the vocal folds (the ends that are together in Figure 6.4) are attached to the **thyroid cartilage.** Figure 6.2 on page 108 shows the arytenoid cartilage and the thyroid cartilage.

The vocal folds are not merely thin membranes or string like structures. Each vocal fold has within it a bundle of muscle tissue known as the **thyroarytenoid muscle.** It is referred to in this way because the two structures to which it is attached are the thyroid cartilage and the arytenoid cartilage.

You should be familiar with one other structure within the larynx. The **epiglottis** is a flexible leaflike structure, the lower end of which is attached to the thyroid cartilage. The upper end is located behind the **hyoid bone.** Figure 6.2 on page 108 shows the epiglottis and hyoid bone. During swallowing, the epiglottis lowers to prevent what we are swallowing from entering the lungs through the opening between the vocal folds.

Vocal Fold Vibration

The vibration of the vocal folds results from the buildup of air pressure below them in the respiratory system and is responsible for making the particles of exhaled air vibrate. The rate (i.e., frequency) at which the vocal folds vibrate is determined by several factors, including their length, mass, and tension. The longer they are, the lower the frequency at which they tend to vibrate. This is why the pitch of male voices tends to be lower than that of female ones. The greater the vocal folds' mass (i.e., thickness), the lower the frequency at which they tend to vibrate. Tumors on the vocal folds, for example, increase their mass and result in a lowering of the pitch of the voice. And the less tense they are (for a given length and mass), the lower the frequency at which they tend to vibrate and the lower the pitch of the voice. Therefore, the lowest frequency would occur with someone with long, thick, less tense vocal folds. Video Clip 6.1, which is described on page 112, shows the vocal folds vibrating.

Arytenoid cartilage
Two small cartilages in the larynx, the movements of which abduct and adduct the vocal folds.

Abduct
To separate, or open.

Adduct
To bring together, or close. Also called approximation.

Thyroid cartilage
A part of the larynx; the bulge in the neck referred to as the Adam's apple.

Thyroarytenoid muscle
The muscle in each vocal fold.

Epiglottis
A leaflike structure in the larynx that lowers during swallowing to prevent what is being swallowed from getting into the lungs.

Hyoid bone
A complex of bones at the base of the tongue and above the thyroid cartilage that supports the tongue and its muscles.

Cricoid cartilage
A cartilage that sits on top of the trachea and forms the base of the larynx.

Laryngoscopic view
The view of the top surface of the vocal folds through a round laryngeal mirror. It is the view of the larynx yielded by indirect laryngoscopy.

Indirect laryngoscopy
A procedure for viewing the top surface and edges of the vocal folds through a laryngeal mirror.

Video Clip 6.1	**Vocal Folds Vibrating**
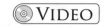	A slow-motion animation of the vocal folds vibrating (UCLA Humanities Web Page Portal, n.d.)

Changing Pitch

We vary the pitch of our voice by varying the tension of the vocal folds. We do this by causing the thyroid cartilage—the bottom of which is attached by two joints to the right and left sides of the **cricoid cartilage**—to move in either an anterior or posterior direction. Because the anterior ends of the vocal folds are attached to the thyroid cartilage, when the cartilage rocks forward, tension on the vocal folds increases. And when it rocks backward, the folds become less tense. Consequently, we raise the pitch of our voice by causing the thyroid cartilage to move in an anterior (i.e., forward) direction.

Looking at the Vocal Folds

The two views of the vocal folds in Figure 6.4 on page 111 are **laryngoscopic views.** The procedure used to obtain these views, known as **indirect laryngoscopy,** is illustrated in Figure 6.5.

The examiner (usually a physician) places a round mirror with a hole in the center over one eye. A light reflected from this head mirror is directed into the patient's mouth and onto the laryngeal mirror, which is placed against the back wall of the patient's pharynx at a 45-degree angle. The light from this mirror is directed into the patient's larynx, allowing an image of the top surface and edges of the vocal folds to be reflected in it.

Figure 6.5	**Indirect Laryngoscopy**

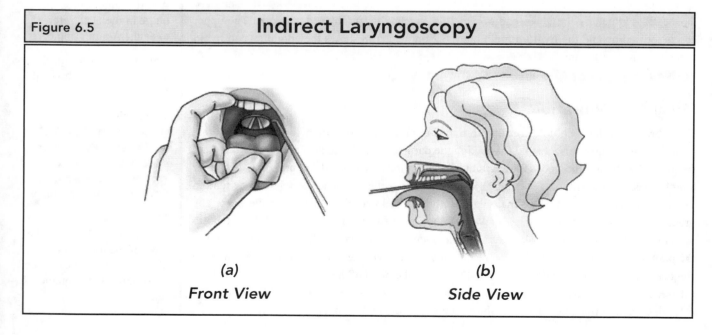

(a)
Front View

(b)
Side View

Opening and Closing of the Vocal Folds

The view in Figure 6.4(a) on page 111 illustrates the configuration of the top surface of the vocal folds during normal respiration—that is, when no attempt is being made to speak. The folds are widely separated, allowing an unrestricted flow of air from the environment to the lungs and vice versa. They do not vibrate, and air flows continuously through the opening between them. This open space is referred to as the **glottis.**

The view in Figure 6.4(b) on page 111 illustrates the configuration of the top surface of the vocal folds while an attempt is being made to speak. During phonation, the vocal folds adduct at the midline of the larynx. Air pressure then builds up below them, causing them to vibrate.

Anything that keeps the vocal folds from approximating normally can produce a voice disorder. To learn more about the role of the larynx in the production of voice, see Borden, Harris, and Raphael (1994), Deem and Miller (2000), and Ferrand (2001).

Voice and Resonance Disorders

There are five major types of voice disorders. Disorders can be related to (1) trauma; (2) problems that have an unknown cause; (3) **congenital** problems; (4) disorders of the brain and/or nervous system; and (5) vocal resonance.

Trauma-Related Disorders

There are three primary causes of trauma to the larynx. Behavioral trauma involves overuse of the voice (i.e., hyperfunction). Mechanical trauma is physical injury from sources either external or internal. Trauma from burns may also cause a voice disorder.

Behavioral Traumas

Either vocal abuse or vocal misuse can cause behavioral trauma to the larynx. Table 6.1 on page 114 list some common ways people abuse and/or misuse their larynges and the possible side effects on the voice. Figure 6.6 on page 115 shows four types of vocal fold growths. The most common of these is vocal nodules which are caused by behavioral trauma.

Mechanical Traumas

Mechanical traumas to the larynx can come from either external or internal sources. External injuries to the larynx occur in several ways. The most common cause of an external injury to the larynx is an automobile accident in which the neck and larynx come into contact with the steering wheel or other part of the car. An external injury to the larynx can also come from other blunt objects striking the larynx with great force, for instance, a child hitting the handlebars of a bicycle; falling on a curb or step; running into a wire; or being hit with a baseball bat.

External injuries that penetrate the larynx usually are caused by a gunshot, knife wound, or an automobile accident. Malpositioning of a **tracheostomy** tube during an emergency procedure, especially in children because of their incompletely developed laryngeal structures, may cause injury to the larynx. Injuries to the larynx caused by internal sources include: (1) an **endoscopic examination** performed improperly, (2) an **endotracheal intubation** during

---

Glottis
The space between the vocal folds.

Tracheostomy
Opening the trachea surgically in order to allow air into the lungs.

Endoscopic examination
Insertion of an endoscope to observe the vocal folds.

Endotracheal intubation
Insertion of a flexible plastic tube through the mouth into the trachea to ensure the passage of air.

Table 6.1	Possible Side Effects of Vocal Misuse and Abuse
Vocal Misuse and Abuse	**Possible Side Effect**
• Yelling, screaming, cheering (which cause vocal folds to adduct with great force)	• Hematomas • Vocal nodules • Breathy, hoarse, or harsh voice
• Strained vocalizations (e.g., children mimicking machine noises or vocalizations made when lifting heavy objects) that cause vocal folds to adduct tightly to trap air	• Vocal fold irritation • Breathy, hoarse, or harsh voice
• Excessive talking	• Vocal fold irritation • Hoarse or harsh voice
• Frequent use of hard glottal attack (adducting the vocal folds, building up air, and releasing it in an explosion)	• Hoarse, harsh, or breathy voice • Chronic laryngitis • Vocal nodules • Vocal polyps • Contact ulcers
• Throat clearing and coughing	• Hoarse voice • Contact ulcers
• Inhaling dust, cigarette smoke, and other pollutants	• Vocal edemas • Carcinoma • Vocal polyps
• Singing with poor technique (too loud, at an inappropriate pitch, or with hard glottal attack)	• Vocal fold irritation • Vocal nodules • Hoarse, harsh, or breathy voice
• Using inappropriately low pitch	• Contact ulcers
• Using inappropriately high pitch	• Vocal nodules • Breathy, hoarse, or harsh voice
• Alcohol overuse	• Vocal edemas
• Untreated infection	• Acute laryngitis

Nasogastric tube
A flexible plastic tube running from the nose, through the esophagus, and into the stomach. It is used to either drain the stomach or to deliver medications and/or nutrients.

surgery that irritates the mucus membrane, or (3) a **nasogastric tube** that causes laryngeal irritation during swallowing, resulting in hoarseness and/or laryngeal pain.

The most severe form of mechanical trauma is when one or both of the vocal folds are removed surgically in a procedure called a **laryngectomy.** If the vocal folds aren't present, they can't vibrate! The primary reason for this type of surgery is cancer of the larynx. The entire larynx may be removed (total laryngectomy), or only the tumor and the tissue surrounding it may be removed (partial laryngectomy). People who have had a laryngectomy usually can have their ability to speak restored by surgery, by the use of a device known as an **electrolarynx,** or by being taught to utilize the musculature of the **esophagus** to set molecules of air into vibration.

Figure 6.6	Laryngoscopic Views of Four Types of Vocal Fold Growths

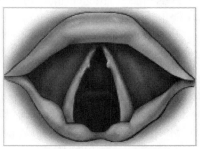

Vocal Nodules

Typically on the anterior
third of the vocal folds

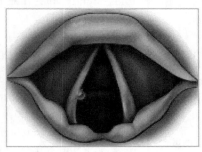

A Vocal Polyp

Typically on one vocal
fold, but can form on both

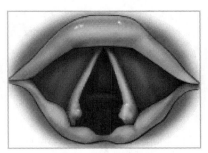

A Contact Ulcer

Typically on the posterior
third of the vocal folds

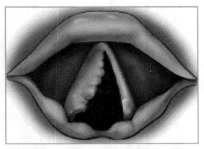

Carcinoma (Cancer) of the Larynx

Typically on the
edges of the vocal folds

Trauma Caused By Burns

Burns to the larynx are either thermal or chemical. Thermal burns, which are seen most often in firefighters and members of rescue teams, may be caused by inhaling hot air or gas. Thermal burns may also be caused by swallowing hot foods or liquids. Thermal burns are painful and cause a hoarse voice; however, if treatment is begun immediately, healing is usually rapid.

Chemical burns to the larynx occur most frequently in children, from swallowing a dangerous substance. They are frequently serious and are accompanied by burns of the esophagus and upper pharynx. Some people may lose their voices altogether, while others may have a hoarse, breathy voice. Because scarring is common, voice quality may not improve with healing.

Voice Disorders of Unknown Cause

Some voice disorders are caused by faulty approximation of the vocal folds that does not result from any known organic cause. Vocal folds can be either overly tense and hyperadducted (held tightly together), or they can be lax and hypoadducted (held somewhat apart). These disorders can range in severity from complete **aphonia** to continuous use of a high pitch.

Laryngectomy
The surgical removal of all or part of the larynx.

Electrolarynx
A small battery-powered electrical device that can enable persons who have had a laryngectomy to produce a voice.

Esophagus
The tube that connects the oral cavity to the stomach.

115

Ventricular folds
A pair of soft, flaccid folds above the true vocal folds that contain little muscle fiber. Also referred to as false vocal folds.

Dystonia
Abnormal muscle tone caused by involuntary muscle contractions.

Basal ganglia
A group of nerve cells at the base of the brain that participate in regulating motor performance.

Ventricular Dysphonia (False Vocal Fold Phonation)

Ventricular dysphonia, a rare voice disorder, occurs when an individual uses the **ventricular folds** (i.e., false vocal folds) to produce voice. Sometimes, a person will hold the true vocal folds slightly apart (i.e., hypoadducted) and use the ventricular folds for phonation. Often the voice that results is lower in frequency than that produced with the true vocal folds.

Conversion Voice Disorders

Conversion voice disorders are so-called because the individual loses all or part of her or his phonatory ability because of emotional distress or a psychological problem. These disorders include complete mutism, in which the individual makes no attempt to phonate. They also include aphonia, in which the person can whisper but the vocal folds do not vibrate, and dysphonia, in which the individual exhibits varying degrees of hoarseness.

Mutational Falsetto

Mutational falsetto is the continued use after puberty of the higher-pitched voice used before puberty, in spite of a larynx that is physically capable of producing the normal lower pitch of adults. This disorder affects boys and girls, although it is more noticeable in boys because their prepubescent voice is about one octave higher than the postpubescent voice. (For girls the difference is only three to four semitones.) Postpubescent boys and men who use falsetto voice often suffer social consequences, which vary from culture to culture.

Spasmodic Dysphonia

Spasmodic dysphonia, a form of **dystonia,** stems from either hyperadduction or hypoadduction. In the hyperadducted form, the vocal folds are so tightly closed that they cannot vibrate for any length of time; in the hypoadducted form, the vocal folds periodically move apart, producing a severely breathy voice. Spasmodic dysphonia is thought to be caused by abnormal functioning in the **basal ganglia.** Spasmodic dysphonia affects slightly more women than men and usually begins in adulthood. Audio Clip 6.2 is an example of spasmodic dysphonia speech.

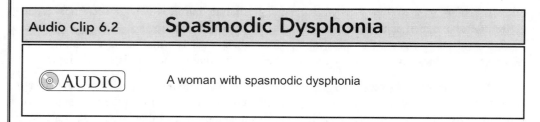

Audio Clip 6.2   **Spasmodic Dysphonia**

AUDIO   A woman with spasmodic dysphonia

Vocal Fold Dysfunction

Vocal fold dysfunction is a closing of the vocal folds even when the person is inhaling, resulting in an airway obstruction. This disorder is chronic and is sometimes mistaken for asthma. There is no consensus regarding its cause, although most recent studies suggest multiple causes. Vocal fold dysfunction produces several nonphonatory symptoms, including tightness in the throat and chest, wheezing, coughing, and shortness of breath. The voice is often breathy or hoarse.

Congenital Dysphonias

Congenital dysphonias occur as a consequence of certain congenital anomalies of the larynx, including airway obstructions. These obstructions cause respiratory difficulties, hoarseness, a weak cry, and **dysphagia.** These congenital abnormalities, which are usually identified in children, are usually treated medically before the SLP becomes involved.

Congenital Mass Lesions of the Larynx

Mass lesions of the larynx include tumors and viral growths, both of which may produce voice symptoms. Although neither type of lesion typically results in voice problems themselves, the most common voice symptom that does occur is hoarseness that appears following the surgical removal of the lesion.

Congenital Structural Anomalies of the Larynx

Sometimes infants have insufficient or delayed calcium depositing in the larynx, which can cause nonphonatory problems. However, a tracheostomy may be performed to allow the symptoms time to disappear. Because the child is unable to produce voice until the tracheostomy has been closed, the SLP may need to monitor the child's developing language and provide alternative communication forms if necessary.

Children with a particular chromosomal **anomaly,** the partial deletion of chromosome number 5, have what is called cri-du-chat syndrome (i.e., cat's cry syndrome). Their voice sounds like a kitten mewing. Children with this syndrome also have other characteristics including developmental disability; small-size head; widely spaced and downward-slanting eyes; asymmetrical eye movements; and speech and language delays. Video Clip 6.2 is an example of someone with cri-du-chat syndrome.

Video Clip 6.2	**Cri-du-chat Syndrome**
⊚ VIDEO	An SLP working with a child with cri-du-chat syndrome

Congenital Laryngeal Webs

A laryngeal web is connective tissue that **occludes** the larynx, either partially or totally. Total laryngeal webs are usually treated immediately at birth in order for the infant to be able to breathe. Laryngeal webs are caused by the failure of the vocal fold tissue to develop during the first trimester of pregnancy. If the web is located at the level of the glottis, the voice can be hoarse, aphonic, or elevated in pitch. Figure 6.7 on page 118 provides a picture of a laryngeal web.

Disorders of the Brain and/or Nervous System

Dysarthrias, or motor speech disorders, are neurogenic dysphonias that result from impairments in the innervation of the respiratory, resonatory, or phonatory muscles used to produce voice; impairments of muscle function; or impairments of motor planning at the neurologic level. The most common way to classify dysarthria is based on a system devised by Darley,

Anomaly
An abnormality.

Occlude
To create a blockage.

Figure 6.7	A Laryngoscopic View of a Laryngeal Web

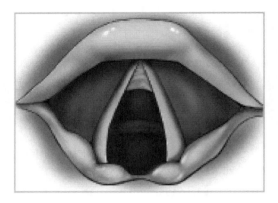

Nasality
Nasal resonance.

Orality
Oral resonance.

Aronson, and Brown (1975) and is still used today. Their system describes six types of dysarthria. Table 6.2 summarizes the types of dysarthria and their voice characteristics.

Disorders of Vocal Resonance

Languages vary in the amount of nasality their consonants use. In English consonants, **nasality** is used to produce only three phonemes: /m/, /n/, and /ŋ/. All other English consonants are produced using **orality,** although some nasality is usually present but not distinctive. Other languages (e.g., French) use more nasality than English, and some United States dialects incorporate more nasal "twang" than others.

Oral resonance is shaped by the oral cavity. The size and resiliency of the pharynx and the postures of the tongue, palate, and lips combine to shape the oral cavity. At the same time the velum and the nasopharyngeal wall close against each other to seal the oral cavity so that no air escapes into the nasal cavity.

To produce nasality, the velum drops down and the pharynx relaxes. This allows air and voice to flow into the nasal cavity to be shaped by their various structures. The resulting voice sounds more nasal than the voice produced when there is no resonance in the nasal cavity.

Hypernasality

Excessive nasal resonance results in **hypernasality,** which usually occurs because the velum has not made sufficient closure between the oral and nasal cavities. Sometimes a structural defect makes it difficult or impossible for the soft palate to seal the oral cavity. This can happen with a cleft palate; a short velum; or surgical or accidental injury to the velum.

Hyponasality

Hyponasality occurs when an individual cannot produce any nasal resonance. The resulting voice sounds like the person has a stuffy nose. Hyponasality almost always stems from an

Table 6.2	**Dysarthrias and Their Voice Characteristics**		
Dysarthria Classification	**Location of Damage**	**Possible Causes**	**Possible Voice Characteristics**
Ataxic	Cerebellum	Degenerative diseases, strokes, TBI, tumors, lead or mercury poisoning	• Harsh • Loud • Dysrhythmic
Flaccid	Nerves that enervate the speech musculature	Muscular dystrophy, myasthenia gravis, ALS, polio, infections secondary to AIDS, surgical trauma	• Weak voice • Hypernasal • Breathy • Monoloud • Monopitch
Spastic	Damage to both the pyramidal and extrapyramidal systems	Stroke, ALS, TBI, brainstem tumor, cerebral anoxia, viral or bacterial infection, multiple sclerosis	• Strained • Harsh • Low pitched • Hypernasal • Bursts of loudness
Hyperkinetic	Extrapyramidal system (basal ganglia)	Essential tremor syndrome, Huntington's disease, dystonia	• Harsh • Strained • Voice stoppages • Hypernasal
Hypokinetic	Extrapyramidal system	Parkinson's disease, Alzheimer's, stroke, TBI, tumors, drug toxicity	• Hoarse • Low volume • Hypernasal • Monotonous • Monoloud
Mixed	Combination of 2 or more dysarthria types	ALS, multiple sclerosis	• Varies based on neurological conditions

organic disorder causing an obstruction in the nasal cavities or nasopharyngeal area (e.g., a chronic sinus infection).

Assimilative Nasality

Assimilative nasality occurs when the nasality of a consonant "leaks" over to a vowel nearby. It is usually associated with an inability to move the **velopharyngeal port** quickly enough.

Faulty Tongue Postures

Resonance problems can occur if the tongue is habitually held high and to the front (i.e., anterior) of the mouth, or deep in the back (i.e., posterior) of the mouth. Because habitual anterior tongue posture is almost always a habit and not the result of any organic condition, it is more likely to be changeable through intervention than the posterior tongue position. Organically based tongue postures are much more resistant to change than those that are not organic.

Stridency

Stridency results when the pharynx is shortened, which raises the larynx and increases the reflective properties of the pharynx. A strident voice is usually harsh, shrill, and strained.

Velopharyngeal port
The soft palate and nasopharyngeal wall.

119

Oncologist
A physician who specializes in the treatment of cancer.

Psychiatrist
A physician who specializes in the diagnosis, treatment, and prevention of mental and emotional disorders.

Because it is the result of habit rather than an organic condition, stridency can be reduced through learning to relax the pharyngeal musculature.

Management

The management of voice disorders depends on a number of variables, including the origin of the disorder (organic or nonorganic; neurological or muscular; congenital or acquired); the contributions of medical professionals; the client's perception of the disorder and commitment to change; and the client's family. The management of voice disorders usually involves a team that includes, at a minimum, an **otolaryngologist** and an SLP. It could also include an **oncologist** and a **psychiatrist** (if a client has hysterical aphonia or is habitually tense).

The first goal in the process of voice rehabilitation is to restore the condition of the vocal folds to normal or, if this is not possible, compensate for whatever abnormality is present. The primary goal of voice rehabilitation following a laryngectomy is restoring the condition of the larynx as much as possible or providing the person with an alternative way to phonate.

If a client has had a total laryngectomy, he or she could use several strategies to set the molecules of air in the oral and nasal cavities into vibration. One involves the use of an instrument known as an electrolarynx, which is pictured in Figure 6.8. This is a small, battery-operated device that can be held in one hand and has a surface that vibrates. When the device is turned on and this surface is not in contact with anything solid (only in contact with air), it produces a relatively low-pitched buzzing sound.

To set the molecules of air in the oral and nasal cavities into vibration, the vibrating surface of the electrolarynx is pressed against the neck. This causes the skin and underlying structures (e.g., muscle fibers) in the neck to vibrate, which in turn causes molecules of air in the oral and nasal cavities to vibrate. The person then forms speech sounds in the usual way—that is, by moving structures in the speech musculature. An example of someone using an

| Figure 6.8 | **An Electrolarynx in Its Charging Dock** |

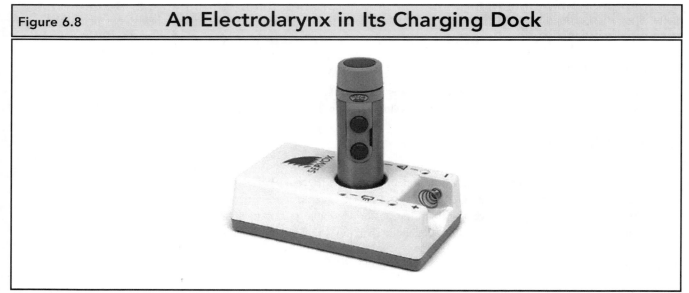

Photo courtesy of Servox

electrolarynx can be heard on Audio Clip 6.3. For further information about laryngectomy rehabilitation, see Bloom, Singer, and Hamaker (1998) and Casper and Colton (1998).

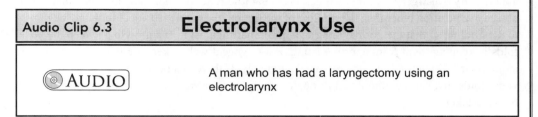

Audio Clip 6.3	**Electrolarynx Use**
AUDIO	A man who has had a laryngectomy using an electrolarynx

Another approach that can be used to set the molecules of air in the oral cavities into vibration is taking air into the esophagus and expelling it in a controlled way. Speech produced in this way is known as **esophageal speech.** Inside the esophagus is a structure, the upper esophageal sphincter, that functions as a valve to prevent the contents of the stomach from being expelled into the oral cavity. This valve opens and closes in a manner somewhat similar to the vocal folds, and is used to control the airflow of esophageal speech.

There are two approaches for injecting air into the esophagus for this type of speech. In esophageal speech, air is injected into the esophagus through the mouth. In **tracheo-esophageal speech,** air is injected into the esophagus from the lungs through a small opening in the wall that separates the trachea and the esophagus.

To get air into the esophagus, the person opens the esophageal sphincter and ingests (i.e., swallows) air. To produce voice, the person then expels this air through the closed sphincter. This action sets the sphincter's edges into vibration, which in turn sets the molecules of air above it (in the oral cavity) into vibration. The person then forms speech sounds in the usual way. Audio Clips 6.4 and 6.5 give examples of people using tracheo-esophageal speech.

For some clients with voice disorders not related to a laryngectomy, a goal could be to produce the best voice possible and/or prevent a recurrence of the laryngeal pathology. If the pathology resulted from vocal abuse, intervention would focus on the person learning how to produce an appropriate voice.

Audio Clip 6.4	**Tracheo-Esophageal Speech Example 1**
AUDIO	A person using tracheo-esophageal speech shortly after having had a laryngectomy

Audio Clip 6.5	**Tracheo-Esophageal Speech Example 2**
AUDIO	A woman who has had a laryngectomy using tracheo-esophageal speech to describe what she has to do to talk

Esophageal speech
A type of speech used by persons who have had a laryngectomy that requires air to be injected into the esophagus.

Tracheo-esophageal speech
A type of speech used by persons who have had a laryngectomy in which air passes from the lungs into the esophagus through a small opening in the wall that separates the trachea from the esophagus.

Sometimes surgery is part of voice management. If the vocal folds are unable to approximate either because they are paralyzed or absent, it may be possible to compensate for the abnormality by surgery. If, for example, one vocal fold functions normally and the other is paralyzed at a position other than the midline of the larynx, the paralyzed vocal fold may be moved to the midline so that the normal one can approximate against it. If a growth between the vocal folds is keeping them from approximating or a laryngeal web is keeping them from vibrating along their full length, it will be removed surgically. If there is a growth or other lesion on the vocal folds that can be eliminated through surgery or vocal rest, either or both processes will be undertaken.

The prognosis in some voice disorder cases is poor because the client may not perceive the disorder as needing change, the client may not be motivated to change, or the client may not have the familial support to carry out the necessary procedures involved in changing vocal habits and patterns. In children, the conditions leading to the voice disorder may not be under their control. The SLP may need to include the family in the intervention process to ensure that any necessary environmental and situational changes can be made and the child can benefit from intervention.

Families also play a major role in the intervention process with adults. Without support and contributions from family members, many adults with voice disorders are unable to follow through on the commitment necessary to effect permanent changes in their voice. To learn more about the management of voice disorders, see Boone and McFarlane (2000), Deem and Miller (2000), and Mathieson (2001).

Speech and Swallowing Disorders Associated with Dysarthria

Chapter 7

Learning Objectives

- Describe the major speech characteristics of dysarthria.

- Describe cerebral palsy and the management of associated dysarthrias in children.

- Describe the classification of acquired dysarthria in adults.

- Describe the management of the major types of dysarthria in adults.

- Describe dysphagia and how swallowing works.

- Describe dysphagia and its management in children.

- Describe dysphagia and its management in adults.

Chapter 7

Introduction

In Chapter 6, the types of voice disorders associated with various types of **dysarthria** were described. Some of the same disease processes that cause dysarthria can also affect swallowing and speech. In this chapter, the speech and swallowing disorders associated with dysarthria in children and adults are addressed. The most common cause of dysarthria in children is **cerebral palsy (CP).** In adults, dysarthria is most frequently associated with neurological or cerebrovascular disease.

Dysarthria

Dysarthrias are neuromuscular disorders that prevent structures within the vocal tract, particularly the oral cavity, from moving properly to produce speech sounds. In their most severe form, they result in paralysis. More often, they keep movement from occurring in a well-coordinated manner.

The specific type of movement disturbance that results from dysarthria is determined by the site of the damage. Predictable sets of symptoms are associated with lesions at various sites in the central and peripheral nervous systems. Consequently, all conditions that damage a particular site will have similar symptomatologies—that is, all of them will result in similar disturbances in the functioning of the **articulators.**

Flaccidity, for example, is the symptom associated with damage to the muscle fibers, **myoneural junctions,** or **lower motor neurons.** A number of conditions can cause such a lesion. The condition responsible most often for damaging muscle fibers is **muscular dystrophy.** This condition usually begins during childhood, appears to be hereditary, and is characterized by a chronic, progressive deterioration of muscle fibers.

The condition most often responsible for damaging the myoneural junctions is **myasthenia gravis.** This condition usually has its onset during adulthood, is progressive in nature, and tends to produce weakness of muscle contractions rather than paralysis. The musculature of the velum is particularly susceptible. In fact, one of the first symptoms a person with this condition is likely to show is **hypernasality.** Medication that augments the functioning of the myoneural junctions can often improve the nasality of persons with myasthenia gravis.

Several conditions can damage the lower motor neurons. One is **trauma,** which can occur during certain surgeries. For instance, the tongue may become paralyzed following an accidental cut to a nerve during heart surgery. Another condition that can damage the lower motor neurons is a viral disease such as **polio,** in which the functioning of the soft palate is frequently affected.

Spasticity is associated with a lesion in the **pyramidal** and **extrapyramidal systems.** Such a disturbance in the control of voluntary movement and reflex activity can limit the extent of an articulatory movement (e.g., elevation of the tongue tip). The range of movement possible may be so limited that the person cannot produce the movement at all. A number of conditions can cause spasticity, including **anoxia** and **stroke.** Audio Clip 7.1, which is described on page 126, provides a sample of dysarthria caused by relatively mild spasticity.

Flaccidity
Paralysis or weakness of muscle contraction resulting from damage to muscle fibers, myoneural junctions, or lower motor neurons.

Trauma
Damage that is usually accidental to the nervous system or other bodily structures.

Polio
A viral disease that damages lower motor neurons and causes flaccidity. The functioning of the velum is frequently affected.

Spasticity
A condition in which certain muscles are continuously contracted. It is the result of a lesion in the pyramidal and extrapyramidal systems.

Anoxia
Oxygen deprivation, which frequently results in destruction of brain cells.

Hemiplegia
A neuromuscular disorder that affects only one side of the body.

	Dysarthria Caused by Spasticity
Audio Clip 7.1	

 AUDIO | Note that the intelligibility of this man's speech is fairly good. This would not have been true if the spasticity had been relatively severe.

Anoxia is an insufficient flow of oxygen to the brain. If this occurs either before, during, or immediately following birth and the pyramidal system is damaged, the person will be diagnosed as having spastic cerebral palsy.

Another condition that can cause spasticity is a stroke. Some strokes damage the pyramidal system on only one side of the brain (right or left), which produces spasticity on the opposite side of the body (i.e., **hemiplegia).** Damage to the pyramidal system on the left side of the brain produces spasticity on the right side of the body.

Dysarthria in Children Caused by CP

Most dysarthrias in children are the result of cerebral palsy, which is the result of an incident that causes anoxia. The lack of oxygen usually occurs **prenatally, perinatally,** or **postnatally.** The resulting damage to the developing brain causes abnormal movements and postures of various muscles, including those involved in respiration, phonation, resonance, and articulation. Cerebral palsy is not progressive, and it is not reversible. It can range in severity from mild to severe, and it can affect one or more parts of the body.

Categories of Cerebral Palsy

Cerebral palsy is categorized in two ways, one to describe the effects and one to describe the types. The three most typical categories for describing the effects of CP are:

1. *Hemiplegia* which affects one side (left or right) of the body

2. *Paraplegia* which affects only the legs and lower trunk

3. *Quadriplegia* which affects all four limbs

Cerebral palsy is usually described by type, which is related to the neurological system(s) involved. Most professionals describe four main types of cerebral palsy:

1. *Spastic cerebral palsy* which is characterized by slow, stiff, and abrupt movements; increased muscle tone; and rigidity of the muscles

2. *Athetoid cerebral palsy* which is characterized by involuntary and uncontrolled movements that are slow and writhing

3. *Ataxic cerebral palsy* which is characterized by a disturbed sense of balance and depth perception, awkward gait, and uncoordinated movements

4. *Mixed cerebral palsy* which is a combination of these types in a person

Speech Problems Associated with Cerebral Palsy

The speech problems associated with CP depend on severity, which parts of the body are affected, and whether there are any associated conditions such as cognitive disabilities. Because the motor system is impaired in CP, children's speech development will be affected by the resulting weakness and incoordination. Children with CP typically have problems with articulation, because it requires rapid, coordinated movements and adjustments in numerous muscles. These children have poor respiratory control, are unable to coordinate respiration with phonation, and produce weak voices. Their ability to produce coordinated speech sounds may be so impaired that their speech is relatively **unintelligible** unless their listener knows the topic. Children with CP have the most difficulty producing the sounds that develop latest in typically developing children, and often experience difficulties into adulthood.

Impaired **prosody** of speech, shortened utterance length, and hypernasality also contribute to lowered intelligibility of speech in persons with CP. Impaired prosody results in a monotonic speech pattern, robbing it of the nuances carried by the melody and intonation associated with various meanings. Children with CP also tend to produce shorter utterances because they do not have the respiratory support for longer sustained phonation. Their speech can also be hypernasal because of an inability to coordinate the muscles of the **velum** and pharynx to seal the oral cavity from the nasal cavities.

Management

Treatment for childhood dysarthria involves increasing muscle tone and strength through structured activities and repetition. The goal is to increase speech intelligibility through improving range and rate of motion. The initial goal for a child with dysarthria may be to develop a stable respiratory pattern to support speech. Once the child has learned to phonate using the stable breathing pattern, the SLP teaches him or her various movements of the articulators that are basic to producing consonants (e.g., closing the lips, blowing, putting the upper teeth on the lower lip). From here, articulation of consonants and vowels is gradually differentiated.

Children whose intelligibility cannot be improved enough for successful communication via speech often learn alternative means for communicating. These may include augmentative/alternative devices such as computers or communication boards that use pictures or words.

Dysarthria in Adults (Acquired Dysarthria)

Dysarthrias in adults are speech disorders emanating from neurological problems that cause impaired muscular control of the speech mechanism. Impaired control may include incoordination, weakness, and/or paralysis. Either the central nervous system or the peripheral nervous system may be involved.

Dysarthria in adults differs from dysarthria in children in two important ways. First, the adult has developed speech and language in a relatively normal fashion, while the child with CP experiences speech and language difficulties throughout the developmental process. Second, children with CP suffer damage to the motor system early in development, while adults with dysarthria develop motor system damage later in life. Some of the most common causes of dysarthria in adults are **Parkinson's disease, Huntington's disease, amyotrophic lateral sclerosis (ALS),** and **multiple sclerosis (MS).** Dysarthrias can also result from the toxic effects of alcohol and/or drugs, or encephalitis.

Prosody
Variations in stress, pitch, and rhythms of speech that carry meaning.

Huntington's disease
A genetic disease resulting in gradual loss of brain cells. Both neurological functioning and intelligence are affected. Also referred to as Huntington's chorea.

Amyotrophic lateral sclerosis (ALS)
A progressive, fatal neuromuscular disorder also known as Lou Gehrig's disease. Causes damage to nerve cells in the brain and spinal cord.

Multiple sclerosis (MS)
A neurological disorder that can affect the functioning of the auditory nerves and other structures within the brain that support motor and sensory abilities. Typical symptoms are weakness, incoordination, paresthesias, speech disturbances, and visual complaints.

Speech Problems Associated with Acquired Dysarthria

Dysarthria in adults can be categorized into six types based on the muscle dysfunction that characterizes the disorder. Table 7.1 summarizes the types of dysarthria and their speech characteristics.

Management

Because the speech disorders related to dysarthria in adults vary considerably, treatment includes a wide range of techniques. Treatment may focus on respiration, phonation, resonance, articulation, or any combination of these processes. Respiration must be sufficient for sustained phonation; phonation must be sustained and of high enough quality to support the production of speech sounds. Resonance must be primarily oral so that the voice and speech do not sound hypernasal. Treatment of articulation includes focus on the muscles used in producing phonemes and modifying speaking rate, prosody, pitch, and loudness.

Table 7.1 Dysarthrias and Their Speech Characteristics

Dysarthria Classification	Location of Damage	Possible Causes	Speech Characteristics
Ataxic	Cerebellum	Degenerative diseases, strokes, TBI, tumors, lead or mercury poisoning	• Slurred and slow • Elongated phoneme and syllable production • Imprecise consonants • Distorted vowels • "Drunken" sounding
Flaccid	Nerves that enervate the speech musculature	Muscular dystrophy, myasthenia gravis, ALS, polio, infections secondary to AIDS, surgical trauma	• Slowed rate • Imprecise consonants • Short phrases
Spastic	Damage to both the pyramidal and extrapyramidal systems	Stroke, ALS, TBI, brainstem tumor, cerebral anoxia, viral or bacterial infection, multiple sclerosis	• Imprecise consonants • Distorted vowels • Short phrases • Slowed rate
Hyperkinetic	Extrapyramidal system (basal ganglia)	Essential tremor syndrome, Huntington's disease, dystonia	• Imprecise articulation • Short phrases • Speech flow breakdowns
Hypokinetic	Extrapyramidal system	Parkinson's disease, Alzheimer's, stroke, TBI, tumors, drug toxicity	• Imprecise consonants • Phoneme repetition • Slowed rate • Moments of freezing
Mixed	Combination of 2 or more dysarthria types	ALS, multiple sclerosis	• Range from barely noticeable to completely unintelligible

Dysphagia

Dysphagia is a disorder of swallowing that can result from an impairment of the musculature used in any of the stages of the eating process. Swallowing disorders affect a person's ability to eat, which poses three types of problems. First, the person may not be able to ingest enough food or liquid for nutrition and hydration, both of which are essential to survival. Second, eating plays an important role in the social fabric of every culture. Difficulties with swallowing effectively prevent people from participating in family rituals and social events. Third, a swallowing disorder removes a person's pleasure in eating and can instead turn eating into an unpleasant and frightening experience. To help you understand dysphagia, the normal anatomy and physiology of eating and swallowing are described in the next section.

How Swallowing Works

Getting food from the mouth to the stomach is a complex process, involving as many as fifty pairs of muscles. The process can be viewed in three phases. The first is the oral phase in which mastication (i.e., chewing) prepares the food for swallowing. In this stage, the tongue collects the food or liquid, and moves the food around in the mouth for chewing. Chewing makes the food the right size to swallow and helps to mix the food with saliva. Saliva softens and moistens the food, which makes the food easier to swallow. The food is then formed into the **bolus,** which can be swallowed.

During the second phase, the pharyngeal phase, the tongue pushes the bolus to the back of the mouth. This triggers a swallowing reflex that causes the food to pass through the **pharyngeal cavity** to the entrance of the **esophagus.** Also, the **epiglottis** closes tightly to prevent **aspiration.**

During the third phase, the esophageal phase, the bolus enters the esophagus and flows through it to the stomach. Passage of the bolus through the esophagus usually takes about three seconds, depending on the texture and consistency of the material.

To learn more about the anatomy and physiology of eating, see Murry and Carrau (2001). You can also visit the National Institute on Deafness and Other Communication Disorders (NIDCD; 2005b) webpage on dysphagia for more information.

Dysphagia in Children

Some children who are born prematurely or who have been diagnosed with cerebral palsy have problems with eating and drinking. Their difficulties could be due to poor posture or head control, or to a neuromuscular impairment of some or all of the oral musculature. Poor lip closure is a common impairment, and is partially responsible for drooling. It is crucial that children's swallowing problems be addressed as early as possible. Speech-language pathologists are often members of teams that have the mission to reduce the severity of feeding problems. SLPs on such teams are likely to collaborate with parents, teachers, **occupational therapists, physical therapists, dieticians,** and **pediatricians.** Members of these teams evaluate and modify child positioning for feeding, provide adapted feeding equipment (e.g., specialized cups and spoons), and recommend optimal food textures.

Bolus
The rounded mass of food formed through chewing and saliva prior to swallowing.

Aspiration
Food or liquid entering the airway.

Occupational therapist
A professional who helps people improve basic motor functions to perform daily living and work tasks.

Physical therapist
A professional who helps those suffering from disease or injury restore function, improve mobility, relieve pain, and prevent or limit permanent physical disabilities.

Dietician
One who is trained in the science of food and nourishment.

Pediatrician
A physician who specializes in the care of infants and children.

Tongue thrust
Thrusting the tongue against the incisors (i.e., front teeth) while speaking and swallowing.

Incisors
The four front teeth in each jaw (i.e., the two central and two lateral incisors).

Myofunctional therapy
Therapy intended to eliminate tongue thrusting.

In addition to treating children who have been diagnosed with feeding impairments, SLPs also treat children who appear to be at risk for developing dysphagia. These are children whose birth and developmental histories suggest that they have a neurological deficit that could result in an oral-motor impairment. Suggestions would be made to parents for improving the strength and functioning of the child's oral musculature.

Tongue thrust is a swallowing pattern that is common in infancy but usually disappears by age 6. During a tongue-thrust swallow, the tongue either pushes against the upper-front **incisors** or protrudes between the upper and lower incisors. (During the normal swallow, the tongue moves up and back in the mouth.) The average person swallows 600 to 2,000 times a day, and each tongue-thrust swallow exerts a pressure on the incisors. Consequently, it is not particularly surprising that a tongue-thrust swallow can be a contributing factor to dental problems (e.g., the upper incisors being pushed forward, resulting possibly in an anterior open bite) and/or malformations of the jaw.

A number of conditions can contribute to the development and/or maintenance of a tongue-thrust swallow. They include thumb sucking; enlarged tonsils or adenoids; allergies; and a high, narrow palate.

A malocclusion that is due, at least in part, to a tongue-thrust swallow may be corrected by an orthodontist. However, the problem is likely to recur if the tongue-thrust swallow is not eliminated. Consequently, many orthodontists refer their patients who have this type of swallow to SLPs to have it eliminated. It is desirable for a tongue-thrust swallow to be eliminated before any orthodontic work is done. However, SLPs often receive referrals from orthodontists for **myofunctional therapy** after they have completed their work.

The goal of myofunctional therapy is to retrain the muscles involved in swallowing and eliminate the tongue thrust. If the client is an adolescent or adult, he or she has swallowed incorrectly millions of times. Consequently, the tongue-thrust swallow is a strong habit and requires a real effort to eliminate. To be successful, a client must be willing to make myofunctional therapy a priority almost every day for three or four months. To learn more about tongue thrust and myofunctional therapy, see Garliner (1976) and Hanson and Barrett (1988).

Dysphagia in Adults

In dysphagia, weak cheek or tongue muscles can make it harder to move food around in the mouth for chewing so at least some of the pieces remain too large for swallowing. Pieces of food too large for swallowing can also enter the pharynx, block the pharynx, and block the passage of air through the **larynx** into the lungs. In addition to this life-threatening risk, other problems that can result with dysphagia include the following:

- The inability to start the swallowing reflex because of a stroke or other nervous system disorder

- Weak pharyngeal muscles that cannot move all the food to the entrance of the esophagus

Dysphagia can cause several problems. One, of course, is an inability to take in a sufficient amount of nourishing food. Another is food or liquid entering the respiratory system (i.e., aspiration) through the larynx that coughing or throat clearing cannot dislodge. Such material remaining in the respiratory system can cause a serious bacterial infection.

Any neurological condition that impairs the functioning of any of the muscles used for swallowing can cause dysphagia. Such conditions include stroke, cerebral palsy, Parkinson's disease, ALS, **traumatic brain injury (TBI),** polio, **dementia,** and side effects of certain prescription drugs.

Dysphagia in adults can occur at any of the three phases involved in swallowing. Disorders in the oral phase involve problems with chewing because of reduced tongue movement; reduced range of jaw movement; poor alignment of upper and lower jaw; and reduced tension in the mouth. Disorders in forming the bolus may occur because the tongue has difficulty moving in a posterior direction; collecting food residue; premature swallowing or aspiration before the swallow; tongue thrust; reduced strength of the oral musculature; and reduced range of tongue movement.

Disorders in the pharyngeal phase are related to the act of swallowing. Disorders in this phase may be caused by a delayed or absent swallow reflex; food that is in the nasal cavities or trachea; aspiration before and after the swallow; pharyngeal paralysis or reduced ability to contract; reduced ability of the base of the tongue to move; and inadequate closure of the trachea.

Disorders in the esophageal phase of swallowing, when the bolus has moved into the esophagus, result from problems with musculature that is not under voluntary control. People may have difficulties during this phase because food has moved back up from the esophagus to the pharynx (i.e., backflow), the esophagus cannot contract enough to move the food through, the esophagus may be obstructed (e.g., by a tumor), an abnormal pouch that collects food may be present, or there may be a hole in the esophagus.

Management

Dysphagia treatment includes medical procedures, direct services, and indirect services. SLPs provide both direct and indirect services but are not involved in the medical procedures used to treat dysphagia. Direct service for clients who have dysphagia includes evaluating the ability to eat and drink, and teaching new ways to swallow. It may also involve teaching the client to eat with the body positioned in a way that facilitates the swallowing process (e.g., with the head turned to one side) or teaching caregivers how to prepare food to facilitate it being swallowed (e.g., a thickener may have to be added to some liquids).

Indirect treatment does not involve food but instead is focused on improving muscle strength throughout the three phases of swallowing. Treatment may include exercises to strengthen weak muscles and/or improve coordination between the various muscles that contribute to swallowing, including those of the lips, tongue, palate, pharynx, larynx (to close the airway), and jaw. Also, treatment can include stimulating the swallow reflex.

In recent years, SLPs have become increasingly involved in providing services to clients with tracheostomies and **ventilator-dependence.** These SLPs typically work as part of a team that includes a variety of health care practitioners, including physicians, nurses, **respiratory therapists,** registered dieticians, and **social workers,** among others. The type of services

Ventilator-dependence
Dependency on a mechanical device (ventilator/ respirator) in order to breathe.

Respiratory therapist
A professional who evaluates, treats, and cares for individuals with breathing or other cardiopulmonary disorders.

Social worker
A professional who helps individuals function their best in their environments; help deal with relationships; and help solve personal and family problems.

provided by SLPs varies from facility to facility. Although assessment and management are highly individualized because of the wide range of conditions presented by clients, certain knowledge and skills are necessary regardless of client or facility. Dikeman and Kazandijan (2004) list these four areas:

- Knowledge of both vocal and nonvocal communication methods

- Knowledge of posttracheostomy anatomy and the potential impact on swallowing of the tracheostomy and ventilator-dependence

- An awareness of other conditions that can affect swallowing function

- Skills with dysphagia assessment, including clinical approaches and instrument management

To learn more about dysphagia and its management, see ASHA (2005g), Hall (2001), and Murry and Carrau (2001).

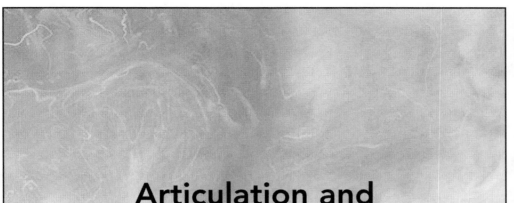

Articulation and Phonological Disorders

Chapter 8

Learning Objectives

- Explain how phonemes are formed.

- Explain how speech sounds are classified.

- Explain how articulation and phonological disorders are similar/different.

- List some possible causes of articulation disorders.

- Explain management for articulation and phonological disorders.

Introduction

People who have an articulation disorder do not produce speech sounds as accurately as most others their age. They do not use their speech mechanism appropriately, at least some of the time. Children with **phonological disorders** have difficulty with the rules for the sound system.

To understand why speech sound errors occur, you first have to understand, at least intuitively, how the speech mechanism—specifically that part known as the **vocal tract**—molds air particles flowing from the lungs into the **phonemes** of a language. Articulation errors result when this physical mechanism does not function as it should. **Speech-language pathologists (SLPs)** have been working with clients on articulation skills since the early years of the profession. Study More 8.1 provides a list of terms used to describe articulation disorders during

Study More 8.1	We Regret to Inform You That Your Child Has...

Sixty years ago all students of speech-language pathology were required to master long lists of Greek and Latin names for speech disorders. Such a name could make a disorder appear to be more debilitating than it was. These terms are rarely used today. The following types of dyslalia (i.e., articulation disorders) were recognized by the Nomenclature Committee of the American Academy of Speech Correction during the 1940s.

- *Asapholalia:* Mumbled speech, in which the patient can usually produce each vowel and consonant correctly by itself or a consonant with a vowel but speaks so rapidly—or moves his lips, tongue or jaw so little—that he sounds as though he was talking with a full mouth

- *Atelolalia:* Delayed development of speech

- *Barbaralalia:* Foreign dialect

- *Bradylalia:* Abnormal slowness of speech

- *Dialectolalia:* Provincial dialect

- *Embololalia:* Adding speech sounds or syllables which do not belong to the word

- *Idiolalia:* Invented language in which the patient uses a language all his own

- *Leipolalia:* Omission of speech sounds or syllables that belong to the word

- *Metalalia:* Transposition of speech sounds, such as "er" for "re"

- *Paralalia:* Mispronunciation or substitution of one speech sound for another

- *Pedolalia:* Baby-talk; a syndrome composed of sound omissions, sound substitutions, and the omission of articles, prepositions, conjunctions, and many pronouns

- *Rhinolalia aperta (hyperrhinolalia):* Functional cleft palate type of speech that includes nasality, nasal fricatives, and the substitution of glottal click or nasals for plosives.

- *Rhinolalia clausa (hyporhinolalia):* Hypernasaity; sounds like speech with a plugged nose.

- *Tachylalia:* Abnormally rapid speech without mumbling

Source: Robbins (1948, p. 121)

Alveolar ridge
A ridged shelf in the upper jaw (i.e., maxilla) behind the upper teeth.

Hard palate
The anterior portion of the roof of the mouth.

that time period. Phonological disorders are a more recent diagnosis that evolved with greater understanding of **phonology** as a rule-based system that governs the use of speech sounds in a language.

Production of Speech Sounds

Air from the lungs is molded into phonemes by the vocal tract, as shown in Figure 8.1. The vocal tract extends from the **glottis** to the lips and nose. The main components of the vocal tract are three air-filled passages: the **pharyngeal cavity,** the **oral cavity,** and the **nasal cavity.**

All vowels and most consonants are produced by vibration of the vocal folds. Some consonants, however, are produced by air that is set into vibration in the oral cavity. During the production of /f/, for example, air is set into vibration by being forced to exit through the narrow passage between the upper **incisors** and lower lip. The production of /s/ is accomplished by pushing air between the tongue and the **alveolar ridge.**

The configuration (i.e., shape) of the cavities in the vocal tract at a particular moment determines which phoneme will be produced. Each phoneme has a unique configuration. Because during every second of conversational speech as many as 14 phonemes are produced (Darley, Aronson, & Brown, 1975), the configuration of the vocal tract is continually in a state of transformation.

The oral cavity is the most important component of the vocal tract for determining which phoneme will be produced. It significantly affects the production of all but one English speech sound (/h/ as in *h*at). The nasal cavity, on the other hand, only affects the production of three English speech sounds: /m/ as in *m*at; /n/ as in *n*o; and /ŋ/ as in si*ng*.

The structures in the oral cavity that affect the configuration of the vocal tract are the tongue, teeth, lips, **mandible, hard palate,** and **velum** (i.e., soft palate). These structures are referred to as **articulators.**

The tongue is one of the most important structures in the oral cavity for determining the configuration of the vocal tract. Either the back or tip of the tongue is involved in the production of

| Figure 8.1 | **Transformation of Air into Phonemes by the Vocal Tract** |

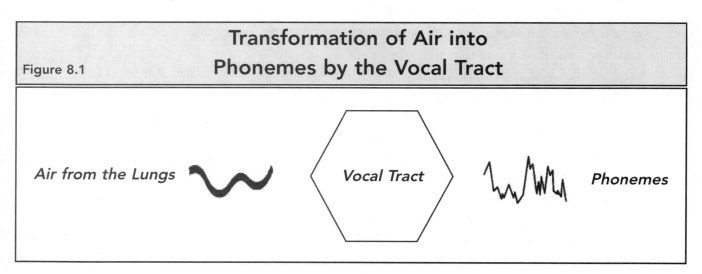

Air from the Lungs   *Vocal Tract*   *Phonemes*

most consonant sounds. Those in which the back is active include /k/ and /g/. Examples of those in which the tip is active are /s/, /z/, /t/, /d/, /n/, /l/, and /r/.

The teeth that are most important for the production of speech are the four front ones in each jaw—the two central and two lateral incisors. They are used with the lower lip to create a constriction for /f/ and /v/. They are also used with the tongue to create a constriction for the two "th" sounds (the ones in *th*ink and *the)*.

Some phonemes are shaped by the lips. For example, closure of the lips is one of the main features of three English speech sounds: /p/, /b/, and /m/. During the production of /u/ as in b*oo*t and /w/, the lips protrude.

The mandible plays an active role in the production of most English speech sounds. It brings together and separates the upper and lower lip, and the upper and lower teeth. Consequently, it is active during the production of all speech sounds that involve these structures, including /f/, /v/, /s/, and /z/. It also plays an active role during the production of speech sounds in which the mouth is open, such as /a/ as in f*a*ther and /k/ as in *k*ing.

The hard palate forms the anterior portion of the roof of the mouth. The anterior three-fourths of the hard palate are a part of the same bone that forms the **maxilla.** Along with the velum, the hard palate separates the oral cavity from the nasal cavity. Behind the upper teeth is a ridged shelf known as the alveolar ridge. The action of the tongue tip in relation to the alveolar ridge contributes to the production of many speech sounds, including /t/, /d/, and /n/.

The velum forms the posterior portion of the roof of the mouth. When the vellum is not elevated, an opening is present in the roof of the mouth and air can flow from the oral cavity into the nasal cavity. When the velum is elevated, it contacts the posterior wall of the pharynx. As a result, the opening in the roof of the mouth is closed and no air flows from the oral cavity into the nasal cavity. This **velopharyngeal closure** occurs to some degree during the production of all English speech sounds except /m/, /n/, and /ŋ/. To learn more about the mechanism responsible for the production of speech sounds, see Zemlin (1998).

Classification of Speech Sounds

Consonant speech sounds have been classified in a number of ways with regard to how they are produced. The most commonly used classification characteristics include presence of voicing, place of articulation, and manner of articulation.

Presence of Voicing

All speech sounds can be classified as either **voiced** or **voiceless.** All the vowel sounds in English are voiced. Some consonants are voiced and some are voiceless. An example of a voiced consonant sound is /z/, and an example of a voiceless consonant is /s/. Actually, the only difference in the configuration of the vocal tract for these sounds is that while /z/ is being produced, the vocal folds are approximated, and while /s/ is being produced they are separated.

Maxilla
Upper jaw.

Velopharyngeal closure
Elevation of the velum to contact the posterior and lateral walls of the pharynx, thereby closing off the opening between the oral and the nasal cavities.

Voiced sounds
Sounds produced when air particles entering the vocal tract are set into vibration by the vocal folds (e.g., /z/ and /v/).

Voiceless sounds
Sounds produced when air particles entering the vocal tract are not set into vibration by the vocal folds (e.g., /s/ and /f/).

Bilabial sound
Sound produced with closure of the lips.

Labio-dental sound
Sound produced with the upper teeth placed on the lower lip.

Lingua-dental sound
Sound produced with the tongue between the upper and lower teeth.

Lingua-alveolar sound
Sound produced with the tongue against the alveolar ridge.

Palatal sound
Sound produced with the tongue against the hard palate.

Velar sound
Sound produced with the tongue against the velum.

Glottal sound
Sound made with an open glottis.

Plosive
A consonant sound that cannot be sustained.

Continuant
A phoneme that can be sustained.

You can feel the presence of voicing by touching the front of your neck at the level of the **larynx** and producing the voiced and voiceless members of a pair. For example, first produce a sustained /z/ and then a sustained /s/. You should feel vibration during the production of /z/, but not during that of /s/. The consonant sounds produced with no voicing and their voiced counterparts are listed in Study More 8.2.

Place of Articulation

Consonant sounds are classified on the basis of where in the vocal tract they are formed. The following terms are used to classify consonant phonemes according to their place of articulation: **bilabials, labio-dentals, lingua-dentals, lingua-alveolars, palatals, velars,** and **glottals.**

Manner of Articulation

Consonants can be described by the way in which the oral musculature works to produce them. For instance, a **plosive** sound is a type of consonant that is produced by impounding air behind an occlusion in the vocal tract and releasing it suddenly. It cannot be sustained. For /p/ and /b/, the closed lips act as the occlusion behind which air is impounded. The contact between the tongue tip and alveolar ridge forms the occlusion for the production of /t/ and /d/. The back of the tongue and the velum form the occlusion for /k/ and /g/.

A **continuant** is a speech sound that can be sustained (e.g., /s/, /f/, and /a/). All vowel sounds are continuants. Continuants can be further described by their quality. **Fricative** sounds are produced by forcing air through a narrow opening in a comparatively prolonged way (e.g., /s/ as in *s*un). **Nasal** sounds are produced by opening the velopharyngeal port to allow some air to resonate in the nasal cavity. The three nasal sounds in the English language are /m/, /n/, and /ŋ/ as in si*ng*. **Liquid** sounds are produced by air passing along one or both sides of the tongue such as /l/ as in *l*ine and /r/ as in *r*ain.

The final two descriptions of manner of articulation are **affricates** and **glides.** Affricates are produced by narrowing an opening for the air to pass through, but in a short burst (i.e., /tʃ/ as in *ch*air and /dʒ/ as in *j*ump). Glides are described as semi-vowels and include the /j/ sound in *y*es and /w/ sound in *w*ell.

Table 8.1 summarizes the classification of all English consonants according to place of articulation, manner of articulation, and presence of voicing. To learn more about the classification of phonemes, see Bernthal and Bankson (1998), Hodson (1997), and Polloway, Miller, and Smith (2004).

Study More 8.2	Voiceless and Voiced Consonants
Voiceless	**Voiced**
/p/	/b/
/t/	/d/
/k/	/g/
/s/	/z/
/f/	/v/

Table 8.1	Classification of Consonants											
	Manner											
	Plosives		Fricatives		Affricates		Nasals		Liquids		Glides	
Place	V	VL	V	VL	V	VL	V	VL	V	VL	V	VL
Bilabial	b bat	p pat					m mat				w win	
Labio-dental			v van	f fin								
Lingua-dental			ð that	θ thin								
Lingua-alveolar	d dip	t toe	z zip	s sit			n no		l lap			
Palatal			ʒ measure	ʃ shoe	ʤ jump	ʧ chair			r rat		j yes	
Velar	g goat	k cat					ŋ sing					
Glottal				h hat								
V= Voiced VL=Voiceless												

From Phonological Analysis Practice: An Electronic Workbook [Computer software], by M. Watson, J. Murthy, and N. Wadhwa, 2003, Eau Claire, WI: Thinking Publications. © 2003 by Thinking Publications. Adapted with permission.

Phonological Disorders

Many children make multiple speech sound errors for which there appears to be no organic cause. The structure and function of their peripheral speech mechanism seem normal, and there is no evidence of a hearing loss or developmental disability. Such children usually are diagnosed as having a phonological disorder. Strictly speaking, **phonological disorders** are language-based disorders rather than speech disorders, because the assumption is made that their speech sound errors are caused by faulty learning on the phonological level of language. Because it is important to be able to differentiate between a phonological disorder and an articulation disorder, phonological disorders are described here rather in the chapter on child language disorders.

From a phonological perspective, spoken English consists of ordered sequences of phonemes that are segmented into words. Phonemes are represented by a notational system called the International Phonetic Alphabet (IPA), which is used to transcribe speech when diagnosing various types of speech disorders. Study More 8.3 on page 140 shows some typical words and how they are represented by the IPA.

The phrase "I love you" is perceived as an ordered sequence of six phonemes (/aɪ l u v j u/) segmented into three words The sequence of phonemes is uttered in the order the rules of the language require. The failure to produce multiple phonemes correctly in appropriate sequences

Fricative
A consonant sound produced by forcing air through a narrow opening.

Nasal sound
Sound produced with air flowing through the nose.

Liquid sound
Sound produced by air passing along one or both sides of the tongue.

Affricate sound
Sound produced by narrowing an opening for air to pass in short bursts.

Glide sound
The two semivowels, /j/ as in *yes* and /w/ as in *well*.

Study More 8.3	**IPA Transcriptions of Selected Words**		
shadow	ʃæɾo	aphasia	əfeʒə
church	tʃɝtʃ	judge	dʒʌdʒ
yesterday	jɛstɚde	pinch	pɪntʃ
satisfy	sərɪsfaɪ	yellow	jɛlo
speech	spitʃ	pathology	pəθɔlədʒi
audiology	ɔdiɔlədʒi	stuttering	stʌɾɝɪŋ
communication	kɜmjunɪkeʃʌn	science	saɪənts
disorders	dɪsɔrdɚz	language	leɪŋgwədʒ

Source: Robbins (1948, p. 121)

Phonological processes
Ways children below the age of 3.5 years sometimes simplify their production of words.

Phoneme collapse
The production of one sound by the child for several different adult target sounds, or the deletion of several adult target sounds in a given position (e.g., /t/ substituted for /f, p, h, θ, n/).

by an age at which most peers can produce them is classified as a phonological language disorder unless it is caused by some abnormality in the structure or function of the peripheral speech mechanism (e.g., dysarthria).

Recall from Chapter 3 that phonological language learning involves two interrelated tasks. The first is learning to produce the various phonemes of one's language. The second is learning the rules that dictate how they can be combined into words, phrases, and sentences.

Children learning to speak do not pronounce many of their words the way that adults do. They simplify them, for example, by omitting and substituting for phonemes they have difficulty producing. As their ability to produce speech sounds improves, their simplifications decrease and their speech becomes more like adults.

When children simplify the production of words, their simplifications are predictable and universal across languages. These simplifications have been observed in the speech of young children in many countries. Speech-language pathologists refer to these simplifications as **phonological processes.** Although there are many phonological processes exhibited by children with phonological disorders, five common ones are described in Table 8.2. By the age of three-and-a-half, most children have stopped using them.

Williams (2003; 2006) describes error patterns in terms of **phoneme collapses,** which are larger rule sets that involve a substitution or deletion error that encompasses several different adult target sounds and can include singletons and clusters from several different sound classes. A phoneme collapse represents a one-to-many correspondence between the child's error and the adult targets. The resulting use of a small number of different phonemes makes a child's speech highly **unintelligible.**

A child who simplifies production of words more than same-age peers is likely to be regarded as having a phonological disorder. Children with these disorders constitute the largest subgroup of clients served by SLPs according to the American Speech-Language-Hearing Association (ASHA; 2004a). Although most preschool children with a moderate-to-severe phonological disorder will improve their speech sound production abilities dramatically by the

	Five Common Phonological Processes Used by Children	
Table 8.2		
Process	**Definition**	**Examples**
Syllable reduction	Child reduces the number of syllables in a word	/bæ/ for basket; /tɛlfon/ for telephone
Final consonant deletion	Child deletes the final consonant in a word	/fɪ/ for fish; /hæ/ for hat
Velar fronting	Child substitutes /t/ & /d/ for /k/ & /g/	/do/ for go; /tʊti/ for cookie
Cluster reduction	Child deletes one or both consonants in a consonant cluster	/nek/ for snake; /bo/ for boats
Gliding	Child substitutes /j/ (yellow) or /w/ for another sound	/jaɪt/ for light; /wop/ for rope

later elementary grades, manifestations of communication disabilities remain for many of these individuals throughout childhood and adolescence, and sometimes even beyond (Felsenfeld, Broen, & McGue, 1992).

Some evidence suggests that children with phonological disorders are likely to have other communication disorders including other types of language disorders, voice disorders, and fluency disorders (Ruscello, St. Louis, & Mason, 1991). To learn more about phonological development, see Gleason (2001). To learn more about how articulation disorders differ from phonological disorders, see Bernthal and Bankson (1998) and Hodson (1997).

Articulation Disorders

People who are regarded as having an articulation disorder make more speech sound errors than their age peers. They may omit speech sounds (e.g., they may say "leap" when they wish to say "sleep"). They may substitute one speech sound for another (e.g., substituting /w/ for /r/ and say "wed" for "red"). Or they may produce a speech sound in a distorted manner (e.g., producing /s/ in a manner that sounds like a whistle). Most people with articulation disorders make some combination of these types of errors. Errors rarely occur on vowel sounds, partly because vowels require less precise movements of the articulators than consonant sounds. Audio Clip 8.1 is an example of a sound omission.

Audio Clip 8.1	**Sound Omission**
◎ AUDIO	The sound /θ/ is omitted in the word *toothbrush*.

Glossectomy
Surgical removal of a portion of the tongue. Such surgery is usually done to remove a malignant tumor from the tongue tissue.

Intelligible
Understandable.

Excised
To remove something surgically (e.g., a tumor).

Prosthodontist
A person who specializes in the part of dentistry pertaining to replacement of missing teeth and tissues with artificial substitutes.

The majority of persons diagnosed as with an articulation disorder are children. However, not all children who make articulation errors have a disorder. Most preschool children, particularly those below the age of 3, make articulation errors. Acquisition of the ability to produce the various consonant sounds correctly tends to follow a predictable developmental sequence, which is summarized in Table 8.3. We ordinarily would not be concerned about a child's inability to produce a particular consonant correctly unless his or her chronological age exceeded the upper age limit given in the table. For example, the failure to produce /g/ correctly would not ordinarily be of concern in children below the age of 4.

The extent to which articulation errors interfere with communication depends on several factors. One factor is the number of errors. The greater the number of articulation errors in a person's speech, the more difficulty listeners are likely to have understanding it. A second factor is the type of error. Sound omissions are more likely than sound distortions to interfere with others' comprehension. A third factor is which phonemes are produced in error. Some phonemes occur more often in English than others and, consequently, producing them incorrectly will result in a greater number of errors. For example, a defective /s/ in English is likely to result in more errors than a defective /w/. To learn more about the characteristics of articulation disorders, see Bernthal and Bankson (1998) and Hodson (1997).

Causes of Articulation Disorders

A number of different conditions can result in articulation disorders. They are often caused by the improper functioning of structures within the vocal tract. Others result from genetic conditions.

Structural Anomalies

If the size, shape, or alignment of one or more of the structures within the vocal tract is abnormal, or if one of these structures is incomplete or missing, it may not be possible for the vocal tract to assume the configuration required for the production of a particular phoneme. Depending on the structure affected and the extent of the anomaly, the result could be anything from a minor sound distortion to a complete inability to produce a particular phoneme. The following are examples of structural anomalies that can cause articulation errors.

Glossectomy

Because the tongue (particularly the tip) influences the configuration of the vocal tract for most consonant sounds, a **glossectomy** will almost always cause articulation errors. In spite of this, speech may remain fairly **intelligible.** The impact of a glossectomy on speech **intelligibility** is largely a function of the amount of tissue **excised** and its location. The greater the amount of tissue excised, particularly from the tongue tip, the poorer speech intelligibility is likely to be. Excision of tissue at the back of the tongue tends to affect the production of vowels more than consonants, and excision at the tongue tip affects consonants more than vowels (Leonard, Goodrich, McMenamin, & Donald, 1992). Video Clip 8.1, which is described on page 144, is of a man with a glossectomy.

Some patients who have had only a partial glossectomy can be helped to improve the intelligibility of their speech. A **prosthodontist**, for example, may be able to make an appliance that attaches to the hard palate. The appliance would provide a surface at a height that can be contacted by the tongue stub. This would enable the person to more closely approximate the vocal tract configuration required for such speech sounds as /t/ and /d/, for which contact between

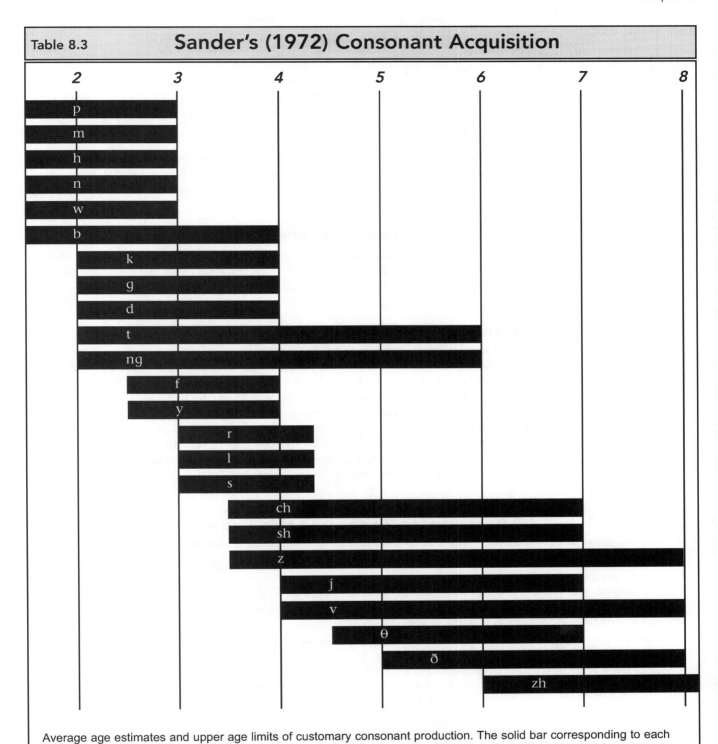

Table 8.3 — **Sander's (1972) Consonant Acquisition**

Average age estimates and upper age limits of customary consonant production. The solid bar corresponding to each sound starts at the median age of customary articulation; it stops at an age level at which 90% of all children are customarily producing the sound.

From "When Are Speech Sounds Learned?" by E. Sander, 1972, *Journal of Speech and Hearing Disorders,* 37, p. 62 ©1972 by the American Speech-Language-Hearing Association. Reprinted with permission.

Ablative surgery
Surgical removal of all or part of a structure (e.g., the lips or mandible).

Prosthesis
An artificial body part.

Lingual frenum
A fold of membrane that extends from the floor of the mouth at the midline to the underside of the tongue.

Tongue-tied
Having a lingual frenum that extends too near the tip of the tongue and, consequently, restricts the ability of the tongue tip to move.

Video Clip 8.1	**Man with a Glossectomy**

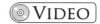 A man who has highly intelligible speech in spite of having a glossectomy. The speech of most persons who have had a glossectomy isn't this intelligible.

the tongue tip and hard palate is essential. Another possibility would be to surgically increase the length of the tongue stub. Both of these approaches partially compensate for the shortening of the tongue and thereby increase intelligibility. For an interesting case involving a man with a partial glossectomy see Study More 8.4.

Acquired Structural Deficits Other Than Glossectomies

Acquired structural deficits ordinarily result from trauma to oral cavity structures or **ablative surgery.** Ablative surgery can involve partial or total removal of the mandible, the lips, or the palate (hard and/or soft). The impact on articulation often can be reduced by reconstructing the affected structure(s) surgically or by means of a **prosthesis.**

Lingual Frenum That Restricts Tongue Movement

If the **lingual frenum** extends too near the tip of the tongue, it can restrict one's ability to move the tongue tip. Sometimes people with this restriction are referred to as **tongue-tied.** At one time it was common practice for physicians to clip a child's lingual frenum if it seemed to be too short—that is, if it seemed to be interfering with tongue tip mobility. This is no longer the case. We now know that people with this condition can almost always be taught to produce the speech sounds that require tongue tip mobility (Bernthal & Bankson, 1998). Also, physicians now hesitate to cut the frenum because of the possibility of hemorrhages, infections, and scar tissue. Occasionally, however, one does encounter a child whose tongue tip movement is so restricted that clipping of the lingual frenum is necessary.

Study More 8.4	**The Case of Johannes the Dumb**

This case, published in Amsterdam around 1650 by Dr. Nicholas Tulp, is interesting because it demonstrates an awareness more than three centuries ago that it is possible for a person to learn to produce intelligible speech following a partial glossectomy. The young man became known as "Johannes the Dumb" after being partially glossectomized as a punishment. Note that most authorities at this time believed that the tongue influenced phonation (i.e., voice) as well as articulation. The term *dumb* referred to a lack of speech.

After experiencing the removal of all the loose part of his tongue for three years he was unable to speak—but recovered his voice, during a tempestuous night after a shock of alarm from a flash of lightning. Him we heard, not only distinctly speaking, but likewise pronouncing accurately one and all of the consonants, the enunciation of which is attributed, by the most sagacious investigators of nature, to the tip of the tongue alone—as far as it is movable the tongue divides the voice into distinct words, and as it strikes against either the teeth, or the palate, or the lips, it is believed, by the learned, to discriminate words accordingly, and to modulate, with fineness, the sounds of speech. And for the same reason is it not wonderful that when the tongue, the genuine instrument of articulate voice, had received injury, the voice itself should have been injured likewise; but, that the same voice, after being mute for three years, should nevertheless have come back to him in perfect state while the tongue remained mutilated just as before, is indeed a thing which exceeds the comprehension of all the learned.

Source: Twistleton (1873)

Dental Anomalies

The teeth, particularly the lateral and central incisors, play an important role in configuring the vocal tract for a few consonant sounds, especially /s/ and /z/. If these teeth are missing, the tongue may protrude through the opening, and the person will substitute /θ/ for /s/. This sound substitution, which is referred to as a frontal lisp, also can occur if there is an **anterior open bite.**

Some people exhibit anterior movement of the tongue during speech and swallowing—that is, they "thrust" their tongue against their anterior incisors while engaged in these activities. The result is called **tongue thrust.** They may also press their tongue against their incisors when they are not speaking or swallowing. The pressure of the tongue on the incisors can cause the teeth to protrude. This condition can result in articulation errors. The speech sound most likely to be affected is /s/. Tongue thrust was discussed in Chapter 7 on page 130. For more information about tongue thrust, visit ASHA's (2005j) webpage.

A dental **anomaly,** such as missing incisors or an open bite, will not necessarily cause articulation errors. Some people with dental anomalies produce all the speech sounds correctly (Bernthal & Bankson, 1998). They compensate by positioning their articulators, particularly their tongue, a little differently than do most people when saying certain sounds.

Cleft Palate

A **cleft palate,** illustrated in Figure 8.2, is **congenital.** This opening connects the oral cavity to the nasal cavity. It results in an abnormal configuration of the vocal tract for all but three English speech sounds: /m/, /n/, and /ŋ/. (These are the only ones for which there is normally a flow of air through the nasal cavity.) An unrepaired or partially repaired cleft palate is highly likely to result in at least a few articulation errors. It may, in fact, result in so many errors that the person's speech is unintelligible.

Anterior open bite
A type of dental malocclusion in which there is a relatively large space between the upper and lower incisors when the jaws are together.

Cleft palate
A congenital disorder in which there is an opening in the hard palate, soft palate (i.e., velum), or both.

Figure 8.2	A Hard and Soft Palatal Cleft

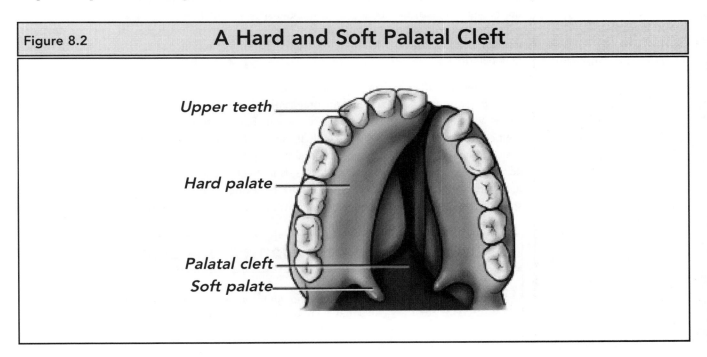

Upper teeth

Hard palate

Palatal cleft

Soft palate

Verbal apraxia
A disturbance in the ability to voluntarily program the oral musculature to produce speech sounds, resulting from damage to the central nervous system. There is no weakness, paralysis, or incoordination of the oral musculature while it is being used for vegetative purposes (i.e., eating and drinking), as there is with dysarthria.

Developmental apraxia of speech (DAS)
A disturbance in the ability to voluntarily program the oral musculature to produce speech sounds resulting from damage to the central nervous system, usually either before, during, or immediately following birth. Also referred to as developmental verbal dyspraxia.

Sensorineural hearing loss
A hearing loss caused by pathology in the inner ear.

Conductive hearing loss
Hearing loss caused by pathology in the outer or middle ear.

Verbal Apraxia

Verbal apraxia, like most types of dysarthria, is a motor speech disorder caused by damage to the central nervous system (CNS). It differs from dysarthria in that a person who has verbal apraxia would have difficulty programming the speech mechanism to produce certain speech sounds, but there would be no weakness, paralysis, or incoordination of the oral musculature while it is being used for manipulating food in the mouth, chewing, and swallowing. With dysarthria, the ability of the oral musculature to perform all these functions would be impaired.

The articulation errors of people with verbal apraxia tend to be inconsistent. Sometimes they produce a speech sound correctly, and sometimes they don't. They have difficulty programming their articulators to produce the sounds they want to produce and are often aware when they haven't been successful. As a result, their speech tends to be slow and effortful because of frequent trial-and-error attempts at the desired articulatory postures and movements (Darley, Aronson, & Brown, 1975).

In children, this condition is called **developmental apraxia of speech (DAS)**. The American Speech-Language-Hearing Association describes DAS as a nervous system disorder that affects the child's ability to produce and sequence sounds, syllables, and words. Children with this disorder know what they want to say but are unable to do so because the brain does not send the correct instructions to the speech musculature. To learn more about this condition, see Bernthal and Bankson (1998), Hall (1992), and Robin (1992). You can also visit ASHA's (2005e) childhood apraxia webpage for more information.

Hearing Loss

To produce speech sounds correctly, speakers have to be able to hear and monitor their speech to tell whether they are producing speech sounds correctly. This can have several consequences. When a child develops a severe hearing loss before beginning to speak, he or she may not be able to learn to produce at least some speech sounds without special training. This is why children who are deaf at birth do not learn to speak in the usual way. If a person develops a severe hearing loss after learning to speak, the ability to produce at least some speech sounds may deteriorate.

A **sensorineural hearing loss** is more likely than a **conductive** loss to cause articulation errors for two reasons. First, sensorineural hearing losses tend to interfere more than conductive losses with self-monitoring of speech. People who have sensorineural hearing losses tend to hear their own speech as relatively soft, while those who have conductive hearing losses tend to hear it as relatively loud. Second, sensorineural hearing losses can be more severe than conductive hearing losses. (Conductive hearing losses cannot cause deafness.) The more severe a hearing loss, the more likely it is to interfere with monitoring speech auditorily. Audio Clip 8.2 is a speech sample from a man who is deaf. Hearing loss is described in more detail in Chapter 10.

Audio Clip 8.2 **Voice of a Man who is Deaf**

 Notice that although his speech contains articulation errors, this man's speech is relatively intelligible.

Cognitive Disabilities

The acquisition of speech sounds tends to follow a predictable developmental sequence (refer back to Table 8.3 on page 143) that is related to intellectual development. Children usually do not learn to produce specific speech sounds until they achieve a certain level of mental maturity. Consequently, children who have a **cognitive disability** usually do not produce the various speech sounds by the ages most children learn to produce them, which means they tend to make more articulation errors than most children their age. To learn more about the etiology of articulation disorders, see Bernthal and Bankson (1998).

Management

The long-term goal for a client who has an articulation or phonological disorder can be any of the following, depending on its etiology. More than one of these goals may be appropriate for any particular client:

- To correct the client's phonological disorder

- To correct the client's articulation error(s)

- To increase the intelligibility of the client's speech

- To augment the client's ability to communicate

Correcting Phonological Disorders

When a child's speech errors are classified as a phonological disorder, remediation focuses on target patterns to be acquired rather than on isolated phonemes. Several different approaches may be followed when remediating phonological disorders.

Hodson and Paden (1991) advocate the use of a **Cycles** Approach when remediating phonological disorders. With this approach, error patterns are identified and treated; individual phonemes are targeted as a means to achieving the end goal (i.e., producing the patterns). For example, the final consonant deletion error pattern may be targeted with word-final /t/ words (e.g,, *boat, hat, boot, dot)* during one cycle and word-final /p/ (e.g., *cup, pipe, rope, mop)* in a subsequent cycle, rather than teaching each sound the child deletes (Buteau & Hodson, 1989). To learn more about the Cycles Approach, see Hodson and Paden.

Williams (2006) recommends the use of multiple contrastive word pairs for children who have moderate to serve speech sound disorders, which result in a one-to-many phoneme collapse of serval adult target sounds for one child error substitute or omission. For example, it is not uncommon for children to substitute /t/ for several adult targets, such as /k, s, ʃ, tʃ/ and clusters, such as /st, tr, kl, kr/. This error substitute results in a 1:8 phoneme collapse of adult target phonemes and clusters. As a result, the child produces words with these different target sounds as homonyms, such as /tu/ for all these words: *two, coo, Sue, shoes, chew, stew, true, clue,* and *crew.* A Multiple Oppositions Approach would direct intervention across the entire phoneme collapse, or rule set, by training up to four target sounds in contrast to the child's error substitute. For example, a Multiple Oppositions Approach could target /t/ in contrast with /k, s, kl, tr/ to induce multiple phonemic splits by directing the child's learning across the multiple homonymous forms that exist as a result of the phoneme collapse. To learn more about the Multiple Oppositions Approach, see Williams (2003, 2006).

Cycle
The time period required for a child to successively focus for two to six hours on each of his or her basic error patterns.

Biofeedback

A process in which a device (usually a computer-based one) is used to give clients feedback about whether they are making movements (e.g., producing speech sounds) correctly.

Correcting Articulation Errors

For children whose articulation errors do not have an organic cause, the goal of intervention is to correct the errors. Most of these children do not have a hearing loss, nor do they have a developmental disability. In addition, there is no dysarthria, verbal apraxia, or structural abnormality that affects the functioning of their vocal tracts. They simply have not learned to produce the sound(s) correctly. Adults can also learn to correct their errors. However, they usually need a higher level of motivation than do children, because they have a longer history of making their errors and, the stronger habit is hard to overcome.

Correcting the errors would also be the goal for children whose articulation errors appear to have an organic etiology that can either be corrected or compensated for. These include some dental anomalies, short lingual frenums, cleft palates, and hearing losses.

There are several strategies that are used for getting clients to produce speech sounds correctly. One is simply to have them imitate the clinician. The clinician makes the sound and the client imitates it. Another is teaching them how to configure the vocal tract for making the sound. This could involve a straightforward description of where to place the articulators. For example, if a client has a lateral lisp (an /s/ distortion in which the air flows between the side teeth rather than the incisors), he or she would be told where to place the tongue so that air will flow between the incisors. An indirect strategy could also be used for getting clients to configure the vocal tract appropriately. For example, if a client has a lateral lisp, he or she could be told to make the voiceless /θ/ while keeping the tongue behind the teeth (rather than placing it between them). Most persons who follow this instruction will produce a fairly normal /s/.

Another strategy that is used for getting clients to produce speech sounds correctly involves the use of **biofeedback.** For example, an adult who was unable to learn to produce /r/ correctly through other approaches may be taught to produce /r/ by speaking into a microphone attached to a device containing a computer. Graphic information is displayed on the computer screen which allows the speaker to judge the correctness of the productions (Schuster, Ruscello, & Smith, 1992). For more information on biofeedback, visit the Arizona Behavioral Health Associates (2005) webpage describing biofeedback.

After the client has learned to produce a misarticulated speech sound correctly in isolation, he or she is taught to produce it in syllables, words, sentences, and finally, conversational speech. Once the client is able to produce a sound correctly during conversational speech in the therapy room, the SLP works to generalize their correct production to situations outside of the therapy room.

Increasing Speech Intelligibility

Correcting the articulation errors is not the primary goal for individuals whose errors are caused by disorders such as dysarthria or verbal apraxia. The prognosis for correcting articulation errors with these etiologies is usually not good. If it is not possible to correct the client's articulation errors either because the vocal tract cannot be made to function normally or it is not possible to compensate for all the abnormalities, the clinician will attempt to increase the intelligibility of the client's speech. The goal will be to make a client's speech understandable to his or her conversational partners. This could involve improving the functioning of the vocal tract as much as possible. For example, if the severity of a client's dysarthria could be reduced by taking a medication, he or she might be encouraged to take it. Increasing the intelligibility of a client's speech could also involve teaching the client to speak in a way that differs somewhat from his or her habitual manners. For example, if a client who has dysarthria is able to speak, but the speech is difficult to understand, it may be possible to improve intelligibility significantly by teaching the client to speak at a slower rate than his or her habitual rate. Audio Clip 8.3 is a speech sample of a person with dysarthria. To learn more about the management of articulation disorders, see Bernthal and Bankson (1998).

Audio Clip 8.3	**Dysarthric Speech**

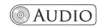 This is a speech sample of someone with dysarthria. Notice that in this case the dysarthria interferes little with intelligibility.

Augmenting the Client's Ability to Communicate

Some clients' vocal tracts are so severely impaired that it is not possible for them to produce much speech that can be understood. This would be the case for most persons who have had a total, or near total, glossectomy. It could also be the case for those who have dysarthria, particularly its most severe form, known as **locked-in syndrome.** Persons whose vocal tracts are severely impaired may only be able to produce a few word approximations that can be understood.

A number of strategies can be used to augment the ability of such persons with a **severe communication impairment** to communicate. These include gestural strategies (e.g., the manual sign system used by the deaf); cardboard communication boards; and electronic, computer-based devices (as pictured in Figure 8.3) that enable a person to transmit messages in printed and/or spoken form. You can read about an augmentative communication approach used with a severe communication impairment in Study More 8.5 on page 150. ASHA's, 2005g webpage on augmentative communication provides more information.

Locked-in syndrome
Severe motoric impairment in which the only muscles that usually aren't paralyzed are those of the eyes. The person may be able to learn to communicate by Morse code by blinking the eyes.

Severe communication impairment
The inability to speak intelligibly enough to meet communication needs. Augmentative communication strategies and devices can enable these clients to meet their communication needs.

Figure 8.3	**An Electronic Computer-Based Communication Aid**

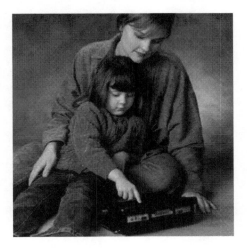

Photo courtesy of the Prentke Romich Company www.prentrom.com

She Talks with Her Eyes

Study More 8.5

How might people communicate who are unable to talk or control most of their muscles but are able to understand speech? Their ability to communicate can be augmented in a number of ways. This excerpt describes an approach that was used with a woman with a severe handicap who could only open and close her eyes.

After 16 months of being totally unable to communicate, I had a great clinician who devised a language system which I could use! I could finally communicate with people! Let me explain how it worked.

I would close my eyes while my clinician would say the letters of the alphabet. When she came to the letter I wanted, I would open my eyes. This was difficult as my reaction time was very slow, and sometimes I would open my eyes too soon, while other times it was too late. My speech-language pathologist was very patient, and together we might complete one sentence during an hour of therapy. With much patience, I became more accurate at opening my eyes on the letter I wanted. The communi-cation methods I used were in sequence as follows:

1. *Word spelling*—Just as I have described it, opening my eyes for the correct letter I wanted.

2. *Yes/No*—Everything had to be phrased to me as a question with a "yes" or "no" answer. I kept my eyes closed for "no" and opened wide for "yes."

3. *Use of parts of speech to construct sentences*—I again would open my eyes for the part of speech I wanted but still had to spell nouns and verbs. This method was faster because of sentence patterns. Not everyone could do this with me as they had forgotten the parts of speech.

From "I'd Rather Tell a Story Than Be One," by J. G. Post and W. R. Leith, 1983, *ASHA, 25,* pp. 23–26. © 1983 by the American Speech-Language-Hearing Association. Reprinted with permission.

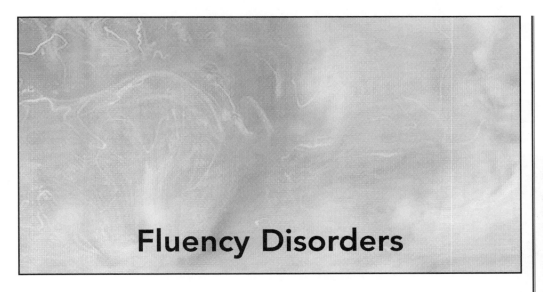

Fluency Disorders

Chapter 9

Learning Objectives

- Describe fluency.

- Describe the difference between normal and abnormal speech fluency.

- Describe the eight types of disfluencies.

- Describe stuttering and its speech characteristics.

- Describe the physiological and psychological symptoms of stuttering.

- Identify the primary theories of what causes stuttering.

- Discuss the relationship between pragmatics and stuttering.

- Describe the characteristics of cluttering, neurogenic acquired stuttering, and psychogenic acquired stuttering.

- Describe the two primary goals for managing stuttering.

- Discuss the difficulty faced by speech-language pathologists designing intervention for people who clutter.

Chapter

Introduction

Fluency is the term used to describe the effortless and smooth production of speech. However, the ability to speak fluently does not mean one's speech is entirely free of **disfluencies.** If you listen carefully to how people speak, you will notice that almost everyone experiences some interruptions in their speech flow. In fact, if you listen to your own speech, you may be surprised at how many interruptions are present.

Recall Van Riper and Erickson's (1996) definition of a communication disorder from Chapter 2, in which they described a communication disorder as having at least one of the following three aspects:

1. There is a perception by others that the person's communication deviates enough from normal hearing, speech, or language that it interferes with communication.

2. The person's communication calls adverse attention to him or her.

3. It causes the person to be self-conscious about it or, as Van Riper and Erickson put it, "maladjusted."

When a person's speech flow deviates from what is considered "normal," when it calls adverse attention to itself, and/or when it causes him or her to be self-conscious or maladjusted, it can be considered to be outside the realm of normal fluency. In the following sections, normal and abnormal speech fluency are discussed, and then stuttering and related disfluencies are explained.

Disfluency
Hesitations, repetitions, mispronunciations, and interjections in one's speech. They may be either normal or symptoms of stuttering or another fluency disorder. Also called moments of disfluency.

Normal versus Abnormal Speech Fluency

Hesitations are a normal part of speaking. Most people hesitate frequently while they are speaking. We all occasionally (particularly when we are tense) repeat sounds, syllables, words, and phrases; interject sounds and syllables between words (e.g., "um"); have abnormally long pauses between words; prolong speech sounds, particularly the initial sounds of words; and stop to correct errors of pronunciation, syntax, and word usage.

If everyone has moments of disfluency while speaking, when is the disfluency abnormal—that is, when is it symptomatic of a speech disorder? This question is not an easy one to answer. Considerable research has attempted to identify differences between normal disfluency behaviors and those resulting from fluency disorders. As you will see, there is considerable overlap in the speech of people with disfluencies and people with normal speech.

Frequency of Occurrence

One of the first areas investigators analyzed for differences between normal and abnormal disfluency behaviors was frequency of occurrence. They thought that although all speakers exhibit such behaviors, those who have fluency disorders may exhibit them more often than those who do not have a fluency disorder. The findings of these studies indicated that while some persons who have fluency disorders are disfluent more often than normal speakers, overlap (sometimes considerable) occurs between the groups. Consequently, there are normal speakers who are disfluent as often as some of those who have a fluency disorder. This overlap between groups appears to be greater for preschool-age children than for adults.

Duration of Individual Moments of Disfluency

If amount of disfluency does not sharply differentiate people who have fluency disorders from those who do not, perhaps the duration of their individual moments of disfluency does. That is, perhaps individual moments of disfluency of people with fluency disorders tend to last longer. Most studies comparing the durations of normal speakers' moments of disfluency to those of persons who have a fluency disorder found the durations to be similar to those for frequency of disfluency. That is, while the moments of disfluency of some persons who have a fluency disorder tend to last longer than those of persons who do not have one, there is overlap between the groups. Some normal speakers can have moments of disfluency that last as long as those of some persons who have a fluency disorder. Again, this overlap between groups appears to be greater for preschool-age children than for adults.

Amount of Tension Present

A third attribute of moments of disfluency that investigators have looked at in an attempt to differentiate normal from abnormal disfluency behavior is the amount of tension present. Normal disfluencies tend to be relatively free from tension or struggle, and are rarely accompanied by facial grimaces or other signs of tension. Almost all people whose moments of disfluency are accompanied by audible or visible signs of tension are considered to have a fluency disorder. However, some individuals who have a fluency disorder do not show such signs, especially preschool children.

Speakers' Awareness of and Attitude towards Moments of Disfluency

A fourth attribute of moments of disfluency that has been investigated is the speakers' awareness of them. Disfluencies are more likely to be labeled abnormal is the speaker appears embarrassed by them. Embarrassment is often communicated nonverbally (e.g., staring at the floor). Having a negative attitude about being disfluent can handicap a person in other ways. For example, it can cause him or her to avoid talking. A person who avoids talking is being handicapped by being disfluent regardless of his or her amount of disfluency. While those who are highly aware of their moments of disfluency tend to be individuals who have a fluency disorder, many do not exhibit such awareness.

Distribution in the Speech Sequence

A fifth attribute of moments of disfluency that has been investigated is their distribution (i.e., loci) in the speech sequence. Does the distribution tend to be random or do moments of disfluency tend to occur more often than would be expected by chance on (or adjacent to) words having certain characteristics? The findings of most studies suggest the latter. Moments of disfluency tend to be more likely to occur, for example, on words having certain grammatical functions. However, this attribute does not differentiate normal from abnormal disfluency behavior. People who stutter, for example, tend to do so on words having the same grammatical functions as those on which normal speakers tend to be disfluent.

In summary, the findings of most studies that have compared audible and visible attributes of moments of disfluency in the speech of typical speakers with those of persons who have a fluency disorder suggest that they have much in common. In fact, the disfluency behaviors of some people who have a fluency disorder seem similar both quantitatively and qualitatively to those of typical speakers. The age group for which this similarity has been reported most often is preschool-age children. However, the relationship between normal and abnormal speech disfluency is not a settled issue, and research on it is ongoing. To learn more about the attributes of disfluency behavior, see Silverman (1996).

A number of protocols have been developed for helping speech-language pathologists (SLPs) decide whether disfluency is abnormal. Most of them consist of criteria for differentiating beginning stuttering from the normal disfluency of preschool children. For descriptions of several of these protocols, see Gordon and Luper (1992a, 1992b) and Onslow (1992).

Types of Disfluencies

All children and adults are disfluent occasionally while they are speaking. Both psycholinguists and speech-language pathologists have conducted considerable research on what happens when this occurs. The psycholinguistic literature refers to such investigations as research on *hesitation phenomena* and the speech-language pathology literature refers to it as research on *disfluency behaviors*. The next paragraphs summarize some of the findings of this research to provide you with a basis for differentiating normal from abnormal disfluency behavior, particularly in young children. Eight types of behaviors may occur in the speech of children and adults while they are being disfluent:

1. **Part-word repetitions** occur when a person repeats sounds or syllables in words. This phenomenon usually occurs at the beginning of words and almost never at the end of them. Though the number of times a particular sound or syllable is repeated can be quite high, it is usually only once or twice. Audio Clip 9.1 is an example of a moment of stuttering containing a part-word repetition.

Audio Clip 9.1	**Part-Word Repetition**
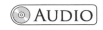	A moment of stuttering consisting of a combination of a part-word repetition and dysrhythmic phonation on the first sound of the word *the*

2. **Word repetitions** are repetitions of entire words, most often single-syllable words. Although a word may be repeated a relatively large number of times, it is usually repeated only once or twice. Audio Clip 9.2 is an example of a word repetition.

Audio Clip 9.2	**Word Repetition**
	A moment of stuttering consisting of a word repetition of the word *can* and an interjection following the word repetition

3. **Phrase repetitions** are repetitions of phrases consisting of two or more words. Phrases are usually repeated only once or twice. Audio Clip 9.3, which is described on page 156, gives an example of a phrase repetition.

Part-word repetitions
Repetitions of sounds and syllables in words.

Word repetitions
Repetitions of entire words. In most cases they are single syllable ones.

Phrase repetitions
Repetitions of units of two or more words.

Interjections
Sounds, syllables, words, and/or phrases added between words.

Revision-incomplete phrases
Disfluencies in which the speaker begins an utterance but does not complete it.

Dysrhythmic phonations
Disturbances in the normal rhythms of words.

Tense pauses
Pauses filled with barely audible heavy breathing or muscle tightening. Also referred to as blocks.

Audio Clip 9.3	**Phrase Repetition**
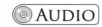	A phrase repetition on the words *the fast brown* and an interjection following the phrase repetition

4. **Interjections** are sounds, syllables, words, or phrases that are added between words. They do not usually perform a linguistic function in messages—that is, their presence does not usually affect the denotative meanings of messages. Examples are *um* and *you know*. Audio Clip 9.4 gives an example of three interjections of *um*.

Audio Clip 9.4	**Interjection**
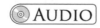	A revision-incomplete phrase and three interjections of *um*

5. The **revision-incomplete phrase** category includes instances in which the speaker becomes aware of making an error and corrects it. The error may be in how a word was pronounced or it may be related to the meaning of the word(s) that was said. Also included are instances in which the speaker begins an utterance but obviously does not complete it. Audio Clip 9.5 gives an example of a revision-incomplete phrase.

Audio Clip 9.5	**Revision-Incomplete Phrase**
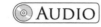	A revision-incomplete phrase and interjection of *um*

6. **Dysrhythmic phonations** are disturbances in the normal rhythms of words. The disturbance may be attributable to a prolonged sound; an accent or timing that is notably unusual; an improper stress; a break (usually between syllables); or any other speaking behavior that occurs within words and is not compatible with fluent speech. Audio Clip 9.6 is an example of a dysrhythmic phonation.

Audio Clip 9.6	**Dysrhythmic Phonation**
	A dysrhythmic phonation (prolongation) on the first sound of the word *noticed*

7. **Tense pauses** are phenomena that occur between words, part-words, and interjections. They consist of pauses during which there are barely audible manifestations of heavy breathing or muscle tightening. The same phenomena within words would be classified as dysrhythmic phonations. Audio Clip 9.7 gives an example of a tense pause.

Audio Clip 9.7	**Tense Pause**

 AUDIO   A word repetition and a tense pause before the word *often*

8. **Unfilled pauses** are abnormally long pauses between words. Although the existence of such pauses is acknowledged by all investigators of speech disfluency, they have not been studied as much as the other seven types because they are difficult to identify reliably. Investigators disagree about how long a pause between words has to be before it can be classified as abnormal.

Audio Clip 9.8 illustrates a moment of stuttering. Which types of disfluency does it contain? Try to identify at least three of the eight disfluency types in it.

Audio Clip 9.8	**A Moment of Stuttering**

 AUDIO   Try to identify at least three of the eight disfluency types in this segment.

Fluency Disorders

Four disorders have abnormal speech disfluencies as a symptom: (1) stuttering, (2) cluttering, (3) neurogenic acquired stuttering, and (4) psychogenic acquired stuttering. Each of these disorders are described in the following sections. However, more emphasis is placed on stuttering since it is the most common of the four.

Stuttering

Stuttering is the most common disorder of fluency. Approximately 1 percent of the United States population has the disorder—almost as many people as live in Los Angeles. Although its onset usually occurs between the ages of 3 and 5, it can begin at any age, even during adulthood. (See Yairi & Ambrose, 1992, and Yairi, Ambrose, & Niermann, 1993 to learn more about the onset and first several months of stuttering development.) More males than females stutter. The ratio between males and females has been reported to be between 3:1 and 5:1. The disorder tends to run in families; some authorities believe this indicates that genetic factors exist that put some people at greater risk for developing it (see Lewis, 1992).

Because stuttering usually has its onset during early childhood, the first professional to be consulted is likely to be a **pediatrician.** The physician may prescribe a treatment regimen for the child, refer the child to a speech-language pathologist for evaluation, or postpone action (a "wait and see" approach). The latter appears to be the most common action (Yairi & Carrico, 1992).

Although the speech of most people who stutter contains a great deal of disfluency, some people who stutter exhibit little disfluency. In fact, some individuals who stutter tend to be more fluent than some normal speakers. Such people who are relatively fluent may be regarded as having a significant stuttering problem because they allow their stuttering to keep them from doing things they want to do—that is, it causes them to be handicapped.

Characteristics of Stuttering

No person who stutters does so on every word he or she says. In fact, few stutter on more than half their words. Both frequency and duration tend to vary on a situational basis. Most people who stutter tend to be relatively fluent in these situations:

- Reading in unison with another person, even another person who stutters

- Speaking to an infant or an animal

- Singing

- Swearing or openly expressing anger

- Speaking in any nonhabitual manner—for example, in an overly loud voice; with objects in the mouth; at a very slow rate; or while engaging in rhythmic physical activity such as dancing, walking, or swinging the arms

There is no agreement on the reason(s) for the relative absence of stuttering in these situations. One hypothesis is that these situations represent ones in which people who stutter do not expect to stutter. People who stutter tend to stutter most in situations in which they expect to stutter and fear doing it. Almost all people who stutter tend to stutter a great deal while:

- Speaking on the telephone (see Study More 9.1)

- Speaking to people they regard as authority figures, such as their parents

- Speaking in situations in which they anticipate stuttering and want to avoid disfluencies

- Speaking to people who are likely to react adversely (e.g., laughing; being impatient; or viewing the speaker as childlike or cognitively delayed)

- Desiring to communicate quickly (e.g., when giving an order to a waitress, answering the question "What is your name?" or experiencing difficulty securing talking time in the midst of a conversational "crossfire")

One reason for relatively high levels of stuttering in these situations is that people who stutter tend to stutter most when they wish to stutter least. Thus, the desire to avoid stuttering appears to influence the amount of it. This does not necessarily mean that if they didn't desire to avoid stuttering, there would be none. There are likely other reasons why it occurs.

The frequency and duration of moments of stuttering vary not only on a situational basis, but also on a day-to-day basis. People who stutter tend to have "good" and "bad" days with respect to the amount they stutter, and the amount they stutter in any given situation is likely to vary considerably from day to day.

Study More 9.1	Coping with Stuttering on the Phone

The following is a response to a question from a stutterer about coping with stuttering on the telephone. It was posted on an Internet listserv (STUTT-L). It has been lightly edited to maintain confidentiality but spelling, content, and grammar were unchanged.

Let me tell u my experience with the phone...When I was young I couldnt even answer the phone...I couldnt even get out hello...and I would hardly ever call anyone...Somhow I just decided hey I am gonna use the phone no matter...no matter how much I stutter...If they hang up cause I cant get it out...I'll just call back and try again...

And I decided it doesnt matter how bad my speech would be...as long as I got what I needed to get out of the phone call...meaning if the goal of the phone call...was to get a dentist appointment, and I did that...no matter how much I stuttered...I considered it a 100% success...and really felt that way after...so i Just started using the phone...

Now I call teachers to discuss my children...I make all my own doctor appointments...I solve everything I need to on the phone myself...and somtimes I am aprehensive again...but it is mild and goes away...

I worked for myself most of my adult life...but found myself not making enough money at one point...and took a job selling tires at company owned Goodyear Store...They had this canned greeting that they all used...it went somthing like this...Good Morning Goodyear number one in sales and service,,Jack speaking how may I help u...

Well thats just too much for me... SO I modified it for myself...I said, Good morning Goodyear Jack speaking how may I help u. The G in Goodyear is hard for me...But most of the time i could say it...and ya know if sometimes I had a block so what...I sold more tires than anyone else at the store, including the manager of 10 years...

It doesnt matter that u stutter as long as u can do the job...and somtimes all of sudden, I might have a bad streak...I would start blocking on goodyear...but I would kinda smile to myself...and say ya know if I keep calm...and just keep on pluggin away...I ll stop blocking again...and sure enough in a few days...I would be saying it fluently...but if I would of panicked...start searching for differnt words...differnt tricks...I am sure it would of got worse...the real trick is to not avoid any words...Pick your greeting and stick with it...be deliberate in what ur gonna say...say to urself no matter how scard I am i mite stutter...I am just gonna say it the way it should be said...I am not gonna search for words to subsitute and all that crap...If I block so what, I stutter...thats what i do...I hope this helps u some...

Source: Silverman (Personal transcript)

The frequency and duration of moments of stuttering are also influenced by certain word characteristics. Those who stutter are more likely to stutter on words they stuttered on previously. This phenomenon is known as the **consistency effect.** They also show a greater-than-chance tendency to stutter on words that are nouns, verbs, adverbs, or adjectives; begin with consonant sounds; are relatively long; and/or occur at the beginnings of sentences.

Most persons who stutter develop strategies to avoid stuttering, although many of these strategies cause them to lose more than they gain. One such strategy is not talking when they expect to stutter. Obviously, they will not stutter if they do not talk. Many school-age children who stutter, for example, refrain from asking or voluntarily answering questions in class. Although this strategy will allow a person who stutters to avoid some stuttering, it also is likely to have another effect—that is, to impede his or her ability to give and receive information and to express feelings. The use of this strategy can be more handicapping than the stuttering it is intended to eliminate.

A second avoidance strategy that those who stutter use is substituting words on which they do not expect to stutter for those on which they do. Most adults and some children are able to accurately predict many of the words on which they are going to stutter. This ability is referred to as the **expectancy phenomenon.** Sometimes the words they substitute are not entirely appropriate, which can interfere with their ability to communicate.

Consistency effect
The greater-than-chance tendency for stutterers to stutter on words that they stuttered on previously.

Expectancy phenomenon
The ability of stutterers to predict moments of stuttering with greater-than-chance accuracy.

Secondary behaviors
Behaviors that accompany moments of stuttering, particularly those of adults (e.g., using interjections or eye blinking). Also referred to as secondaries.

Starters
A device that stutterers use to avoid stuttering. They inject sounds, syllables, words, or phrases they believe they can say without stuttering before words on which they expect to stutter.

A third strategy that people who stutter use to avoid a moment of disfluency is **secondary behaviors** (i.e., secondaries). Secondary behaviors include speaking in a nonhabitual manner, using interjections, increasing vocal pitch, or a making a movement of some type. For example, people who stutter may speak at an abnormally slow rate or with an accent, or they may use **starters**. Persons who stutter believe that by using starters they can give their speech mechanism a "running start." An example of a starter is a person who wants to say, "I like coffee with cream" but says, "I mean I was going to say I like coffee with cream." Movements that a person may make to avoid a moment of disfluency include looking away from the listener, making jerking movements of the head, blinking the eyes, and facial contortions.

Why do secondary behaviors accompany moments of stuttering? The most widely held explanation is that they began as devices for avoiding disfluencies or reducing their severity. If a person who stutters anticipates stuttering on a word, he or she may attempt to avoid it by doing something prior to saying the word. Or if the person begins to stutter on a word, he or she may attempt to do something to reduce the duration of the disfluency. A person who stutters is likely to continue using the device until he or she no longer believes that doing so will keep disfluencies from occurring or reduce their duration. By this time, the behavior has become a learned component of the moment of disfluency. Thus, such behaviors may accompany stuttering either because they are currently being used as devices for coping with them, or they are ones that were used for this purpose in the past that no longer "work" but have become habitual. To learn more about stuttering, visit Judith Kuster's Stuttering Homepage (Kuster, 2005c).

Physiological and Psychological Symptoms of Stuttering

The symptomatology of stuttering is not limited to audible and visible aspects of speaking behavior. Stuttering also has physiological and psychological aspects.

Physiologically, the speech mechanism functions abnormally during moments of stuttering. That is, moments of stuttering are accompanied by abnormal physiological events that intermittently influence the processes of respiration, phonation, and articulation. These events are not the same for all people who stutter. For some there are attempts to speak on intake of air; for others this rarely (if ever) occurs. For some individuals who stutter, excessive muscle tensing may occur somewhere in the **larynx** and/or **oral cavity**. The specific sites where this abnormal tensing occurs for a particular person who stutters may change from time to time. It is important to know, however, that these abnormal physiological events do not necessarily cause the stuttering. In fact, they may be the result of the same processes that cause the stuttering.

Stuttering also can have psychological components. One is discomfort or embarrassment—signaled to listeners by behaviors like staring at the floor while speaking, blushing, or turning the head away. Most people are uncomfortable being around others who seem uncomfortable with themselves. Listeners often do not know how to act or respond. Consequently, people who stutter may feel rejected—not because of their disorder, but because their listeners feel uncomfortable around them. Speech-language pathologists help people who stutter to modify their behavior so they are less likely to communicate their embarrassment or discomfort. For example, SLPs work on helping clients develop more normal eye contact while stuttering.

Another psychological component of stuttering can be a poor self-concept, which affects many people who stutter. A poor self-concept is likely to both interfere with interpersonal relationships and increase stuttering severity.

What Causes Stuttering?

Many theories have been advanced during the past two thousand years to explain why people stutter. Although no single theory is currently accepted by all authorities on stuttering, a number are accepted by at least a few such authorities. Most theories fall into one of four broad categories: (1) breakdown, (2) repressed need, (3) anticipatory struggle, and (4) motor speech. To learn more about theories that have been advanced to explain stuttering and the lack of agreement among authorities about its etiology, see Bloodstein (1993), Hahn (1956), Silverman (1996), Van Riper (1971), and Wingate (2002).

Breakdown Theories

Breakdown theories regard stuttering as a breakdown of speech because of some type of pressure. That is, applying a certain type of pressure causes a person to stutter. Where these theories disagree is on the kind of pressure that can cause a person to stutter, and whether all persons are equally likely to stutter if exposed to a particular pressure—that is, whether some psychological or organic factor makes some people more susceptible than others to speech breakdown if exposed to a certain type of pressure. Such a factor, if it were shown to exist, would be said to be a **predisposing cause** of stuttering.

What types of pressure do these theories suggest can cause stuttering? It was argued during the early part of the last century that stuttering can be caused by a traumatic experience—one that causes shock or fright, such as an experience associated with an illness or injury. However, few contemporary authorities believe that stuttering can be caused solely by such an experience.

Emotional stress is another type of pressure that some theories suggest can cause stuttering. Such stress can undoubtedly increase the amount of hesitation in a person's speech and contribute indirectly to precipitating stuttering. However, it is doubtful that it alone can cause a person to begin to stutter.

A number of authorities accept one aspect of many breakdown theories: certain psychological or organic conditions, if present, can increase the risk of becoming a person who stutters. These conditions are predisposing rather than precipitating causes of stuttering, which means that they cannot by themselves cause a person to stutter.

Repressed Need Theories

Repressed need theories view stuttering behavior as a means of satisfying or fulfilling some type of unconscious neurotic need. These theories were formulated during the first half of the last century by Freudian psychoanalysts. Some of these theories maintain that stuttering behavior fulfills the need for oral or anal gratification.

These theories are based on what is known as the **medical model.** Stuttering, according to the medical model, is a symptom in much the same way as a fever is a symptom. Just as one would treat a fever by eliminating the underlying infection, those who accept such theories would treat stuttering by resolving the underlying emotional problem through psychotherapy.

The repressed need perspective on stuttering is no longer widely accepted, one reason being that therapy based on it does not seem to work. The results of Freudian-based psychotherapy that have been reported suggest that it rarely, if ever, eliminates stuttering.

Predisposing cause
A psychological or organic factor that makes some persons more "at risk" than others for developing a disorder.

Medical model
Abnormal behavior (e.g., stuttering) is viewed as a symptom of some underlying disorder. Treatment focuses on what is assumed to be the underlying disorder rather than on the abnormal behavior (i.e., symptom).

Diagnosogenic theory
An anticipatory struggle theory for stuttering that states that the disorder is precipitated by parents (or others) diagnosing normal childhood syllable repetitions as stuttering and encouraging the child to avoid repeating them.

Anticipatory Struggle Theories

Anticipatory struggle theories have been among the most widely accepted since the mid-1940s. They view stuttering as learned behavior. According to these theories, persons do not have to differ from their peers physiologically or psychologically to develop the disorder. On the contrary, they indicate that anyone can develop stuttering by being exposed to a particular set of circumstances. These theories differ, however, concerning the nature of these circumstances.

The term *anticipatory struggle* is used to describe these theories because they state that anticipation of stuttering and the desire to avoid it somehow cause it to occur. According to them, people who stutter have learned to anticipate stuttering and to behave in particular ways when it is anticipated and while it is occurring. People who stutter may, for example, close their eyes when they anticipate stuttering because they believe that doing so will allow them to avoid stuttering or reduce its severity. They may continue doing this after they have stopped believing that it helps them speak fluently because it has become a habit.

These theories suggest another type of learning that contributes to stuttering behavior, one that causes a person who stutters to respond to certain speaking situations and to certain words with anxiety. This type of learning is referred to as *classical conditioning,* which the Russian psychologist Pavlov first demonstrated when he trained dogs to salivate when they heard the sound of a bell. Like salivation, anxiety is controlled by the autonomic nervous system. People who do not stutter, when they speak while experiencing high levels of anxiety, are also likely to be less fluent than usual, as occurs in stage fright.

An anticipatory struggle theory that was accepted by many speech-language pathologists during the last half of the twentieth century is known as the **diagnosogenic theory.** This theory was formulated during the 1940s by Dr. Wendell Johnson, a professor of speech-language pathology at the University of Iowa. Almost all children between the ages of 3 and 5 go through a phase during which they repeat sounds, syllables, and one-syllable words. According to the theory, if nobody reacts adversely to these repetitions, the child will pass through the phase and become a normal speaker. However, if somebody (particularly a parent) diagnoses this repetition as "abnormal" and communicates this judgment to the child, he or she is likely to become fearful about repeating and will try to avoid doing it. Trying to avoid normal repetition leads to struggle behavior—stuttering. The theory is known as diagnosogenic because it states that the diagnosis of normal repetition as abnormal causes stuttering.

The most compelling evidence supporting this theory is an experiment that was done more than 60 years ago (known as the "monster study") in which normal speaking children were reported to have been inadvertently turned into persons who stutter by telling them that their normal syllable repetitions and other disfluencies were abnormal. To learn more about the monster study and the diagnosogenic theory, see Halvorson (1999), Johnson and Associates (1959), and Silverman (1988b, 1996). You can also read an online description of the monster study on the Milwaukee Journal Sentinel's website, JS Online (2005).

Motor Speech Theories

A more recent theory of what causes stuttering is that it is a motor speech disorder; that is, it is a disorder based on a dysfunction of the central nervous system's sensorimotor control mechanism (Caruso & Strand, 1999). One explanation by Smith (2005) is that, for people who stutter, the motor areas of the brain cannot easily generate muscle command signals if there is:

- A high demand for linguistic processing

- High emotional arousal

- A high memory load

Specifically, when the neural signals that produce coordinated movements in the respiratory, vocal, and articulatory systems are disrupted because of these factors, stuttering results. What this suggests is that stuttering can be reduced and/or alleviated through systematic reductions in the linguistic, emotional, and/or memory demands on the speaker. Another implication of this theory is that intervention should begin early so the child can learn to change the motor speech patterns that produce stuttering. Research is currently underway to test these hypotheses (Weber-Fox, 2005).

Relationship between Pragmatics and Stuttering

Some clinicians believe that because the period of greatest language development (i.e., ages two-and-a-half to five) is also the period of greatest risk of developing stuttering, stuttering should be considered within the context of a child's language development (see Bloom & Cooperman, 1999). One of the areas of language development affected by stuttering is pragmatics.

Disfluencies disrupt both the rhythm of the person's speech and his or her ability to keep up with the pace of taking turns with conversational partners. For instance, disfluencies add to the time required to complete an utterance or phrase. Because turn taking in conversations is partly based on the amount of time each person takes per turn, the person who stutters is perceived as taking longer turns and slowing the pace of the conversation. In addition, his or her conversational partners must alter their pacing in order to accommodate the person's elongated turns. The person who stutters may perceive that his or her conversational partners are interrupting—beginning to speak before he or she has finished his or her turn. The quick give-and-take of multiple turns gives way to a slower conversation with fewer turns.

Some people who stutter have developed habits during speaking that interfere with their ability to monitor their conversational partners' understanding and participation. For example, if individuals who stutter close their eyes or look at the floor during a disfluency, they are unable to see how their conversational partners are responding. Bloom and Cooperman (1999) teach their young clients how to wait for their turn before talking, listen to what the other person is saying, and maintain the topic the other person is talking about.

Cluttering

Cluttering (i.e., tachyphemia) is a condition that has an abnormal amount of hesitation as one of its components. People with this condition tend to speak very rapidly. They frequently repeat syllables and words, and the overall rhythm of their speech is abnormal. In addition, they have problems in language formulation as well as fluency. Their articulation tends to be slurred, and they tend to invert words in sentences; use improper syntax; and choose inappropriate words and expressions.

Cluttering
A fluency disorder in which the person speaks very rapidly and hesitates a great deal because of doing so. Also referred to as tachyphemia.

Neurogenic acquired stuttering
A fluency disorder, usually acquired during adulthood, that is caused by damage to the central nervous system (e.g., a stroke or head trauma).

The hesitations of clutterers appear to differ from those of people who stutter in several ways. The first concerns their level of awareness of the hesitations. People who stutter are usually aware of their hesitations, but clutterers are not. In fact, clutterers seem to be unaware that their speech is abnormal in any way, which may be why very few clutterers seek help from SLPs or other professionals.

Clutterers, like those who stutter, tend to be more fluent in some situations than in others. However, the impact of some situations on their fluency levels varies. While people who stutter tend to become less fluent when they feel it is important to be fluent, clutterers tend to become more fluent in this circumstance. For example, people who stutter tend to be less fluent with authority figures than with animals, and clutterers tend to be more fluent with authority figures than animals.

Asking clutterers to pay attention to their speech usually results in less syllable and word repetition because they monitor their speech more carefully, speak more slowly, or both. (When people attempt to monitor their speech, their speaking rate almost always becomes slower.) Asking people who stutter to attend more to their speech almost always results in increased stuttering.

Although the etiology of cluttering is not well understood, it almost always begins during childhood. Clutterers usually have normal intelligence, but their speech and language development tends to be delayed. Their articulation and use of grammar is usually immature, and they tend to have difficulty with reading and writing. It is not surprising, therefore, that some authorities view cluttering as a component of a **specific language impairment (SLI).** To learn more about the symptomatology and etiology of cluttering, see Arnold (1965), Daly (1986, 1993), Kuster (2005a), Meyers and St. Louis (1992), Silverman (1996), Speech Rehabilitation Institute (n.d.), and Weiss (1964).

Neurogenic Acquired Stuttering

A number of case descriptions have been recorded of people who acquired stuttering after childhood, following damage to the central nervous system. Most of these descriptions pertain to people who had no history of stuttering and whose onset of the disorder (which usually was sudden) was associated with a neurological event. The neurological events associated with their stuttering included **strokes,** head traumas, and tumors. Their disorder is referred to most often as **neurogenic acquired stuttering.** Other terms used are neurogenic stuttering, acquired stuttering, neurological disfluency, cortical stuttering, and stuttering of sudden onset. The types of abnormal disfluency behaviors observed in the speech of people with this disorder include repetitions and/or dysrhythmic phonations. The specific symptomatology is determined, in part, by the neurological condition with which the disorder is associated.

Neurogenic acquired stuttering appears to differ from ordinary stuttering and cluttering in several ways. First, most people with this type of fluency problem develop it as an adult rather than as a child. The development of stutterlike hesitations in an adult who has been a normal speaker can be an early symptom of a neurological condition.

A second way in which neurogenic acquired stuttering differs from ordinary stuttering and cluttering is that it varies little (if at all) across situations—the amount of disfluency is approximately the same in all situations. People with this disorder, for example, are quite disfluent even when they read in unison with someone, while almost all people who stutter are completely fluent under this condition. There may be no condition under which people with neurogenic acquired stuttering are normally fluent. To learn more about neurogenic acquired stuttering, see Silverman (1996) or visit Judith Kuster's (2005b) website describing neurogenic acquired stuttering.

Psychogenic Acquired Stuttering

There are a number of reports of stuttering acquired during adulthood at least partially as a reaction to acute or chronic psychological disturbances. These cases involve people who did not have a childhood history of stuttering, and the onset of their disorder—which was sudden and could not be accounted for on the basis of central nervous system damage—appeared to be associated with some form of psychological stress. One young man, for example, suddenly began to stutter after his ship received a direct missile hit during the Korean conflict. Another suddenly began stuttering during an acute anxiety attack. A third is reported to have started stuttering when his marriage began to experience difficulty. Their disorder is referred to most often as **psychogenic acquired stuttering.**

The abnormal disfluency behavior exhibited by people with this disorder usually consists primarily of repetition of initial or stressed syllables, and there may be no situation in which it is absent—that is, in which the person is normally fluent. With this disorder, as with neurogenic acquired stuttering, the person does not become fluent when reading in chorus. Furthermore, the person may have an indifferent attitude toward the disfluency. He or she may not exhibit any of the typical avoidance behaviors, such as avoidance of sounds, words, or speaking situations. To learn more about psychogenic acquired stuttering, see Roth, Aronson, and Davis (1989) and Silverman (1996).

Management

Stuttering

Many theories have been advanced over the years to explain why people stutter, and many different management techniques have been used as well. Study More 9.2 on pages 166–167 is an unedited letter describing the "therapies" dispensed to one man during the first half of the twentieth century.

Although authorities still do not agree about the cause(s) of stuttering (and, consequently, about the best way to manage it), almost all of them try to accomplish two goals when working with someone who has the disorder. These are to (1) reduce the amount of stuttering and (2) decrease the negative effects the stuttering has on the person's life.

The prognosis for curing stuttering is considerably better for young children than it is for older children and adults. Nevertheless, strategies are available that can enable people who stutter at any age to reduce the severity of their stuttering. One strategy used with older children and adults is bringing the disorder "out into the open." Because people who stutter tend

Psychogenic acquired stuttering
A fluency disorder, usually acquired during adulthood, that is caused by an acute or chronic psychological disturbance.

Study More 9.2	Folk Remedies for Stuttering

Dear Sir:

When I was about eight or nine years old someone told my mother that if she did cook a black cat the night of Friday the 13th, and let me eat it at twelve o'clock sharp the same night I would be completely cured of my speech impediment. But this cat shouldn't have not even one white hair on it, and it should be a male, and not over two years of age. One day she found such a cat and cooked as she was instructed. At about eleven thirty in the night she woke me up stating that she had something good to eat. Well, at twelve o'clock sharp I began to eat my cat stew and believe me it wasn't so bad. But when I woke up the next morning I was stammering as usual. Then my mother told me all about the cat meat, and what it was suppose to do. You see I was not supposed to know what I was eating till next day.

About a year later or so, somebody else suggested to my mother that if she let me drink twice a day about half a glass of urine from a virgin mare not over eighteen months old, for thirty days, it would cure my stuttering because this urine contains a certain something in it that would quiet down the nerves in my tongue and cause me to speak freely. Later on my mother found a neighbor who had such a mare and I began my thirty day cure. At the end of the thirty days I was stammering as much as I had before I drank the filthy stuff. I will never forget the awful smell of it.

Well sir, a few months passed away since the above incident and I was stammering as badly as ever. One day my mother and my aunt had a little chat about me. Trying to figure out a way to stop me stammering. My aunt told my mother that she knew a certain old lady who was living in another town, and that this old lady was pretty good in mixing medicines, in fact she had cured many, many people with different sicknesses, and that it was worth while to try her medicines. In fact she was sure that this old lady would fix me.

Well sir, it might seem foolish to you. But after that people began to say that the reason nothing could cure my speech defect was because I either had an evil spirit or the devil himself incarnate into me. So one day someone told my father that he knew a certain old man who was very good in chasing bad spirits away from anyone who had one in him. So one summer day I and my father went to see this old gaffer and asked him if he really thought that I had an evil spirit in me if he would be so kind as to advise us what to do if I did have one hiding under my skin. He was a very kind old gaffer with white whiskers and he might have been a hundred years old for all I knew. Anyway he looked me over from head to foot, and began to make funny faces and noises like a man who was eating a lemon and has an awful stomachache. Finally he said, It is really shame that such a nice young boy like you should be infected with a bad spirit such as this one. But this is a case, he said, where my personal service is absolutely no good. The best I can do is to tell you what to do, and if you follow my instructions, I believe that we can get rid of him

in no time. So he told me that on a certain Friday night when the moon was three quarters full, I should cut down a certain tree named Chiuppo. Cut of a little stick about the size of my middle finger and about eighteen inches long, and put it away so that I can take it home with me. Then chop down the rest of the tree to small pieces so that I could use it for wood. Leave this wood there till the following Friday night and go home carrying the little stick with me, riding an unsaddled black horse. Well sir, on the following Friday night I would return there on the same unsaddled black horse carrying my little magic stick with me, build a circle about six or seven feet in diameter with the wood that I already had prepared from the Chiuppo tree. Spread some kerosene all over the wood, and at twelve o'clock sharp set it afire with a special match that he gave me himself. No other match would do the trick. Then I would have to jump in the circle with my little stick, get in the center of it, get on my knees and pray the good Lord to chase the bad spirit away from me. At the same time I would have to hold the stick between my hands, so that the Lord could bless it. After that I would have to circle the stick around my body thirty times, and every time I would have to say something like. Bad spirit go away and leave me in peace for the rest of my days. After that I would have to wait till the flames died away. Then jump out of the fire circle, hit the black horse with my little blessed stick and drop the stick at the same time. When the black horse carrying the evil spirit away from me, was far enough away, then I could ride any other horse and go home and right to bed, without speaking to anyone, and completely cured of my speech impediment, and carrying my good spirit when I woke up in the morning. Well, I did all of that like the old man told me. But it so happened that when I woke up in the morning, the bad spirit must have been with me yet, because I was stammering as usual.

Well sir, few days after the above incident, my father went to see the old man again, to tell him that we did everything just the way he told us to do it, but that nothing happened. The old man shook his head and told my father that the damned spirit was an awful bad one, and very hard to get rid of, and that it calls for a more severe treatment. But that he would like to take another look at me before he decided another method of chasing him away from me. Well, one day I and my father paid him another visit. The old gaffer looked me over again from head to foot like if I was a young horse to sell and he wanted to buy me. Finally once again he began to make funny faces and noises like if someone stuck a knife through his belly, and said, for the love of God young man you sure have an awful bad spirit in you. I wonder where and how did you get it. But don't worry he said, we will get rid of him this time. I didn't understand this terrible demon the first time I saw you. But I do now and I know just what to do. But if I fail again, he said, I will give up. Young man, he said, I want you with your father's help to get the sex organ of a black bull not over two years old and stretch it till it becomes eighteen inches long, and hang it in the sun for three days and three nights. Then it will be dry enough to look like a little wooden stick. Then on a particular Friday night when the moon is full you must soak this stick in olive oil for a couple of hours before you go to a certain Church riding a black horse and carry your little stick with you. Behind this church is a Chiuppo tree when you get there you must go under this tree get on your knees and pray like you never prayed before, and ask your good Lord to chase this evil spirit away from you, then at twelve o'clock sharp you give your father your stick to beat you up with it till you pass out, and don't howl or make any kind of noise while your father is beating this awful demon away from you.

After that, when you revive, you must take the blessed stick again and hit the black horse with it as hard as you can and drop the stick at the same time. Then your father can put you on another horse and take you home and put you to bed. When you wake up in the morning you will be cured of your stammering because the evil spirit who make you stammering will be gone for ever.

Well, at this point my father asked him if anyone else could beat this spirit away from me beside himself. Because he didn't believe he had the nerve to do it. The old man began to pull his whiskers. Finally he said. No, you don't have to do it, let either one of his Grandfathers do it for you. I forgot the name of the Church he mentioned, but it was an abandoned old Church about two or three miles away from town where at one time monks and nuns were living. Behind this church was a good sized garden with an old Chiuppo tree in the center of it. My father didn't want to go through with the whole rotten thing. But finally one day he convinced my Grandfather. On that particular Friday night he got himself half drunk, and we went through with the whole rotten thing. Next morning when I woke up the whole family was around my bed to see if that damned evil spirit had left me. But just as soon as I opened my mouth to say something and I began to stammering worse than ever. We all knew that the dirty old spirit must have been with me yet. Well anyway, they all bust out crying like little babies and wished me better luck next time. Because although I wasn't cured of stammering, I was pretty well cured of believing in what those no good superstitious people had to offer for cure, and I cursed everyone of them and the day I listened and believed their dirty and useless

word... So my mother went to this old lady and explained to her everything about me. She gave her five or six different kinds of herbs and told my mother to cook the whole thing in about three gallons of water till it was reduced to about a quart. Then drain the juice out and let me take a tablespoon three times a day. This medicine was the worse one I ever took in my life. It was so bitter and sharp that it seemed to cut my tongue and throat, and make me shake like a leaf every time I took it. When I got done taking all of this medicine I was stammering as ever. But I was very glad there wasn't any more of it.

Well, a few more months passed away without experimenting. Till one day a very wise lady told us that the only way to cure my speech defect was to catch a particular snake named Vipera kill it and cook it on a particular Friday night when the moon was half full, and let me eat it at midnight sharp. This snake has a broken spine by nature and is very poisonous. So my father had a special made cage to keep this snake in when we should catch one. So one day we saw a middle sized one and after some trouble we caught it and kept it in the cage till we were ready to kill it. One night the moon was half full and my mother made a pot full of very delicious stew using the snake for me. In the morning I wasn't suppose to stammering any more, but I did as usually, anyway.

As I am writing this I still have my speech impediment, and although I do not stammering as bad as I did when I was young I do stammering bad enough yet to keep me well conscious of my speech defect every time I try to open my trap and say a peep. But I sincerely wish that all those other unfortunate kids with speech impediment will not be as unfortunate and stupid as I was and believe anything that some uneducated and cruel people have to offer for cure, and go through the same foolish and unscientific things that I went through. Well, sir, my experiences might seem ridiculous and unbelievable to you. But I swear that they are the God's truth. I remain

Respectfully yours

(Name withheld)

From "Letter to the Editor" by C. Pedrey, 1950, *Journal of Speech and Hearing Disorders, 15,* pp. 266–269. © 1950 by the American Speech-Language-Hearing Association.

to stutter most severely when they attempt to conceal it, encouraging them to acknowledge their stuttering can reduce its severity.

Another strategy is teaching them speech control techniques for reducing the severity of their stuttering. Unfortunately, although such techniques usually bring about an almost immediate reduction in stuttering severity, few people who stutter use them consistently over time because speech tends to become a fluent "flat drone," and the techniques require so much concentration that users have little working memory left to think about their message (Perkins, 1992).

In addition to therapy on their speech, intervention intended to reduce young children's stuttering severity usually involves some counseling with their parents. Study More 9.3 gives advice for parents of children who may be beginning to stutter. See The Stuttering Foundation of America (2002–2005) and Zebrowski and Schum (1993) for more information to provide to parents. Fluency intervention may also involve counseling with a child's classroom teacher and classmates (e.g., see Cooper & Cooper, 1992).

The amount that people are handicapped by stuttering is determined by how much it keeps them from doing what they want to do. Viewed in this way, some people who stutter a great deal are handicapped very little by the disorder, and others who stutter only occasionally are handicapped a great deal by it. The degree of handicap can usually be reduced through counseling. To learn more about how stuttering has been treated and the outcomes obtained, see Silverman (1996) and Van Riper (1973). Visit the National Stuttering Association (2005) website for information on self-help for stuttering.

Cluttering

Authorities appear to generally agree that people who have this disorder are abnormally disfluent because they do not monitor their speech adequately and are usually unaware of their disfluency or the fact that they are talking rapidly. To reduce their speaking rate and disfluency, therefore, it is necessary to get them to monitor their speech more carefully.

One problem that is frequently encountered when working with people who clutter is lack of motivation. They do not believe their speech is difficult to understand. Almost all are seen by SLPs because someone (usually a parent, teacher, or employer) insists that they need therapy. The prognosis for reducing their speaking rate and disfluency will, of course, be poor if they do not take therapy seriously. To learn more about the management of cluttering, see Arnold (1965), Daly (1986, 1993), Meyers and St. Louis (1992), Silverman (1996), and Weiss (1964).

	Reacting Appropriately
Study More 9.3	to a Child's Stuttering

How should one react to stuttering, particularly to a child's stuttering? The following advice is usually given to the parents of children who may be beginning to stutter.

• Give your child your undivided attention when he or she is speaking to you.	• Do not react to moments of disfluency in your child's speech.
• Speak at a slower rate.	• Do not tell your child how not to stutter (e.g., "slow down").
• Simplify your language patterns.	• Avoid demand speaking (e.g., "Tell Grandma about your new cat.").
• Do not interrupt your child when he or she is speaking.	

Neurogenic Acquired Stuttering

Because neurogenic acquired stuttering results from abnormal function of one or more structures in the central nervous system, it is sometimes possible to reduce the amount of disfluency by having the person modify his or her habitual speaking behavior—for example, by slowing down speech. It also may be possible to do so by "normalizing" the functioning of the central nervous system (CNS)—for example, through the use of drugs or by implanting electrodes that allow parts of the CNS to be stimulated electrically (Silverman, 1996). To learn more about the management of neurogenic acquired stuttering, see Silverman, (1996).

Psychogenic Acquired Stuttering

The appropriate treatment of clients who have this disorder is usually psychotherapy. Consequently, SLPs almost always refer these clients to clinical psychologists or psychiatrists. To learn more about the management of psychogenic acquired stuttering, see Roth, Aronson, and Davis (1989).

Part 4

Hearing Disorders

Part 4 contains two chapters that address hearing disorders. Chapter 10 provides the background necessary for understanding hearing disorders: a description of sound; the anatomy and physiology of the hearing mechanism; and the types and causes of hearing disorders.

Chapter 11 describes the assessment and management of hearing disorders in children and adults. The chapter includes a description of the major types of hearing testing and an overview of the primary approaches used to help people with hearing disorders regain some or all of their hearing, capitalize on their residual hearing, and learn alternative methods for communicating.

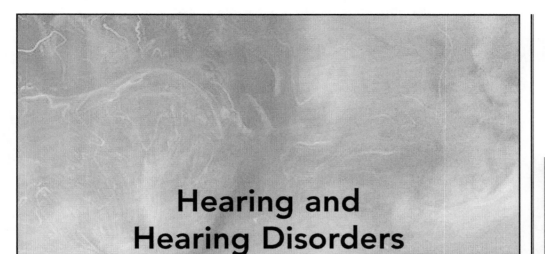

Hearing and Hearing Disorders

Chapter 10

Learning Objectives

- Describe how sound is generated.

- Identify the characteristic waveform associated with different types of sounds.

- Define *pure tone.*

- Define *hertz.*

- Define *decibel.*

- Describe the anatomy and physiology of the outer, middle, and inner ear.

- Describe the etiology and characteristics of a conductive hearing loss.

- Describe the etiology and characteristics of a sensorineural hearing loss.

- Describe a mixed hearing loss.

- Describe hearing difficulties associated with central auditory disturbances.

- Describe the etiology and characteristics of a functional hearing loss.

Introduction

According to the American Speech-Language-Hearing Association (ASHA; 1993), a hearing disorder is the result of impaired auditory sensitivity of the physiological auditory system that may limit the development, comprehension, production, and/or maintenance of speech and/or language. The demographics of hearing loss indicate that:

- Children who are hard of hearing will find it much more difficult than children who have normal hearing to learn vocabulary, grammar, word order, idiomatic expressions, and other aspects of verbal communication (National Information Center for Children and Youth with Disabilities, 2004).

- The number of children with disabilities, ages 6–21, served in the public schools under the Individuals with Disabilities Education Act (IDEA) Part B in the 2000–01 school year was 5,775,722 (in the 50 states, Washington, DC, and Puerto Rico). Of these children, 70,767 (1.2 percent) received services for hearing disorders. However, the number of children with hearing loss and deafness is probably higher because many of these students may have other disabilities as well (United States Department of Education, 2002).

- Overall estimates of the prevalence of newborns with **congenital** hearing loss in the United States are between 1 to 6 per 1,000 newborns (Cunningham & Cox, 2003; Kemper & Downs, 2000). Most children with congenital hearing loss have hearing impairment at birth and are potentially identifiable by newborn and infant hearing screening. However, some congenital hearing loss may not become evident until later in childhood (Cunningham & Cox).

- The average age of detection of significant hearing loss is approximately 14 months (Taskforce on Newborn and Infant Hearing, 1999).

- About half of the cases of childhood hearing loss are believed to be from genetic causes (Canalis & Lambert, 2000).

- The prevalence of genetic hearing loss has been calculated at approximately 1 in 2,000 (Canalis & Lambert, 2000).

- In about 30 percent of babies with a hearing loss, the loss is part of a syndrome, meaning that these babies have other problems. There are more than 400 syndromes that can cause hearing loss (National Center on Birth Defects and Developmental Disabilities, 2003).

Physics of Sound

Sound is generated by the movement of air molecules. The products of their movement are referred to as sound waves. Sound waves are invisible, but they can be detected by instruments and displayed graphically.

Waveforms

The way particles of air move determines which sound will be generated. Each sound has a unique movement pattern, or **waveform.** As you can see in Figure 10.1 on page 176, the waveform for the vowel /a/ differs considerably from that for middle C played on a piano and the

Waveform
The manner in which particles of air that are perceived as sound vibrate. There is a unique vibration pattern for each speech sound.

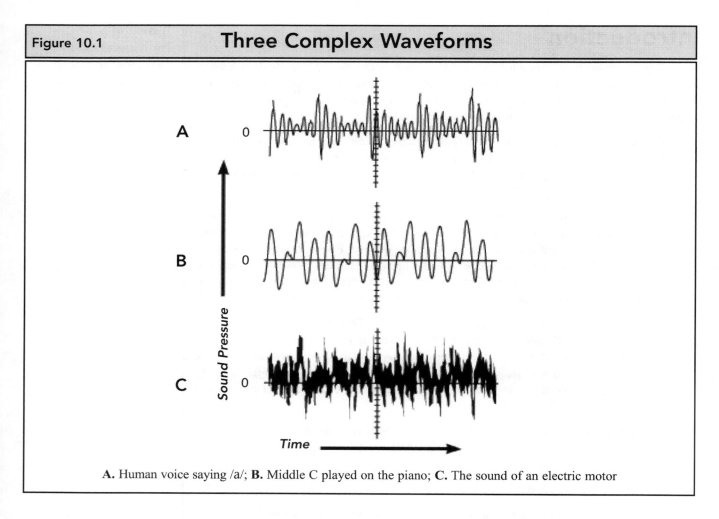

Figure 10.1	Three Complex Waveforms

A. Human voice saying /a/; **B.** Middle C played on the piano; **C.** The sound of an electric motor

Pure tone
A sound in which particles of air vibrate at a single frequency.

Sine wave
The waveform for a pure tone.

Hertz (Hz)
The unit of measurement for the pitch of sounds. The higher the pitch, the larger the number.

noise produced by an electric motor. Furthermore, the waveform for the vowel /a/ differs from that for every other vowel and consonant sound.

The movements of particles of air that cause sounds to be generated can be classified as either simple or complex. Those classified as simple—which are referred to as **pure tones**—produce a waveform known as a **sine wave** and a tone containing acoustic energy at a single frequency (hence, one that is "pure"). The waveform at the top of Figure 10.2 (labeled 100 Hz) depicts a single sine wave (also known as a single cycle), and the two in the middle (labeled 300 Hz and 500 Hz) depict a series (or a number of cycles or replications) of sine waves. The number of sine waves (or the number of cycles) that occur each second determines the pitch of a pure tone—the larger the number, the higher the pitch. This number is designated in a unit of measurement known as **hertz (Hz).** A 500 Hz pure tone has more cycles per second and consequently a higher pitch than a 300 Hz tone (see Figure 10.2). Tuning forks are one of the few instruments that can generate pure tones. The size (i.e., mass) of the fork, rather than the force used to strike it, determines the pitch of the tone.

Almost all the sounds we hear are complex because particles of air in the real world rarely vibrate at a single frequency, and, therefore, they do not have a sine wave waveform. Complex

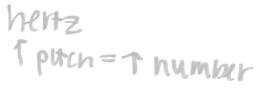

sounds are of two types: periodic and aperiodic. The waveforms for individual cycles for periodic sounds are complex but repeat themselves. Complex periodic tones consist of combinations of pure tones. The waveform at the bottom of Figure 10.2 illustrates how pure tones combine to produce complex periodic tones. The waveforms for all three sounds displayed in Figure 10.1 are complex periodic ones, as are those for all vowel sounds.

Many sounds (e.g., those produced by a book dropping or production of the consonant /s/) are complex in that they consist of more than one frequency, but they are aperiodic because their waveforms over time do not consistently (i.e., periodically) repeat themselves. The waveform of a complex aperiodic sound, like that of a complex periodic one and a pure tone, determines what will be heard.

Intensity (Loudness)

Sounds are differentiated from each other not only by the nature and periodicity of their waveform, but also by height (i.e., amplitude) of the waveform. The amplitude of a waveform determines the relative intensity (i.e., loudness) of the sound it generates. The unit of measurement for the loudness of sounds is the **decibel (dB).** The louder a sound (i.e., the higher its number on the decibel scale), the greater the amplitude of the waveform that produced it. The amplitude of the waveform for the 300 Hz tone in Figure 10.2 is greater than that for the 500 Hz one. Consequently, people with normal hearing would perceive the 300 Hz tone depicted

Decibel (dB)
The unit of measurement for the loudness of sounds. The louder the sound, the larger the number.

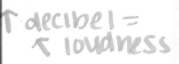

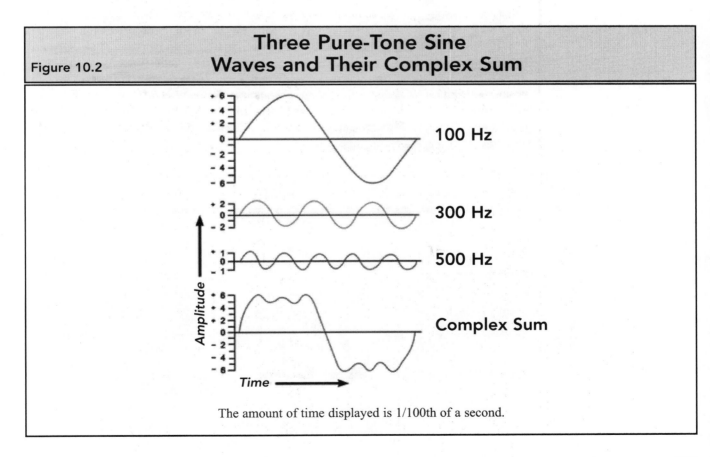

| Figure 10.2 | **Three Pure-Tone Sine Waves and Their Complex Sum** |

100 Hz

300 Hz

500 Hz

Complex Sum

Time

The amount of time displayed is 1/100th of a second.

Auricle
The largely cartilaginous, projecting portion of the outer ear. Also referred to as the pinna.

External auditory meatus
The part of the outer ear that is also referred to as the ear canal.

Cilia
Small hairs on the inner surface of the external auditory meatus.

Ceruminous glands
The glands that secrete cerumen.

Cerumen
Ear wax.

Tympanic membrane
The eardrum.

in this figure as being louder than the 500 Hz one. To learn more about the physics of sound, see Borden, Harris, and Raphael (1994); Ferrand (2001); and Speaks (1999).

Anatomy and Physiology of the Hearing Mechanism

Almost all hearing disorders are caused by damage (on one side or both sides) to the outer ear, middle ear, inner ear, auditory nerve, or brain—specifically that part of the brain referred to as the **central auditory nervous system (CANS).** The functions of these structures are represented in Figure 10.3. To understand why damage to these structures results in a predictable type of hearing deficit, you have to know something about their functions, or physiology. When one or more of these structures functions abnormally, the result is a problem with hearing. The specific type of problem is determined by the anatomical location of the damage rather than its cause (i.e., etiology). All conditions that damage a particular structure in the ear, auditory nerve, or CANS produce the same type of hearing problem (i.e., all exhibit the same symptomatology). Figure 10.4 illustrates the anatomy of the ear. The outer ear, the middle ear, and the inner ear are briefly described in the following sections.

Outer Ear

The largely cartilaginous external portion of the outer ear is referred to as the **auricle.** (See site 1 in Figure 10.4.) This is the only part of the ear we can fully observe without using instruments. The auricle acts like a funnel to direct sound-induced vibration of air particles into the **external auditory meatus.** (See site 2 in Figure 10.4.) On the inner surface of this tubelike structure there are small hairs called **cilia,** and **ceruminous glands** that secrete **cerumen.** Cilia and cerumen help to protect the **tympanic membrane** (See site 3 in Figure 10.4.), which is situated at the end of this canal, from being damaged by dirt, insects, or other foreign objects. The tympanic membrane separates the outer ear from the middle ear. It is conical in shape with the tip of the cone facing inward.

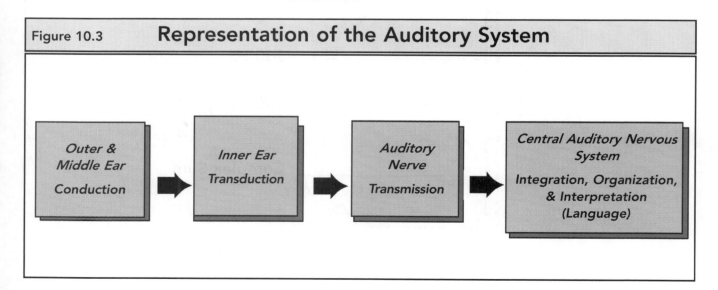

Figure 10.3	**Representation of the Auditory System**

Outer & Middle Ear Conduction → *Inner Ear Transduction* → *Auditory Nerve Transmission* → *Central Auditory Nervous System Integration, Organization, & Interpretation (Language)*

Middle Ear

The middle ear consists of a small air-filled cavity containing a chain of three tiny bones—the **malleus** (i.e., hammer), the **incus** (i.e., anvil), and the **stapes** (i.e., stirrup)—known as the **ossicular chain.** (See site 4 in Figure 10.4.) The size of the cavity is about that of a garden pea. The stapes is the smallest bone in the human body, about the size of a grain of rice. The malleus is attached to the tympanic membrane. When the tympanic membrane vibrates, it causes the malleus to vibrate, which causes the incus to vibrate, which, in turn, causes the stapes to vibrate. The stapes is attached to a membrane known as the **oval window.** (See site 5 in Figure 10.4.) The oval window is located in the bony wall that separates the middle ear from the inner ear.

The middle ear is connected to the nasopharynx (in the back wall of the throat) by a hollow structure that is referred to as the **eustachian tube.** (See site 7 in Figure 10.4.) Its function is to aerate the middle ear so that the air pressure behind the tympanic membrane equals that in front of it. Equal air pressure is necessary for the membrane to vibrate freely. When you are at a high altitude (e.g., in an airplane or on top of a mountain) and experience pain or a feeling of fullness in an ear, the eustachian tube is not allowing enough air out of the middle ear cavity to equalize the pressure on both sides of the tympanic membrane. Yawning, chewing, or swallowing sometimes can relieve this condition because they cause the end of the eustachian tube in the nasopharynx to open, allowing air to pass into or out of the middle ear cavity. The eustachian tube provides the route by which infections travel from the throat to the middle ear cavity, causing earaches.

Malleus
The first of the three tiny bones in the middle ear.

Incus
The second of the three tiny bones in the middle ear.

Stapes
The third of three tiny bones in the middle ear.

Ossicular chain
The three tiny bones in the middle ear.

Oval window
The membrane that separates the middle ear from the inner ear.

Eustachian tube
A hollow structure that connects the middle ear to the back wall of the throat.

Figure 10.4	**Anatomy of the Ear**

The numbered sites indicate where lesions or abnormalities can cause hearing loss.

1. Auricle
2. External auditory meatus (ear canal)
3. Tympanic membrane (eardrum)
4. Ossicles
5. Oval window
6. Cochlea
7. Eustachian tube
8. Auditory nerve

Outer Ear *Middle Ear* *Inner Ear*

Semicircular canals
The structures in the inner ear responsible for the detection of rotation.

Vestibule
The structure in the inner ear responsible for the detection of linear acceleration and gravity.

Cochlea
The structure in the inner ear responsible for hearing.

Transduce
Convert energy from one form into another. The inner ear transduces sound-induced vibration into a form of electrochemical energy.

Auditory nerve
A branch of the VIIIth cranial nerve that transmits electrochemical energy generated by the inner ear to the central auditory nervous system (CANS).

Bilateral conductive hearing loss
A conductive hearing loss in both ears.

Inner Ear, Auditory Nerve, and Central Auditory Nervous System

The inner ear contains the **semicircular canals,** the **vestibule,** and the **cochlea.** (See site 6 in Figure 10.4 on page 179.) Each of these structures is filled with fluid. The semicircular canals and vestibule are responsible for balance and equilibrium. The cochlea is responsible for hearing. The cochlea contains many microscopic structures that **transduce** sound-induced vibration into a form of electrochemical energy. Vibrations are conducted from the middle ear to the cochlea by way of the stapes and oval window. The **auditory nerve** (See site 8 in Figure 10.4 on page 179.) transmits electrochemical energy generated by the cochlea to the CANS.

Summary of Sound Vibration Transmission

The process by which sound-induced vibrations are conducted from the outer ear to the inner ear can be summarized as follows, with the numbers corresponding to Figure 10.4 on page 179. The sound waves enter the outer ear at the auricle (1) and are conducted along the external auditory meatus (2) to the tympanic membrane (3). The sound waves set the tympanic membrane into vibration, which in turn sets the three little bones in the middle ear (4)—the malleus, incus, and stapes—into vibration. The vibration of the stapes sets the oval window (5) into vibration, thereby conducting sound-induced vibrations to the cochlea in the inner ear (6). Electrochemical energy from the cochlea is then transferred to the auditory nerve (8) and then the CANS. To learn more about the anatomy and physiology of the hearing mechanism, see Zemlin (1998).

Types and Causes of Hearing Disorders

People who have a hearing disorder have some degree of difficulty understanding speech and/or hearing environmental sounds (e.g., automobile traffic noise). The severity of the disorder can range from occasional difficulty localizing the sources of sounds to being unable to hear anything (i.e., being totally deaf).

A number of conditions (e.g., diseases, congenital abnormalities, types of trauma) can result in children and adults being unable to hear and understand speech as well as their peers. People can have one or more of these conditions, each of which contributes uniquely to a hearing disorder.

Conductive Hearing Loss

People who have **conductive hearing losses** have a bilateral (i.e., both sides) or unilateral (i.e., one side) lesion or abnormality in the outer and/or middle ear. (See Figure 10.4 on page 179.) Those who have a **bilateral conductive hearing loss** experience speech and other sound as being relatively "soft." How soft depends on the severity of the loss. They experience what you experience if you listen to a radio with the volume set very low. You only understand what is being said if you concentrate very hard and the room is relatively quiet. Individuals with a bilateral conductive hearing loss may have lost the ability to equalize air pressure on both sides of the tympanic membrane, which impedes the membrane's ability to vibrate and conduct vibrations to the inner ear.

People with a **unilateral conductive hearing loss** ordinarily experience speech and other sound as being adequately loud unless the sound is soft and on the same side as the impaired ear. Their main problem usually is localizing—finding the source of a sound. The brain needs information about the relative intensity of a sound at both the right and left sides of the head to localize it in space. Consequently, if the ears are not equally sensitive to sound, the brain cannot accurately interpret differences in loudness as reflecting differences in distances between the sound source and the right and left ears. Localization errors occur as a result.

A conductive hearing loss, by itself, cannot cause a person to become deaf. This is true even if the structures of both the outer and middle ear are missing bilaterally, because sound energy can also be conducted to the inner ear through vibration of the bones of the head.

Etiology

Conductive hearing losses are caused by a lesion or abnormality in the outer or middle ear. (See Figure 10.4 on page 179.) This lesion or abnormality prevents sound-induced vibrations from being conducted normally into the inner ear, which is why this type of hearing loss is referred to as conductive. Several types of lesions and abnormalities can interfere with the conduction of sound-induced vibrations from the outer ear to the inner ear. Some of these are described in the paragraphs that follow.

Cerumen Impaction

Cerumen impaction occurs when an overabundance of cerumen partially or totally blocks the external auditory canal. This impedes the conduction of sound-induced vibrations. Cerumen is a less efficient medium for conducting vibrations from the auricle to the eardrum than air. When the excess cerumen is removed (preferably by a physician), hearing level should return to normal.

Congenital Atresia of the Outer Ear

A child may be born with a **congenital atresia.** The auricle may also be absent or deformed. This abnormality can occur in one or both ears and it is present from birth. The explanation for why congenital atresia causes a conductive hearing loss is similar to that for cerumen impaction—bone or fibrous tissue is a less efficient medium than air for conducting sound-induced vibrations from the auricle to the eardrum. If it is possible for a plastic surgeon to construct an auricle and external auditory canal, the hearing loss should either be reduced in severity or eliminated—provided the structure and function of the ear are otherwise normal.

Otitis Media

Otitis media is an inflammation of the middle ear—the space between the tympanic membrane and the oval window—in one or both ears. (See Figure 10.4 on page 179.) It may be the result of a eustachian tube malfunction, or bacterial or viral infection. The space becomes filled with a fluid, which impedes the vibration of the ossicles. As a result, the vibrations that reach the oval window are weaker than normal. Both children and adults can develop otitis media. It can be a chronic or recurring condition, and it may lead to a perforation of the tympanic membrane. Fluid in the middle ear can often be eliminated through medical treatment if it is caused by a bacterial infection—for example, administering antibiotics to eliminate the infection producing the fluid. Once the fluid has been eliminated, the magnitude of the vibration of the ossicles increases and hearing improves.

Unilateral conductive hearing loss
A conductive hearing loss in only one ear.

Cerumen impaction
An overabundance of ear wax.

Congenital atresia
A partial or complete absence or blockage of the external auditory meatus.

Otitis media
An inflammation in the middle ear that can cause a conductive hearing loss.

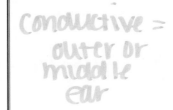

Conductive = outer or middle ear

Cholesteatoma
A type of tumor that can occur in the middle ear and cause a conductive hearing loss.

Otosclerosis
A disease in which the stapes (the third bone in the ossicular chain) becomes fixated in the oval window, thereby causing a conductive hearing loss.

Ossicular discontinuity
One of the three tiny bones that form the ossicular chain in the middle ear breaks or somehow becomes disconnected from the other two. The result is a conductive hearing loss.

Dhooge (2003) reports that otitis media is the most frequently diagnosed disease in infants and young children. Seventy-five percent of children experience at least one episode of otitis media by their third birthday. Almost half of these children will have three or more ear infections during their first three years (National Institute on Deafness and Other Communication Disorders, 2002a). Health costs for otitis media in the United States have been reported to be $3 to $5 billion per year (Alsarraf, Jung, & Perkins, 1998). For more information on otitis media, visit the otitis media webpages of the National Institute on Deafness and Other Communication Disorders (NIDCD; 2005g, 2005c).

Cholesteatoma

A **cholesteatoma** is an abnormal accumulation of a fibrous material that can occur in the middle ear. It may be **congenital** or acquired, and it can damage the ossicles. The effect of a cholesteatoma on the conduction of vibration in the middle ear is somewhat similar to that of otitis media—the fibrous material lessens the magnitude of vibration of the ossicles. The effect on the magnitude of these vibrations (and thereby on hearing) tends to be greater if the ossicles are damaged.

Otosclerosis

Otosclerosis is a disease in which the third of the little bones in the middle ear, the stapes, becomes immobilized in the oval window. Because the stapes cannot move normally, it cannot conduct noise-induced vibrations normally to the oval window. The fixation of the stapes can sometimes be corrected through surgery. To learn more about otosclerosis, visit the NIDCD website (2005h).

Ossicular Discontinuity

The three ossicles bridge the space between the eardrum and the oval window. If one of the bones breaks or separates from the other two, vibration can no longer be conducted through them to the oval window. **Ossicular discontinuity** can result from a number of conditions, including severe head trauma. To learn more about the symptomatology and etiology of conductive hearing loss, see Martin (2000).

Sensorineural Hearing Loss from Inner Ear Abnormality

People with a lesion or abnormality in the inner ear (See Figure 10.4 on page 179.) have a **sensorineural hearing loss.** Those who have a loss in both ears (i.e., bilateral) experience speech and other sound as distorted and usually as relatively soft. The sound distortion occurs because the ability of the inner ear to transduce sound-induced vibrations into electrochemical energy is not impaired to the same degree for all frequencies. It tends to be more impaired for transducing relatively high frequencies than for transducing relatively low ones. Consequently, the higher the pitch of a sound, the more difficulty a person with a bilateral sensorineural loss is likely to have hearing it.

When people with this type of hearing loss listen to someone speak, they tend to hear certain speech sounds less well than others. They are particularly likely to have difficulty hearing sounds that contain a great deal of high-frequency energy, such as the consonant /s/.

Study More 10.1 demonstrates how a person with a bilateral sensorineural hearing loss may hear certain words. If their hearing loss is extremely severe, they will be unable to hear any sounds (except possibly those that are very low pitched) and will be referred to as deaf.

What is it like listening to distorted sound? You can simulate the experience by listening to your favorite music through the loud speaker on a small, inexpensive radio or on a low-end laptop computer. A loud speaker is a transducer that converts electrical energy into acoustical energy. Because the small speakers in such radios and laptops are not equally sensitive to all sound frequencies, they will reproduce some frequencies louder than others, thereby distorting the music. You probably will not like what you hear!

If your ability to hear has ever been impaired temporarily after being exposed to loud noise (e.g., at a concert), you have had firsthand experience with a hearing loss of this type. You have experienced what is known as a **temporary threshold shift.**

Some people who have a sensorineural hearing loss experience **tinnitus.** In some cases the noise is described as a diffuse roaring or rushing sound, with its source somewhere in the head. In others the source is localized in one or both ears. To learn more about tinnitus, see Tyler (2000). Audio Clip 10.1 illustrates the internal sound that someone who has tinnitus might hear constantly. For more information on tinnitus, visit the NIDCD website (2005f).

Temporary threshold shift
A temporary hearing loss after being exposed to loud noise that affects the functioning of the inner ear.

Tinnitus
A constant or almost constant ringing, whistling, or roaring sound that appears to the person experiencing it to be located in one or both ears or somewhere in the head.

Loudness recruitment
An abnormally rapid growth of loudness with an increase in intensity.

Audio Clip 10.1	Tinnitus
⊚ AUDIO	An example of an internal sound that someone who has tinnitus might hear constantly

Another phenomenon that persons with a sensorineural hearing loss may experience is known as **loudness recruitment.** In an ear in which there is recruitment, an increase in the intensity of a sound will tend to produce a greater increase in the person's perception of loudness than would be the case for a normal ear. Loudness recruitment must be considered when fitting a person with a hearing aid. If the person can hear loud sounds normally (or nearly so) without amplification, such sounds can be too loud with amplification and can produce physical discomfort.

Study More 10.1	Sensorineural Hearing Loss	
Word Said		**Word Heard**
sold		old
slate		late
smile		mile
trucks		truck
sink		ink
books		book
house		how
place		play
grocer		grower
since		in

Presbycusis
Sensorineural hearing loss resulting—directly or indirectly (e.g., long-term exposure to noise)—from the effect of the aging process on the inner ear.

Etiology

As stated above, a lesion or abnormality in the inner ear can produce a sensorineural hearing loss. The inner ear converts the vibrations conducted to it by the middle ear into electrical signals that are sent to the brain through the auditory nerve. (See site 8 in Figure 10.4 on page 179.) A transducer changes, or transforms, one form of energy into another form of energy. The inner ear transforms mechanical energy into electrochemical energy. If the inner ear is functioning normally, it will convert the information contained in the vibrations it receives from the middle ear into electrochemical signals without distorting them. However, a lesion or abnormality in the inner ear can cause the information contained in the vibrations to be distorted when they are transduced into an electrochemical signal. The part of the inner ear mechanism responsible for transducing relatively high-frequency mechanical energy into electrochemical signals appears to be more vulnerable to damage than that responsible for transducing relatively low-frequency mechanical energy.

If the mechanism of the inner ear is severely damaged, little (or none) of the information contained in noise-induced vibration will be transduced into electrochemical signals and sent on to the brain. When the mechanisms of both inner ears are severely damaged or destroyed, little or no information is sent on to the brain, and the person is referred to as deaf. Hence, the greater the damage to the inner ear, the greater the distortion of the information in the vibrations conducted to it. A number of conditions can cause the mechanism of the inner ear to function abnormally.

The Aging Process

Sensorineural hearing loss resulting from the effect of the aging process on the inner ear is referred to as **presbycusis.** Aging ordinarily damages rather than destroys the inner ear. Hence, patients with presbycusis usually complain of an inability to understand speech (because they cannot hear certain consonant sounds) rather than an inability to hear. They report that it sounds to them like people are mumbling. The NIDCD presbycusis web page (2005i) provides additional information regarding presbycusis.

Drugs

Ingesting certain drugs can damage the inner ear or cause it to function abnormally. The resulting hearing loss is usually bilateral and of approximately the same magnitude in both ears. One drug that can produce a sensorineural hearing loss when ingested in high doses is aspirin—the hearing loss may disappear when use of the drug is discontinued. There is also some evidence of moderate to profound hearing loss following prolonged use of certain prescription painkillers that combine hydrocodone and acetaminophen. If hearing improves after the use of a drug is discontinued, the effect of the drug on the inner ear probably was to cause it to function abnormally rather than to damage it.

Loud Noise

Brief exposure to extremely intense noise—such as that produced by a loud explosion—can damage the inner ear. Trauma to the ear caused by brief exposure to extremely intense noise usually affects hearing almost instantly. Also, prolonged exposure to loud noise can damage the inner ear or cause it to function abnormally. An immediate hearing loss does not occur from trauma caused by prolonged, or chronic, exposure to loud noise. The effect of such trauma is insidious; a person can work in a noisy environment for many years and be unaware of developing a hearing loss because this type of trauma initially damages a part of the inner ear mechanism that transforms relatively high frequency information—that at a frequency of approximately 4,000 Hz—into electrical signals. Several explanations as to why noise-induced hearing losses tend to affect frequencies around the 4,000 Hz range are given in Study More 10.2. The loss of acoustic information at this frequency ordinarily does not interfere with understanding speech. However, as the trauma process continues, portions of the inner ear mechanism are affected that transduce information above and below this frequency. Eventually, the damage becomes so widespread that the person experiences difficulty understanding speech. Unfortunately, the person does not become aware of the problem until considerable damage has occurred.

Which types of noise can cause acoustic trauma and result in a noise-induced hearing loss? Almost any loud noise that a person is exposed to repeatedly can do this. A firefighter can develop a loss over time from the noise he or she is exposed to while riding in a fire engine. A musician can develop a loss by playing frequently with a "heavy-metal" rock band. And anyone can develop a loss by frequently attending concerts or by frequently playing very loud music through headphones. Study More 10.3 on page 186 explains why musicians are moving toward hearing conservation.

Noise loud enough to damage the inner ear sometimes produces a temporary hearing loss before producing a permanent one. Such a loss is referred to as a temporary threshold shift, which means the threshold of hearing has shifted upward. If, after leaving a very noisy environment, your ears felt "stuffy" and/or you had tinnitus, you experienced a temporary threshold shift.

Study More 10.2	**Why 4,000 Hz?**

You may have wondered why noise-induced hearing losses tend to affect hearing initially at frequencies in the vicinity of 4,000 Hz. Several possible explanations are indicated in the following.

Approximately 10 million people in the United States have developed hearing loss as a result of high level noise exposure. Demographic studies of occupational noise-induced hearing loss as well as controlled laboratory studies have shown that, for a given exposure level, the greatest amount of hearing loss occurs in the 3 to 6 kHz [thousand hertz] range, with the peak loss typically occurring at 4 kHz. Several different mechanisms may make the auditory system more vulnerable to hearing loss in the 4 kHz region. One hypothesis is that the anatomical structures of the inner ear associated with the 4 kHz region are simply more susceptible to acoustic trauma.

Another factor that appears to contribute to the hearing loss in the 4 kHz region is the outer ear transfer function. The pinna and ear canal selectively amplify mid-frequency sounds as they pass from the free field environment to the tympanic membrane...The amplifica-

tion provided by the external ear is due in large part to the resonant frequency of the ear canal [which is a function of its length]...The predicted resonant frequency for the ear canal is approximately 3,270 Hz. Given that the maximum hearing loss occurs approximately one-half octave above the exposure frequency, it is not surprising that the maximum hearing loss occurs near 4 kHz. If the length of the ear canal is artificially increased by inserting a longer tube into the external auditory meatus [canal], the resonant frequency decreases and the frequency of maximum hearing loss shifts to a lower frequency.

Finally, the middle ear acoustic reflex may influence the pattern of hearing loss. When the middle ear muscles are activated by high level sounds, the transmission of sound energy into the cochlea is reduced at low frequencies but unaffected at high frequencies.

From "4000 Hz Noise Damage," by R. J. Salvi, 1993, *American Journal of Audiology, 2*(1), p. 21. © 1993 by the American Speech-Language-Hearing Association. Reprinted with permission.

Study More 10.3 | **Musicians Turn to Hearing Conservation**

Many youngsters turn a deaf ear to their parents when they admonish, "Turn your music down. It's too loud!" over the sound surging from home stereos, boom boxes, and Walkmans. After all, rock and roll is supposed to be loud, frenzied, and forceful, according to its enthusiasts.

But when rock legends like Pete Townshend of the Who announce that excessive exposure to loud noise has caused them irreparable hearing damage, fellow artists and fans take heed.

Today, there is a growing movement among musicians, fans, sound engineers, music producers, critics and others involved in the entertainment business toward hearing conservation. It's quite a change from the earth-shaking mind-set that has permeated every rock venue from Woodstock to the Los Angeles Forum over the last 25 years.

A new consciousness is evolving as more and more musicians come forward and announce the hearing problems they have acquired as a result of high-volume musical careers. Townshend, who described his struggle with tinnitus during a press conference before his group's 1989 reunion tour, stated, "The real reason that I haven't performed live for a long time is that I have severe hearing damage. It's manifested itself as tinnitus, ringing in the ear at the frequencies that I play the guitar. It hurts, and it's painful, and it's frustrating when little children talk to you and you can't hear them."

From "Musicians No Longer Turn a Deaf Ear to Hearing Conservation," by R. Trace, 1992, *Advance for Speech-Language Pathologists and Audiologists, 2* (19), p. 9. © 1992 by Merion Publications. Reprinted with permission

---

Ménière's disease
A disease of the vestibular system (part of the inner ear) that has a sensorineural hearing loss as one of its components.

Viral Infections

Several types of viral infections can damage the inner ear. The measles virus, for example, can produce enough extensive damage to both inner ears to cause a severe sensorineural hearing loss. Measles was one of the main causes of childhood deafness prior to the development of vaccines, which became available in 1963. The mumps virus can also produce a severe sensorineural hearing loss. This loss differs from that caused by measles in that it usually affects only one ear (Zarnoch, 1982).

Tumors

Acoustic tumors are almost always benign. But as the tumor grows, it can apply pressure to nerve fibers in the inner ear, thereby damaging them. The resulting sensorineural hearing loss usually is unilateral.

Ménière's Disease

The primary symptom associated with **Ménière's disease** is vertigo, or dizziness. People who have Ménière's disease also experience tinnitus. These disturbances are ordinarily episodic rather than constant, and they can last anywhere from a few minutes to several hours. Patients can remain symptom-free for weeks, months, or even years. The hearing loss associated with this disease is usually unilateral.

Trauma

Injuries to the skull can damage the inner ear. Such injuries can result from accidents; bullet wounds or blows to the head; and surgery (particularly mastoid surgery). The hearing loss associated with trauma is usually unilateral. To learn more about the symptomatology and etiology of sensorineural hearing loss, see Martin (2000).

Sensorineural Hearing Loss from Auditory Nerve Damage

Acoustic neuroma
A tumor that impedes the functioning of the auditory nerve by pressing on it.

Acoustic neuritis
Inflammation of the auditory nerve.

The right and left VIIIth cranial nerves are components of the peripheral nervous system. Each has two branches, one of which is the auditory nerve. The other—the vestibular nerve—controls the mechanism for balance and equilibrium, which is located in the inner ear. The auditory nerve transmits nerve impulses from the inner ear on each side to the parts of the brain that make up the CANS. Its function is similar to that of an electrical wire, or cable—that is, to convey electrical energy signals from one point to another. If an auditory nerve is severed or otherwise made inoperable, electrical information will not be sent from the inner ear on that side to the CANS, and the person will be deaf in that ear. If an auditory nerve is damaged (not destroyed), the information sent to the CANS will be incomplete, and what the person hears will be abnormally soft, distorted, or both.

Disorders of the auditory nerve, like those of the inner ear, result in hearing losses that are classified as sensorineural. Two common early symptoms of auditory nerve disorders are a hearing loss that is greater for speech sounds containing considerable high-frequency energy (e.g., /s/) and tinnitus. If a sensorineural hearing loss is unilateral, the cause is more likely to be damage to the auditory nerve than to the inner ear.

Etiology

Lesions of the auditory nerve can occur as a result of trauma, disease, irritation, or pressure on the nerve. One of the most common causes is a tumor that impedes the functioning of an auditory nerve by pressing on it. Such tumors (usually referred to as **acoustic neuromas**) are usually benign and unilateral. Two other conditions that can interfere with the functioning of this nerve are **acoustic neuritis** and **multiple sclerosis.** To learn more about the symptoms and etiology of hearing loss from auditory nerve damage, see Martin (2000). For more information on multiple sclerosis, see the National Institute of Neurological Disorders and Stroke (NINDS; 2005a).

Mixed Hearing Loss

A person with a mixed hearing loss has a lesion or abnormality in either the outer or middle ear and the inner ear or auditory nerve. He or she exhibits a combination of the symptoms associated with conductive and sensorineural hearing loss. If conductive components predominate and the loss is bilateral, the deficit will be primarily one of speech being perceived as too soft. If sensorineural components are predominant with such a loss, the deficit will be one of speech being distorted and probably also perceived as too soft.

Any of the causes for conductive and sensorineural hearing loss that have been discussed can contribute to the etiology of a mixed hearing loss. Damage to the inner ear may predate that to the outer or middle ear, or the reverse could be true. To learn more about the symptomatology and etiology of mixed hearing loss, see Martin (2000).

Auditory agnosia
A disorder of the central auditory nervous system in which the person has difficulty separating figure from background noise.

Hearing Difficulties from Central Auditory Disturbance

Information conducted to the inner ear and changed by it into electrical signals is sent to the brain via the auditory nerve for integration, organization, and interpretation. The brain cells that perform this function—which are located in the brain stem, medulla, midbrain, thalamus, and cerebral cortex—make up the CANS. This system, like that of the ear, is discussed here from the perspective of what it does rather than how it does it. Central auditory disturbances do not cause a loss of hearing; rather, they cause difficulties with how sounds are processed.

Damage to the CANS can disturb the ability to localize sound and understand speech in a variety of ways. The characteristic symptoms caused by a CANS lesion is determined by its location. Lesions at specific locations in the CANS tend to produce predictable symptoms regardless of their cause. This is a consequence of localization of function within the brain, which makes some parts of it more important than others for mediating specific functions. The following paragraphs discuss some disturbances in hearing that can result from lesions in the CANS. For further information about such disturbances, see Chermak and Musiek (1992).

Disturbed Localization Ability

Information from both ears is integrated in the CANS in a way that enables the source of a sound to be located. Someone who has a lesion in the brain cells responsible for mediating this function would have difficulty locating the source of sounds like a car horn while driving, someone's voice if they're not in immediate view, or the sound of an emergency vehicle in traffic.

Disturbed Bilateral Synthesis Ability

The CANS does not usually receive exactly the same information from both ears. (It can only be identical if its source is equidistant from each ear). The function of some cells in the CANS is to synthesize this information. Consequently, a person whose bilateral synthesis ability was severely disturbed probably would not perceive stereo music normally.

Disturbed Ability to Separate Figure from Background

People who have this condition, which is sometimes referred to as **auditory agnosia,** have difficulty concentrating auditorily. What they have trouble listening to is the figure (i.e., target sound) rather than all the other sounds present in the environment (i.e., the background). For example, a student may not be able to listen to a teacher's lecture because the air conditioner noise is distracting him or her.

If our CANS is functioning properly, we usually have the ability to concentrate on what somebody is saying without being distracted by sounds in the environment. In fact, we may not even be aware of them. Have you ever been in a building, such as a doctor's office, where there is music playing and not be consciously aware of it until you have been there for a while? People whose CANS is intact only have difficulty concentrating auditorily when the degree of separation between figure and background is quite small. This might occur where there is considerable background noise—for example, at a party. If several conversations are going on near you at such a party, you may have difficulty concentrating on one and ignoring the others because they all compete for your attention at once.

Short Auditory Memory Span

People with this condition have difficulty remembering what they hear as well as other people their age can remember. (The ability to store and recall what one hears increases with age during childhood.) People with a short auditory memory span may answer questions incorrectly (particularly relatively long questions) because they cannot remember them. They also may fail to follow instructions accurately for this reason.

Disturbed Ability to Segment Phonemes

Conversational speech consists of strings of **phonemes** uttered one after the other. You must be able to segment this string of sounds into words to understand what you are hearing. People with this condition have difficulty understanding speech because they have less than normal ability to segment sequences of phonemes into words. The process involved is analogous to that in segmenting this sequence of letters into words: *disturbedabilitytosegmentphonemes.*

Disturbed Ability to Relate
Heard Words to Units of Experience

Words consist of groupings of phonemes arranged in particular sequences. When we listen to words being spoken in a language that we do not understand, we hear groupings of phonemes, but these groupings seem meaningless. We cannot relate them to **units of experience.** A lesion in the CANS can disturb the ability to relate heard words to units of experience. This condition is called **Wernicke's aphasia** and was discussed in Chapter 5 on pages 92–93.

Abstract-Concrete Imbalance

A lesion in the CANS can disturb the ability to categorize and generalize. Persons who have such a disability tend to be overly concrete; that is, they tend "to lose the forest for the trees." This imbalance can interfere with their ability to understand speech because it prevents them from relating some of the words they hear to a sufficiently broad unit of experience. They may visualize only apples when they hear the word *fruit.* Or when they hear the word *chair,* they may think only of an upholstered chair, not also a rocking chair, a beanbag chair, or a metal folding chair. Again, this condition is considered a language disorder rather than a hearing disorder.

Etiology

Central auditory disturbances are caused by damage to the brain—specifically, those parts of the brain that make up the CANS. Any condition that can damage the brain can produce a central auditory disturbance. The following are several such conditions.

Insufficient Blood Flow to the Brain

Brain cells require oxygen to live. Oxygen is carried to brain cells by the blood traveling through arteries. If the flow of blood to any part of the brain is disrupted, the cells in that part will be deprived of oxygen, a condition known as **anoxia.** This is likely to result in their injury or destruction if the disruption lasts for more than a few minutes.

A number of conditions can disrupt the flow of blood to the brain. A **thrombus** can form on an arterial wall, cutting off the flow of blood to a part of the brain. An **embolus** can obstruct

Units of experience
The objects and events to which words refer.

189

Brain abscesses
Walled-off cavities containing dead or dying white blood cells.

Cerebral arteriosclerosis
A thickening of the walls of cerebral arteries resulting in a slower rate of blood flow through them.

Functional hearing loss
A condition in which persons do not respond appropriately to speech or other sound and there does not appear to be an abnormality or lesion in their ears, auditory nerves, or CANS. Also referred to as psychogenic hearing loss, pseudohypacusis, and idiopathic sudden deafness.

an artery, thereby restricting the flow of oxygen-rich blood to brain tissue. An artery in the brain could also rupture—the resulting **hemorrhage** can prevent oxygen from reaching brain cells. For more information on emboli, visit Fact Monster's webpage (2005).

Trauma

Several types of injuries to the skull can damage the brain. In one type, a penetrating wound, something (e.g., a bullet) penetrates the skull, producing brain damage in the path of entry. A second type of trauma in which the skull is not penetrated is known as a cranial blow. The brain may be lacerated at the point of impact, or the blow may cause intercranial hemorrhaging that can damage brain tissue.

Tumors

Tumors (i.e., neoplasms) are abnormal growths within the brain. They may be malignant (i.e., cancerous) or benign (i.e., not cancerous). These can disturb the functioning of the various structures within the CANS, including the auditory nerve. They can destroy brain tissue directly as they increase in size. They can also destroy brain tissue indirectly by pressing on cranial arteries, thereby decreasing blood flow through them.

Infections

Bacterial and viral microorganisms can cause an inflammation of brain tissue known as encephalitis. One possible complication of encephalitis is the formation of **brain abscesses.** These cavities can destroy brain tissue as they expand.

Degenerative Changes

Several other conditions can cause the gradual loss (i.e., degeneration) of brain cells, one of which is the aging process. With increasing age there is a slow, progressive degeneration of brain tissue that can result from reduced blood flow as a consequence of the thickening of the walls of the cerebral arteries. The thicker the wall of an artery, the smaller the diameter of the opening in it and, hence, the slower the rate of blood flow through it. This thickening of the walls of cerebral arteries is known as **cerebral arteriosclerosis.**

Another condition that can result in the gradual degeneration of brain cells is a disease such as **Huntington's disease.** To learn more about the symptoms and etiology of hearing difficulties resulting from damage to the central auditory nervous system, see Martin (2000).

Functional Hearing Loss

People who do not respond appropriately to speech or other sound and who do not appear to have an abnormality or lesion in their ears, auditory nerves, or CANS tend to be classified as having a **functional hearing loss.** This type of hearing loss has also been referred to as psychogenic hearing loss, pseudohypacusis, and idiopathic sudden deafness. Females appear to develop it more frequently than do males (Matsuki, 1989). People who are suspected of having it usually are referred for a psychiatric evaluation.

Functional (i.e., nonorganic) hearing losses are so-called because they do not appear to have an organic cause. This does not necessarily mean that there is no organic cause. There may well be one that has not yet been discovered. To learn more about the symptoms and etiology of functional hearing losses, see Martin (2000).

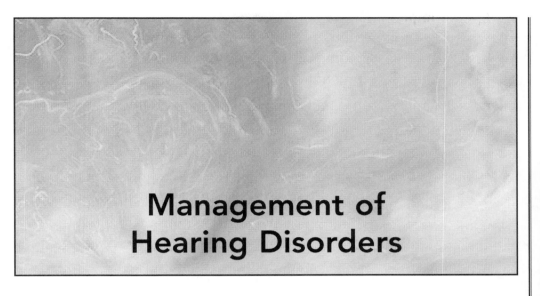

Management of Hearing Disorders

Chapter 11

Learning Objectives

- Describe the use of the pure-tone audiometer to measure hearing acuity.

- Describe the relationship between the decibel and an audiogram.

- Discuss why it would benefit a client with a hearing loss to learn speechreading.

- Describe how an assistive listening device helps modify a listening environment.

- List three types of alerting devices.

- Compare and contrast American Sign Language with Signing Exact English.

- Describe a basic telecommunication device for the deaf.

- Describe telecommunication relay services.

Chapter

Introduction

There are three basic components of managing hearing disorders. Before you can be helpful to a person who has a hearing disorder, you have to identify the reason(s) for it, which was the topic of Chapter 10. Second, the person's hearing mechanism and function must be assessed to determine the type and degree of disorder. And, third, depending on the nature and type of hearing disorder, assistive and/or augmentative systems and devices may be developed by the audiologist and/or the speech-language pathologist (SLP).

Hearing Testing

The approach you use to manage a hearing disorder will be based on the hypotheses you develop about its etiology. To develop a hypothesis about this, clinicians take a case history and administer hearing tests. The **audiometric** tests that are administered most often utilize an instrument known as a **pure-tone audiometer.**

A pure-tone audiometer, such as the one shown in Figure 11.1, is a device for measuring hearing and compiling information needed to answer such questions as:

- Is the client's hearing ability within normal limits?

- If the client's hearing ability is not within normal limits, how severely impaired is it?

- What is the cause of the client's hearing impairment?

Audiometric
Used to measure hearing.

Pure-tone audiometer
An instrument for measuring hearing using pure tones.

Figure 11.1	**An Audiometer**

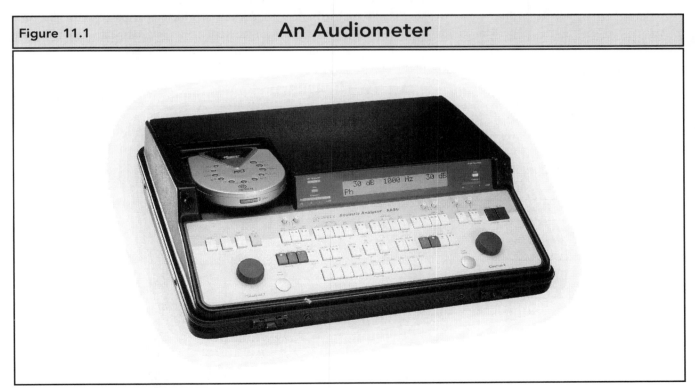

Photo Courtesy of Starkey Laboratories

Threshold
The lowest intensity level (in decibels) that a person hears for a frequency.

Audiogram
A graph for plotting the results of a hearing test that was administered with a pure-tone audiometer.

A pure-tone audiometer is an electrical device for generating sounds. The kinds of sounds it generates are known as pure tones, because the acoustical energy in them consists of only one frequency. The pure tones generated are at frequencies within the range of human hearing— approximately 20 to 20,000 **Hertz (Hz).** The higher the frequency of a pure tone, the higher its pitch; hence, a pure tone of 1,000 Hz would have a higher pitch than one of 500 Hz. Most pure-tone audiometers can only generate tones at the following frequencies within the 20 Hz to 20,000 Hz range: 125 Hz, 250 Hz, 500 Hz, 1,000 Hz, 2,000 Hz, 4,000 Hz, and 8,000 Hz. The tones can be presented through earphones or loudspeakers at many loudness levels. Audiometers have a switch that causes a tone of a specified frequency and intensity to be generated.

A pure-tone audiometric hearing test determines the softest tone that a person can detect in each ear at certain frequencies. The lowest intensity level heard (measured in **decibels,** or **dB**) is the person's **threshold** for that frequency in that ear. These thresholds are plotted on an **audiogram.** Figure 11.2 is an example of an audiogram. The threshold for each frequency tested in the left ear is indicated by an *x* and that in the right ear by an *o*.

The person whose hearing thresholds are plotted in this audiogram has a mild to moderate conductive hearing loss in both his right ear and his left ear. If his hearing ability had been within normal limits, the *x*'s and *o*'s would have clustered around the 0 dB hearing threshold level. The farther below this level a threshold falls, the greater the degree of hearing loss at that frequency. This person has a greater degree of loss in his right ear than in his left at a frequency of 8,000 Hz.

When looking at Figure 11.2, you probably noticed another set of markings that look like this: < and >. These marks are used to chart the levels at which a person can hear the same pure tone frequencies as those presented through the headphones or loudspeakers, but they are

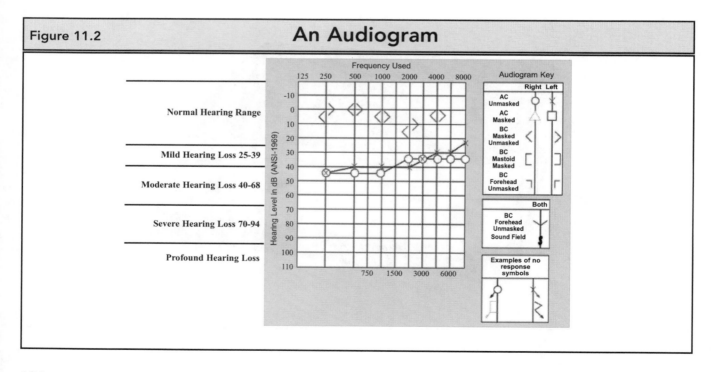

Figure 11.2   **An Audiogram**

delivered through an oscillator that is placed on the mastoid bone behind each ear. Called **bone conduction** testing, this procedure is used to determine the degree to which the inner ear is functioning. The audiogram in Figure 11.2 depicts normal inner ear functioning since the bone conduction results clustered around the 0 dB level.

The test described above is among the most basic done with a pure-tone audiometer. It provides the data needed to answer the first two questions of whether the person's hearing is within normal limits, and, if not, how severe the loss is.

Additional audiometric test data are needed to fully answer the question regarding the cause of the hearing loss. One type of testing that is routinely used is **tympanometry,** in which the examiner determines how well the tympanic membrane is functioning in response to air pressure. If the tympanic membrane is less responsive than expected, the clinician can hypothesize that the **ossicular chain** is not moving properly or that the middle ear is filled with fluid, either of which can result in a conductive hearing loss.

Most hospitals in the United States now offer neonatal hearing screening testing to identify infants with hearing loss. Using advanced technology, hospitals can test day-old infants who have high risk factors for hearing loss such as:

- Family history of hearing loss

- Perinatal infection

- Craniofacial anomalies

- Low birth weight

- Bacterial meningitis

- Characteristics known to be associated with syndromes that include a hearing loss

To learn more about hearing testing, including pure-tone audiometry, see Martin (2000).

Augmenting Hearing and Communication

Medical and Surgical Procedures

One approach for reducing the severity of hearing disorders is attempting to correct the cause medically or surgically. If a person had a conductive hearing loss because of a middle ear infection (i.e., otitis media), an attempt would be made to clear it up, possibly with an antibiotic. On the other hand, if a person had a conductive hearing loss because the footplate of the stapes was fixed (i.e., unmoving) in the oval window, an attempt might be made to surgically correct this **anomaly.** It is possible in some cases to restore the auditory system to normal (both anatomically and physiologically) through medical intervention. If this is done, the person will no longer have a hearing disorder and further intervention will be unnecessary.

In other cases, it is not possible to completely restore the system to normal through medical or surgical intervention. An example would be treating profound, bilateral sensorineural

Bone conduction
The conduction of sound to the inner ear through the bones of the skull.

Tympanometry
The measurement of the energy of a sound signal reflected by the tympanic membrane at different levels of air pressure.

Cochlear implant
A surgically implanted inner ear prosthesis that can enable persons who are deaf to hear some sounds.

Hearing aid
A portable amplifier that can improve the ability of some persons who have a hearing loss to understand speech.

Speechreading
Using visual information to augment hearing for understanding speech. Less accurately called "lipreading."

hearing loss (i.e., deafness) by surgically inserting **cochlear implants** in the patient's inner ears. Cochlear implants can be considered a form of hearing aid since they attempt to make speech audible and understandable. However, cochlear implants have typically used more sophisticated signal processing than **hearing aids;** they use electrical currents to stimulate remaining auditory nerve fibers. Furthermore, cochlear implants are surgically implanted, and their success is less dependent on the degree of hearing loss than conventional hearing aids. Even persons with total hearing loss can usually perceive sounds with cochlear implants. However, neither conventional hearing aids nor cochlear implants restore hearing to normal (Tyler, 1993). According to Tyler,

> Some patients [who have had cochlear implants] receive only minimal benefit, with limited improvement in their lipreading ability and environmental sound recognition. Others, however, obtain very high levels of word recognition. They can converse on the telephone and communicate face-to-face as if they had a mild hearing loss. (p. 29)

To learn more about the medical and surgical management of hearing loss, see Martin (2000) and Waltzman and Cohen (2000). For specific information about cochlear implants, visit the National Institute on Deafness and Other Communication Disorders cochlear implant webpage (NIDCD; 2005a).

Hearing Amplification and Speechreading

The goal of nonmedical treatment for people who have a hearing disorder is to both augment their ability to hear and to reduce the negative impact the disorder has on their life. One of the most common ways to augment a person's ability to hear is to fit him or her with a hearing aid. For this to be helpful, the person must have some usable residual hearing (Osberger, Maso, & Sam, 1993). Audio Clip 11.1 illustrates the speech of a woman with a severe sensorineural hearing loss whose speech was improved by wearing a hearing aid.

Audio Clip 11.1 Sensorineural Hearing Loss

 This woman's ability to speak intelligibly has been increased by wearing hearing aids. Although her speech is abnormal, it is highly understandable.

Less frequently used is a tactile aid that consists of a microphone to pick up sound and an amplifier that turns the sound into a vibration delivered to the person's chest, back, or arm. Tactile devices are not as precise as hearing aids, primarily because our skin's ability to discern tactile vibrations is much less precise than our ear's ability to discern sound. As a result, speech is difficult to understand, especially without visual and/or contextual cues.

Another way to augment a person's ability to hear is to teach him or her to do a better job of **speechreading.** (See Pichora-Fuller & Benguerel, 1991, for a description of a contemporary approach to teaching speechreading.) We all use visual information to help us "hear" better, particularly in noisy environments. If you don't believe it, the next time someone is speaking to you in a noisy environment look away from the person and observe the difference in your ability to understand what he or she is saying to you.

Modifying Listening Environments

Different environments shape and modify sound in a variety of ways. For instance, a room with soft surfaces such as carpets, drapes, and cloth furniture alters sound much less than a room with hard surfaces. Sound waves reverberate and reflect against hard surfaces, which interferes with the original sound. Think about how much easier it is to understand speech in a room with soft surfaces than in one with hard surfaces, particularly when many people are talking at the same time.

People with hearing disorders have a more difficult time understanding sound if it reflects and reverberates against surfaces. For this reason, modifying the environment is sometimes used to increase their ability to hear and understand speech. Most public school classrooms do not offer ideal listening characteristics for children with hearing disorders and need to be altered so they offer less interference.

Ideally, the best way to modify such environments is to reduce background noise and eliminate sound reverberation and reflection. However, such a modification is not always possible. Think of a school cafeteria that is also used as an auditorium—installing carpeting on the floor would be disastrous! However, it is possible to increase a student's ability to hear specific voices (e.g., the teacher) through the use of what is called an **assistive listening device (ALD)**. Some of these devices are used with individual students, and others can be hooked up to several students simultaneously.

Augmentative Systems and Devices

People with severe to profound hearing loss benefit from a range of augmentative systems and devices. Two that are currently being used for facilitating telephone communication are instruments known as **text telephones (TTYs)** and **telecommunication relay services (TRS)**. Alerting devices are another type of tool used to help hearing impaired individuals.

The TTY enables deaf people to communicate with others who have a TTY. Users type their messages and responses on a keyboard. TTYs are basic, dedicated microcomputers that have a modem and telecommunication software built into them. The designation *dedicated* implies that, unlike most microcomputers, they are designed for (i.e., dedicated to) a single task—in this instance, telephone communication. Figure 11.3 on page 198 shows a TTY device.

Telecommunication relay services enable people who are deaf or severely hard-of-hearing to communicate on the telephone with persons who do not have a TTY. TRS also enable persons who cannot speak clearly enough to be understood on the telephone to communicate with others via the telephone. A relay call can be initiated either by the person who has the communication impairment, or by someone who wants to communicate with him or her. The relay call is initiated by contacting the relay service (usually by dialing an 800 number). A person with a hearing impairment would make the call with either a TTY or a standard microcomputer with a modem and appropriate communication software. A person who wants to communicate with the deaf person would use an ordinary telephone.

Assistive listening device (ALD)
A device that captures sound at its source (e.g., through a microphone) and delivers it directly to the listener (e.g., through earphones).

Text telephone (TTY)
A device used by deaf persons to communicate over telephone lines. Both messages and responses are keyboarded. Also referred to as telecommunication device for the deaf (TDD).

Telecommunication relay services (TRS)
Organizations that provide telephone services to persons who do not hear or speak well enough to use a standard telephone. They were mandated by the Americans with Disabilities Act of 1990.

Figure 11.3   A TTY Device

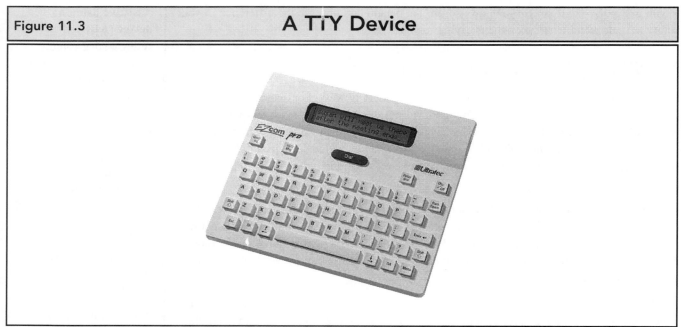

Photo Courtesy of Harris Communications

Oral method
The method used to teach individuals with hearing impairments to communicate through speech.

The operator, known as a communication assistant (CA), will ask for the number the person wants to call. The CA will then dial this number and wait for a person to answer, then ask the one who initiated the call for the first message. The CA will then relay this message—either by keyboarding it with a TTY or by saying it—to the person being phoned. The recipient will then be given an opportunity to respond, and the response will be relayed by the CA. The conversation can continue in this manner for as long as the parties desire.

The information conveyed cannot be divulged to anyone because it is treated as confidential by law. The call will cost no more than a regular call between the two points. For information about accessing the TRS in your state, contact your local telephone company. For more information about TRS in general, visit the NIDCD webpage on the topic (2005d). To learn more about the augmentation of residual hearing, see Hull (2001), Martin (2000), Sandlin (1991), and Silverman (1999b).

Alerting devices are designed to do what their name implies: to alert a person with a hearing loss to important sounds, such as a doorbell, a baby crying, a fire alarm, or an emergency. Some of the devices are mechanical and provide visual signals (e.g., flashing lights) or sound in the person's hearing range. Assistive dogs, called hearing dogs, are used by many people with hearing loss to alert them to these sounds and other emergencies, such as fire, an intruder, unexpected water, high heat, or extreme cold.

Communication Strategies

There are two major strategies used to develop effective communication systems for individuals with a severe-to-profound hearing loss. The **oral method** of communication focuses on teaching individuals with hearing impairments how to use speech effectively; **manual communication systems** teach individuals to communicate using nonspeech communication systems.

Oral Communication

Children with some residual hearing are often taught communication through what is called the oral method, in which the focus is on using the child's residual hearing to acquire communication and language. Many families prefer this method, because they believe that the world is primarily oral, and their children must be able to communicate in that world. How well the oral method works is directly linked to the amount of residual hearing the child has. Advocates of the oral method do not believe in using sign language because they believe deaf children can catch up to their hearing peers if they are given the appropriate intervention through the oral method.

Manual Communication Systems

Children with severe-to-profound hearing loss are at high risk for not developing language unless a functional communication system is developed—as early as possible—for the child and his or her family. The primary goal is for the child to acquire the linguistic and associated cognitive processes necessary to develop a complete language system. Because the oral approach has not been effective for most deaf children with severe-to-profound hearing loss, several manual communication systems have evolved. Some manual systems use manual gestures associated with spoken English; another type, **American Sign Language (ASL),** is a manual-visual language based on gestures and movements of the head, neck, hands, arms, shoulders, and torso.

Perhaps the most widely used manual communication system based on spoken English is **Signing Exact English** (**SEE;** Gustason, 1983). SEE uses a system that links a manual sign to each individual English morpheme that is spoken. For example, in the sentence "I am going home," all morphemes (including -*ing)* are signed. The speaker also speaks at a normal rate. One of the disadvantages of SEE is the high number of signs associated with each English word and the necessity for children to understand the concept of *morpheme* in order to use the system.

American Sign Language does not mirror the English language, or any other spoken language. ASL evolved as a combination of French Sign Language, brought to the United States at the beginning of the 19th century, and a sign language already in use by deaf people in the United States. ASL has its own grammar, although its vocabulary overlaps considerably with English. In contrast to SEE, ASL does not follow standard English rules; rather, it is considered a language with its own syntactic rules. People who use ASL consider themselves to be members of a unique culture, who become bilingual and bicultural when they learn to read English and to communicate with hearing people who rely on English.

A component of ASL is the American Manual Alphabet, shown in Figure 11.4 on page 200. The American Manual Alphabet is used to spell words that have no exact sign and to communicate with hearing people who know the alphabet.

Children who grow up seeing and responding to ASL from an early age develop language and cognition just as easily and fluently as hearing children develop spoken language unless they have other problems in addition to hearing loss. Difficulties arise when children who are deaf grow up in hearing families and are not exposed to ASL. However, hearing children born to deaf parents using ASL develop fluency in ASL and in spoken English, becoming bilingual and bicultural.

American Sign Language (ASL) The visual-gestural language used as a primary mode of communication by people with hearing loss. It is recognized as a natural language and is the native language of deaf people and deaf culture.

Signing Exact English (SEE) A manual communication system based on spoken English.

Figure 11.4	**American Manual Alphabet**

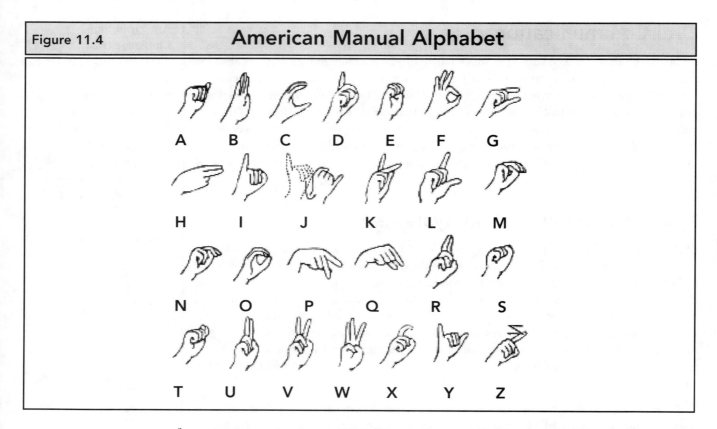

Many people who are deaf utilize services provided by professional interpreters for the deaf when it is necessary to communicate with hearing persons who do not know ASL or when they are attending public events. In addition, interpreters are used in classrooms, business meetings, doctor's appointments, and during court appearances. You can obtain further information about this profession from organizations for the deaf in your state or by visiting the Registry of Interpreters for the Deaf website (2005).

Aural Rehabilitation

People who experience hearing loss, particularly adults, face significant changes to their lives. These include the emotional stress of frequent communication breakdowns; adjusting to medical and/or surgical procedures and their results; and increased strain on family relationships. Aural rehabilitation focuses on:

- Helping people understand how hearing works and how their hearing loss has affected their hearing mechanism

- Teaching people about their medical and/or surgical procedures and what to expect afterwards

- Teaching people how their hearing aids work and how to maintain them for maximum effectiveness

- Developing effective communication strategies following the hearing loss

In addition to focusing on communication abilities, clinicians can help people with impaired hearing through counseling. Clients may need to reduce the extent to which their attitudes toward their disorder keep them from doing what they want to do—that is, attitudes that cause them to be handicapped. Some persons who could benefit from wearing a hearing aid refuse to wear one, and some restrict their activities more than necessary because of embarrassment about having a hearing loss. Unless these attitudes can be changed, their hearing loss will be a handicap rather than a condition that can be remedied.

Part 5

Communication Sciences
and Disorders: The Profession

The profession of communication sciences and disorders encompasses a wide range of specialties, all of which aim to understand the normal processes of communication and to assist people whose communication abilities are impaired in some way. Throughout Part 5, the term *clinician* is used to include both speech-language pathologists (SLPs) and audiologists.

Chapter 12 provides a brief history of the treatment of communication disorders and of the emergence of the profession of communication sciences and disorders in the early twentieth century. Chapter 13 describes the professional roles, work settings, and professional issues associated with communication sciences and disorders.

Chapter 14 focuses on one of the most important aspects of the profession of communication sciences and disorders—the clinical relationship. This therapeutic relationship is defined and discussed. Chapter 15 focuses on the areas of assessment, evaluation, and diagnosis. Chapter 16 addresses the issues and processes associated with providing intervention to people with communication disorders, including how to establish goals, design intervention programs, document progress, and terminate therapy. Finally, Chapter 17 provides some perspective on the clinician's responsibilities in providing clinical services, including the obligation to function as a clinical researcher.

Where Did Communication Sciences and Disorders Come From?

Chapter 12

Learning Objectives

- Describe how an awareness of the history of communication sciences and disorders can help you become a more effective clinician.

- Describe two people who lived prior to the twentieth century who had a speech, language, and/or hearing disorder and who were treated successfully.

- Discuss how historical cultural perceptions of the cause of abnormal communication behavior influenced how communication disorders were treated at different points in history.

- Describe why a therapy that was found to be ineffective in the past can be "rediscovered" by a new generation of clinicians.

- Discuss how to avoid jumping on a bandwagon in assuming that a new and fashionable therapy approach is necessarily better than an existing one.

Introduction

The profession of communication sciences and disorders emerged as a profession in the early twentieth century. Although the profession is relatively young, attempts to help people with communication disorders have existed for thousands of years. Some of those attempts have been more successful than others and have endured, some have disappeared entirely, and some reappear periodically.

Why is it important to be aware of the history of the profession? In other words, why should you spend your time reading about it? First, if you aren't aware of the mistakes others have made in their attempts to help people with communication disorders, you are more likely to make them yourself. If you are familiar with what others have attempted and why those attempts failed, you can spend your time more effectively pursuing approaches that have been shown to work.

Second, some approaches have disappeared because they were ineffective. Many of the intervention strategies that were tried in the past were rejected for good reason. Research and/or clinical experience may have failed to yield evidence that the interventions did what they were intended to do or, for that matter, anything else worthwhile. Or they may have been effective in doing what they were intended to do, but their unpleasant **side effects** discouraged their use.

Conversely, other approaches that were discontinued because they were not effective are periodically rediscovered, only to be discarded once again when they are demonstrated to be ineffective or even harmful. Along the same lines, knowledge of history will help you be less likely to assume that what is claimed to be new is really new. Instead, you will be able to recognize an approach that has been used in the past, regardless of what it may be called or how it may be marketed.

Third, to be maximally effective as a clinician, you will need to be able to distinguish between **intervention strategies** that are simply not effective and those that could be effective if used with a different type of client and/or for accomplishing a different goal. For example, an intervention strategy that was used for a particular purpose with preschool-age children and found to be ineffective may be effective for accomplishing the same goal with older children or adults. Or, an intervention strategy that wasn't particularly effective for accomplishing its intended goal may have a side effect that makes it usable for accomplishing a different goal.

Fourth, understanding how clinical practice has developed will help you be less likely to reject out of hand clinically relevant information that is more than 25 years old. Similarly, you are less likely to assume that just because an approach is new, it is necessarily better than approaches that have been around longer.

The fifth and last reason to study the history of the profession is that you will be aware of how cultural factors impact trends regarding etiology and management of any given impairment at a particular point in time. You will see how cultural influences can alter the way any particular approach is viewed and the degree to which the approach can be successfully utilized.

Side effect
Something an intervention strategy changes other than what it's intended to change. A side effect can be physiological, psychological, desirable, or undesirable.

Intervention strategy
The approach used to try to achieve an intervention goal (i.e., to be helpful to the client).

Appian Way
A road in ancient Rome that had cavelike apertures in the rocky outcrop on both sides, in which people who had mental handicaps, deformities, and communication impairments were caged to provide entertainment for travelers.

Milestones through History

Attitudes about society's responsibility to people with communication disorders (or other physical or mental disorders) have evolved considerably during the past 4,000 years. In early Rome during the seventh century B.C., for example, along the **Appian Way** there were cavelike apertures on the rocky outcrop on either side of the thoroughfare. Persons who were mentally handicapped, deformed, and communicatively impaired (particularly ones who stuttered) were caged there to provide entertainment for travelers (Eldridge, 1968). In some ancient cultures, many children born with physical deformities, like **cleft palates** were murdered by their fathers because they were regarded as useless and likely to bring bad luck to their families. Those who were not murdered were often sold and trained to be prostitutes or beggars (Eldridge). This behavior was condoned by society because such disorders were regarded as an expression of the wrath of a deity.

The history of the treatment of communication disorders has involved contributions from people residing in many countries and practicing many professions. The chronology here contains only a small sample of these contributions.

This chronology could not have been compiled without consulting and paraphrasing portions of the writings of Margaret Eldridge (1968) and G. M. Klingbeil (1939a, 1939b). Their writings deal with the history of the treatment of communication disorders. To learn more about this subject, see their work, as well as those of Benton (1964, 1981), Benton and Joynt (1960), and O'Neill (1980).

2000 B.C.

A word that is possibly the first written reference to a speech disorder appeared in a papyrus of the Middle Egyptian Dynasty. The word has been translated as "to speak haltingly" or "to walk haltingly with the tongue, as one who is sad" (Eldridge, 1968, p. 4). This is believed to refer to **stuttering.** The hieroglyph thought to depict this disorder is shown in Figure 12.1. An analysis of this symbol can perhaps provide some insight into the way people in ancient Egypt may have viewed the disorder.

According to the Merriam-Webster online dictionary (2005), Egyptian hieroglyphic characters were for the most part **pictographic.** The hieroglyph in Figure 12.1 appears to portray a person who has one hand on the ground and the other on his or her face. In the previous edition of this book, Silverman (2004) interpreted this hieroglyph as a tremor—an earthquake—being conducted from the ground to the face. If this is so, then it is likely that the Egyptians used the earthquake as a metaphor for the moment of stuttering.

If Silverman's interpretation of the hieroglyph is correct, their choice of the earthquake as a metaphor could have been an attempt to describe the moment of stuttering and/or explain it. If it were merely an attempt to describe the moment of stuttering, they may have chosen the earthquake as a metaphor because they regarded the tremors and other explosive movements during moments of stuttering as being somewhat similar to those of objects during an earthquake. And if they chose this metaphor to both describe and explain moments of stuttering, they may have done so because they regarded the disfluencies, like earthquakes, as being acts of gods.

Figure 12.1	An Egyptian Hieroglyph Thought to Depict Stuttering

1300 B.C.

In the Bible, Exodus IV:10,11 refers to Moses as having a speech disorder, probably stuttering. Jewish folklore includes this explanation of Moses' stuttering: One day when Moses was a young child and sitting on Pharaoh's lap, he grabbed Pharaoh's crown and placed it on his own head. Pharaoh's astrologers were horror-struck. "Let two braziers be brought," they counseled, "one filled with gold, the other with glowing coals, and set them before him. If he grasps the gold, it would be safer for Pharaoh to put the possible usurper to death." When the braziers were brought, the hand of Moses was stretched out toward the gold, but the angel Gabriel guided it toward the coals. Moses plucked out a burning coal and put it to his lips and, as a consequence, for life remained "heavy of speech and heavy of tongue."

400 B.C.

Thucydides, the Greek historian, described a condition that was probably **anomic aphasia.** He reported that many who suffered from the plague in Athens found that, on recovery, they had not only forgotten the names of their friends and relations, but also their own names (Klingbeil, 1939a).

Handicapped people in ancient Greece and Rome were often known by the names of their afflictions—for example, the squinter, the blind, and the dumb. **Balbus** was a surname given to someone with a speech disorder. Sometimes the whole family was included in the name (Eldridge, 1968).

Herodotus, the Greek historian, records the treatment of a young man named Battus, in the fifth century B.C., for a speech disorder that appears to have been stuttering. According to Herodotus, "When he came to man's estate he went to Delphi to enquire of the prophetess concerning his voice." This was the reply: "Battus, thou askest a voice; but the king, ev'n Apollo, sends thee to found thee a home in Libya, the country of sheepfolds." He took the advice and established a kingdom in Libya. We are not told whether he continued to stutter. Battus apparently thought his stuttering resulted from angering the gods and that in order to overcome it he had to placate them (Eldridge, 1968).

Balbus
A surname given to some persons in ancient Greece and Rome who had a speech disorder.

As early as this time period, people were attempting to understand the brain and its functions. Hippocrates, "the father of medicine," appears to have been aware that disorders of speech result from lesions in the left cerebral hemisphere (Benton, 1981).

350 B.C.

Demosthenes, the Greek orator, was treated for a speech disorder by means of speech exercises in which some pebbles were placed in his mouth. Demosthenes may have been the first to combat stuttering through the use of speech exercises (Klingbeil, 1939b). Study More 12.1 describes the case of Demosthenes. To learn more about how Demosthenes is believed to have overcome his stuttering, visit the Wikipedia website (2005).

Aristotle, the Greek philosopher, suffered from a lisp, which may have been what motivated him to study speech disorders. Aristotle felt that stuttering was due to defective movements of the tongue. He stated that stutterers find it difficult to change the position of their tongue when they have to utter a second sound (Eldridge, 1968). He also wrote about voice disorders, including those associated with deafness. He stated in this regard that there was no possibility of teaching the deaf to speak.

A.D. 25

Celsus, "the Hippocrates of the Romans," considered faulty functioning of the tongue to be the cause of most speech disorders. The following excerpt from his treatise on medicine, *De Medicina,* describes an approach he recommended for improving tongue functioning:

> When the tongue is paralyzed, either from a vice of the organ or as a consequence of another disease, and when the patient cannot articulate, gargles should be administered of a decoction of thyme, hyssop, pennyroyal; he should drink water, and the head and neck and mouth and the parts below the chin be well rubbed. The tongue should be rubbed with lazerwort, and he should chew pungent substances such as mustard, garlic, onions, and make every effort to articulate. He must exercise himself to retain his breath, wash his head with cold water and then vomit. (Eldridge, 1968, p. 19)

A.D. 685

St. John of Beverly is reported by the Venerable Bede to have helped a deaf boy acquire speech. The saint, then a bishop, sent for him and:

> When he had come he ordered him to thrust forward his tongue out of his mouth and show it to him. Then, taking hold of him by the chin he made the sign of the Holy Cross on his tongue. This done he told him to draw it back again into his mouth and to speak—immediately, his tongue was loosed. He said what he had been ordered. The bishop added the names of the letters: "Say, A," and he said it; "Say, B," and he said this too. And, when he repeated the names of the letters as the Bishop said them, one by one, the latter went further and gave him syllables and words to say; and when, in all instances, he at once replied, he told him to say longer sentences and he did so. (Eldridge, 1968, pp. 18–19)

Study More 12.1	The Case of Demosthenes

Many men and women during the past 2,500 years have met the challenge of a communication disorder by becoming their own therapist. Perhaps the most famous of these was Demosthenes, who lived in Greece more than 2,000 years ago. Margaret Eldridge, a British speech-language pathologist, describes in this excerpt how Demosthenes met this challenge.

The story of Demosthenes must surely be, in its essentials, the story of many a man and woman called upon to face the challenge of a speech disorder. After more than 2000 years he is still held up to us as an example of "mind over matter"; certainly his success in overcoming his handicap, if so far as he did overcome it, was due to patience, determination, and strength of character.

To appreciate his problems and his triumph we should consider his background. His father was a prosperous and respected man. He died when Demosthenes, his only son, was barely eight years old. Demosthenes and his sister, three years his junior, were overprotected by their widowed mother, who forbade her son (a boy of poor physique, thin and sickly) to take part in the gymnastic exercises and the sports which were an important part of the education of every young Athenian. Inevitably he was ridiculed by other boys; unable, physically and probably temperamentally unwilling to fight his way into their good graces, he turned within himself to seek satisfaction. Here he found ambition. Lacking companionship he probably read more than most boys of his age, and so discovered the magic of words. But it was not until, as a youth, he heard the orator, Callistratus, that he knew the full glory of speech. He was spell-bound at the power of speech to evoke emotion, to sway opinion and to win applause. He decided to become an orator; not just an orator, but a great orator; the greatest orator in Athens. His lisping, breathless, hesitant speech would not stop him. Nothing would stop him. He set to work to correct his speech defect.

It was at this stage of his life that he inherited his estate; only to find that, owing to the fraudulent transactions of his guardians, only one twelfth of its value remained. Already a hard, clear-headed man of business, old for his years and tinged with bitterness that spoiled his later life, Demosthenes prepared to take his case to court. He studied forensic oratory with Iseaus, a skilled practitioner who specialized in cases of disputed inheritance, and applied himself, whole-heartedly, to improving his speech. When all was ready he sued the four fraudulent guardians separately but, as a result of trickery, a situation was established in which he could not hope for redress.

The case became a "cause celebre" in Athens. Demosthenes was like an avenging god; nothing would stop him in his pursuit of justice. Eventually, in a case which was his first public triumph, he won his suit. It is said that, in the five speeches he delivered, and which are still existent, his attack earned him the name of "Argas," a venomous spirit.

It is probable that his triumph, in this instance, was the result of a tidal wave of emotion; a violent protestation against the injustice to which he and his family had been subjected. Certainly, when he embarked upon his public life it was a very different story. His first appearance before the Assembly was an appalling fiasco. No doubt he was master of his subject: his oration would have been prepared with precision, down to the last detail. But, the moment he began to speak, his fate was sealed. His weak, breathless voice and his lisping utterances and, worst of all, his hesitance, were too much for his critical audience. He was greeted with shouts of laughter; cat-calls of derision assailed him. This happened so often that every appearance before the Assembly must have been a torture to him.

In his distress he sought the help of the actor, Satyrus, and under his instruction embarked on a rigorous course of exercises in breath control, articulation, and voice production. He built himself an underground room into which he retired every day; sometimes he remained there for weeks, or even months, at a stretch. He shaved one half of his head in order that he might more easily resist any temptation to leave his lonely sanctum. Standing before a long mirror he corrected his gestures, and learned to deliver many lines in one breath. He is said to have put pebbles under his tongue—although the reason for this practice is not clear, unless it was with the object of improving his articulation by developing tongue control. Alternatively his aim may have been to relieve his stammer. In a generally accepted theory of the time the tongue was cited as being responsible for all abnormalities of speech; even Hippocrates, who emphasized the importance of the brain as the governing and controlling organ of the body, seems to have subscribed to the theory—which may account for the fact that it persisted through the ages until less than 100 years ago. We are told that Demosthenes treated his voice problem by striding alone on the sea shore at Phalerum, and trying to shout above the roar of the breakers; a small lonely figure challenging, with his weakest weapon, the mighty force of nature.

For years Demosthenes contented himself with writing orations for others to deliver. As his speech improved he appreciated, ever more keenly, the importance of making fluent speech a part of himself, so that he would, at all times, and under all conditions, be able to speak freely, intelligibly, and spontaneously. Recognizing spontaneity as an essential characteristic of normal speech he set himself to acquire it. It is doubtful if he was completely successful…It was not until after the outbreak of the Phoenecian war that he rose to his full stature as an orator and as a man. When the freedom of Greece was assailed by Philip of Macedon and his son, Alexander (later, "Alexander the Great") Demosthenes gathered himself together and took up the defense of the Greeks. Courageous Demosthenes, afire with the power of words.

Obturator
A prosthetic device used to close an opening in the body.

This account indicates an awareness that deaf persons can be taught to speak and that Aristotle's pessimism may not have been warranted.

A.D. 1000

Abu Ali Hussain Avicenna, a court physician of Arabia, blamed the tongue for causing stuttering. He also suggested other causes including lesions of the brain and nerves, and a spasm of the epiglottis, which he advised should be treated by taking a deep inspiration before speaking (Eldridge, 1968). This advice has been given and acted upon periodically since then—even during this century—though it rarely, if ever, produces any lasting benefits.

A.D. 1500s

Ambroise Paré, a French physician, published the first description of an **obturator** for treating palatal clefts. This description is reproduced in Study More 12.2. To learn more about Ambroise Paré, visit John Leinhard's website (2005).

Pedro de Ponce, a Spanish Benedictine monk, was the first to systematically attempt to educate the deaf. We are told that some of those he taught acquired not only reading and writing, but speech as well (Eldridge, 1968).

A.D. 1600s

Juan Pablo Bonet, a Spanish monk, recommended the use of "the language of signs" with congenitally deaf persons (Eldridge, 1968). He taught the deaf sons of Spanish noblemen to read and speak using a one-handed alphabet, and wrote the first book on deaf education.

Lord Francis Bacon, the English philosopher, wrote a comprehensive treatise on speech disorders and blamed coldness of moisture of the tongue, or occasionally its dryness, on all the disorders (Klingbeil, 1939b).

Study More 12.2

Treatment of Cleft Palate During the Sixteenth Century

Ambroise Paré, a French army barber-surgeon who lived between 1510 and 1590, published what appears to have been the first description of the use of an obturator to fill in an opening in the hard palate and, thereby, reduce hypernasality. Paré had been asked to treat persons who had part of their hard palate shot away. This excerpt was taken from a report that he published in 1541 in which he described his use of obturators. These devices are still used to treat some persons with cleft palates.

Many times it happeneth that a portion or a part of the bone of the palate, being broken by the shot of a gun, or corroded by the virulency of the Lues Venerea, falls away, which makes the patient to whom this happeneth that they cannot pronounce their words distinctly, but obscurely and snuffling; therefore I have thought it a thing worthy of the labour to show how it may be helped by art. It must be done by fill-	ing the cavity of the palate with a plate of silver or gold, a little bigger than the cavity itself—on the upper side, which shall be turned toward the brain, a little sponge must be fastened, which, when it is moistened with the moisture distilling from the brain, it will become more swollen and puffed up, so that it will fill the concavity of the palate, that the artificial palate cannot fall down.

Source: Gould and Pyle (1937)

Dr. Nicholas Tulp, of Amsterdam, published a case study of a young man known as "Johannes the Dumb," who learned to speak following a partial glossectomy (Eldridge, 1968). An excerpt from this case study is reproduced in Study More 8.4 on page 144.

Attempts were made by several persons, including an English physician named John Bulwer, to teach **lipreading** to deaf persons (Eldridge, 1968). A timeline from 1000 B.C. to A.D. 1816 that shows the development of approaches for teaching deaf people to communicate can be found at ASLinfo.com (2005). You can learn more about John Bulwer's attempts to teach sign language (including illustrations of some of the signs he developed) from the University of California at Santa Cruz Perceptual Science Laboratory website (2005).

A.D. 1700s

Abbé de L'Epée, a French priest, was the first to educate persons with **congenital** deafness regardless of their social or financial status. He also was the first to found an institute for deaf education. He advocated the teaching of manual sign rather than oral speech (Eldridge, 1968).

An important medical procedure related to the field was developed during this time period. Le Mounier, a French dentist, performed the first successful operation for closing a cleft of the soft palate (Eldridge, 1968).

Several different theories regarding the cause of stuttering were developed during the 1700s. Johann Konrad Amman, a Swiss physician, believed that stuttering was due simply to a vicious habit (Klingbeil, 1939b). This belief was a precursor of the theory currently advocated by many authorities that stuttering is a learned behavior.

Johann Gottfried von Hahn, a German physician, laid the blame for stuttering on the hyoid bone (Klingbeil, 1939b). His idea is a forerunner of a contemporary theory that views stuttering as resulting from some type of laryngeal malfunction.

Moses Mendlessohn, a Jewish philosopher, believed that the chief reason for stuttering was not physical, but psychical—a collision among many ideas flowing simultaneously from the brain. The therapy he recommended was slow reading aloud, the succeeding words being covered, so as not to be seen until they were required to be enunciated (Klingbeil, 1939b).

A.D. 1800–1850

In the early 1800s, again much focus was on stuttering causes and intervention. Erasmus Darwin, an English physician and naturalist, believed that emotions, such as awe or bashfulness, caused stuttering. He advocated constant practice of the sounds on which stuttering occurs, with as much softening as possible of the initial consonants of words (Klingbeil, 1939b). Some speech-language pathologists still advise stutterers to produce the initial consonants of words with a "light contact."

J. M. G. Itard, a French physician, believed that stuttering was caused by a general debility of the nerves that stimulate the movements of the **larynx** and tongue. He recommended that a gold or ivory fork be placed in the cavity of the lower jaw to support the tongue, and that systematic "gymnastics" of the articulators be done against this obstacle. Doing so was supposed to strengthen the tongue (Eldridge, 1968; Klingbeil, 1939b).

Lipreading
An older term for speechreading. Using visual facial information to augment hearing for understanding speech.

Yates, a New York physician, believed that stuttering was caused by a spasm of the glottis, and treated it by advising stutterers to raise the tip of the tongue to the palate and hold it there while speaking (Klingbeil, 1939b). This is another precursor of the theory that stuttering is caused by some type of laryngeal malfunction.

Colombat de L'Isere classified persons who stutter into two groups: (1) those in which the blockings resulted from spasms of the lips and tongues and (2) those in which the spasms occurred in the larynx and respiratory muscles. He advocated the use of breathing exercises and vocal rhythms, including the pacing of speech with a metronome device he invented (Eldridge, 1968). There was a revival of interest in training stutterers to pace their speech with miniature metronomes during the 1970s.

Johann Frederick Dieffenbach, a German surgeon, believed that stuttering was caused by a spasm of the glottis and could be cured by surgery. His operation consisted of removing a triangular wedge from the root of the tongue. The operation was performed on hundreds of people, some of whom died following surgery (Eldridge, 1968).

Another important first during the early 1800s was that the first **laryngectomy** was performed. In 1859 the first artificial larynx for laryngectomized persons was produced (Eldridge, 1968).

1851–1900

During the late 1800s, English physician William John Little presented one of the first comprehensive descriptions of **cerebral palsy.** Cerebral palsy then became known as Little's Disease. Unfortunately, he felt it was hopeless to habilitate children with this disorder, a theory now disproved (Eldridge, 1968).

This time period proved much more positive for persons with hearing impairments. Alexander Graham Bell moved to the United States from Scotland and contributed significantly to the teaching of speech to individuals with hearing impairments. A summary of his contributions is presented in Study More 12.3. Helen Keller, who was deaf and blind, was taught by Annie Sullivan to communicate using the manual alphabet. She also learned to produce intelligible speech and to understand speech by touching the lips of speakers (Eldridge, 1968).

Another view on stuttering emerged during this time period. Klencke, a German physician, believed that stuttering reflected the need of stutterers for psychological help—for treatment of their whole personality (Eldridge, 1968). Some contemporary authorities view stuttering as a symptom that should be treated by psychotherapy.

In the late 1800s the profession of communication sciences began to emerge. The Berlin School of Speech and Voice Therapy, founded by the Gutzmans (father and son), began a training center for teachers wishing to specialize in the treatment of speech disorders (Eldridge, 1968). This was one of the first attempts to train nonmedical persons to work with those having such disorders. In Hamburg, Germany, speech therapy for stuttering was provided in elementary schools (Eldridge). This was one of the first attempts to offer speech therapy services in elementary schools. Also, the first association for teachers specializing in speech-language pathology was formed in Germany. It was called (in translation) The Association of Teachers of Remedial Speech Training (Eldridge).

Study More 12.3	Alexander Graham Bell

Alexander Graham Bell is best known for the invention of the telephone. He also made significant contributions in another area—the teaching of oral speech to deaf persons. This excerpt summarizes his contributions.

The man who probably has had more influence than anyone else in the world on the speech education of the deaf was Alexander Graham Bell (1847–1922). His name and his fame live on, primarily as the inventor of Bell's Improved Telephone but sometimes we forget that he belonged to the third generation of a family which was professionally and vocationally devoted to speech. His grandfather, Alexander Bell, was a teacher of elocution in Edinburgh; Alexander Melville Bell, of the second generation, also taught elocution in Edinburgh, and evolved a system of symbols, showing the position of the speech organs when making sounds.

In 1870 Graham Bell and his father went to the United States. Here the name of Bell became famous. The invention of the telephone brought fortune as well as fame to Graham Bell, and his whole-hearted philanthropy prompted him to use a large part of his fortune to found the Volta Bureau, an organization devoted to promoting and diffusing knowledge of the problems of the deaf; and later to found the Volta-Bell Fund, dedicated to oral teaching of the deaf. His technical skill was of incalculable value in the development of hearing aids. All of his work for the deaf was directed towards encouraging the use of oral speech... There is no doubt that the charming personality of this brilliant and most humane man did much to forward the acceptance of his views on the importance of oral speech.

From *A History of the Treatment of Speech Disorders* (pp. 45–46), by M. Eldridge, 1968, Edinburgh, Scotland: Livingstone. © Livingstone. Reprinted with permission.

1901–1924

During the early 1900s, virtually the only treatment available to people with speech handicaps in the United States was that offered by privately owned commercial schools specializing in the treatment of stuttering. Patients paid large fees (in advance) for "guaranteed cures" (Eldridge, 1968). However, during this time period, many other intervention options were developed.

Centers for treating school-age children with speech disorders were established in school systems in the United States, Germany, Denmark, and England. Speech correction services were offered in the public schools of a number of American cities, including New York, New Haven, and Philadelphia. Treatment centers for people with communication disorders were also established at several U.S. universities, including Columbia, the University of Pennsylvania, and the University of Wisconsin (Eldridge, 1968).

During World War I, hospitals for the treatment of people with brain injuries were established in various parts of the world, particularly Germany. Work done with soldiers with brain injuries resulted in the first large-scale attempt to rehabilitate people with aphasia. Charles K. Mills, a Philadelphia physician, published the first paper in English describing the successful treatment of people with aphasia (Sarno, 1981).

A marked tendency had developed to incorporate psychotherapy, particularly **psychoanalysis,** in the treatment of stuttering. Psychoanalysis, at this time, was viewed as a cure for many mental ills (Eldridge, 1968).

It was also during this time period that the International Association of **Logopedics** and **Phoniatrics** held its first convention in Vienna. This is still the only international association for medical and nonmedical practitioners who work with persons who have communication impairments (Eldridge, 1968).

Psychoanalysis
A system of psychotherapy developed in the late 1800s by Sigmund Freud.

Logopedics
The study of speech disorders.

Phoniatrics
The study of voice disorders.

License
A permit issued by a governmental entity (usually a state) to practice a profession.

1925–1945

The communication science professions grew rapidly during the mid-1900s. The American Academy of Speech Correction was formed in 1925. Currently known as the **American Speech-Language-Hearing Association (ASHA),** it is the national professional association for American speech-language pathologists and audiologists. To learn more about the founding and early history of ASHA, see Paden (1970).

The first issue of the *Journal of Speech Disorders* was published by ASHA. It was the first journal in English that allowed practitioners to share information on services for people with communication handicaps.

Congress authorized the United States Commission of Education to match the amounts spent by cities and states to defray the extra cost of educating "Speech Defectives" and children with other physical handicaps. The availability of this funding motivated many school systems to provide speech therapy services and, thereby, created a need for more SLPs to provide them. Many colleges and universities began training programs to meet this need.

Students training to become SLPs had to learn long lists of Greek and Latin names for communication disorders, as described in Study More 8.1 on page 135. As the field evolved away from a strict medical orientation, these names were used less frequently.

Audiology began as a separate profession during these decades—an outgrowth of treatment programs established at Veterans Affairs (V.A.) hospitals for World War II veterans with hearing impairments. Audiometers were designed to test hearing.

World War II also increased services for those with brain injuries. Several army hospitals in the United States established special programs for soldiers with aphasia resulting from brain injuries. Following the war, such programs were established in many V.A. hospitals. A number of approaches currently used for treating people with aphasia are based on knowledge gained from these programs.

1946–2005

After World War II, the United States experienced considerable growth in the professions of speech-language pathology and audiology. The number of training programs and practitioners more than tripled. The minimum level of academic training for American Speech-Language-Hearing Association certification was first raised from a bachelor's to a master's degree for both speech-language pathologists and audiologists, and then to a professional doctorate (AuD) for audiologists. States began to require a **license** to practice both speech-language pathology and audiology. The **scope of practice** (i.e., what a professional is legally and ethically permitted to do) for both speech-language pathologists and audiologists expanded considerably. And a knowledge explosion occurred that improved treatment approaches for most types of communication disorders. Similar growth, incidentally, occurred in both professions in most industrialized countries.

Some of the people who had the most impact on speech-language pathology early in this period were Charles Van Riper, Wendell Johnson, Elise Hahn, Mildred Templin, Helmer Myklebust, Doris Johnson, and Mildred Berry. Influential people later in the period included

Laura Lee, Raymond Carhart, Leo Doerfler, James Jerger, Margaret Lahey, and Lois Bloom. For more complete descriptions visit Duchan's website (2001a), where she describes the history of speech-language pathology.

Social Influences on Intervention

Culture can have an impact on how communication and its disorders are viewed. The management of communication disorders is also affected by cultural perceptions of the cause of what is considered "abnormal" behavior. For instance, in ancient Rome (as well as in a number of other ancient societies) mental and physical impairments were regarded as punishment for sin or otherwise angering the gods. The appropriate treatment was to seek the gods' forgiveness through prayer or deed. This view influenced how communication disorders were treated in these societies.

One of the main influences on the treatment of abnormal behavior at the end of the nineteenth century and during the early part of the twentieth century was Freudian psychoanalysis. Psychoanalysts considered abnormal behavior to be an overt manifestation (i.e., symptom) of an unconscious, unresolved conflict or repressed need. The appropriate treatment was to help the patient identify and deal with the conflict or need through the process of psychoanalysis, which was used during this period for treating several communication disorders.

During the 1960s, the prevailing view in psychology and psychiatry was that almost all abnormal behavior is learned. Consequently, the appropriate treatment was thought to be helping the client unlearn the behavior through application of what were called laws of learning. This approach was then used to treat almost all communication disorders that were not considered to have an organic etiology.

When pragmatic theory was introduced into the field in the 1970s, attention shifted from the behaviorally based learning model used in the previous decade to one emphasizing the social interactions surrounding and permeating communication. Therapy, particularly for children with language disorders, focused on helping them engage in socially meaningful and relevant communicative interactions.

Most recently, professional attention has centered on **evidence-based practice,** which is an effort to develop intervention based on practices that are demonstratably effective and that have a proven "track record."

Two salient conclusions can be drawn from reviewing the history of the profession. First, what may be marketed as a "new" or "revolutionary" approach may actually be a reappearance of a technique or approach that was utilized in a previous time. Second, new is not necessarily better. Because something is touted as new does not mean that it will work better than an approach that has existed for some time. What is important is to determine whether there is evidence to support the use of any given approach for any given client.

Evidence-based practice (EBP)
Basing decisions about the care of individual clients on the best evidence available about what works. In EBP, clinicians integrate their clinical expertise and judgment with the best available external clinical evidence derived from systematic research.

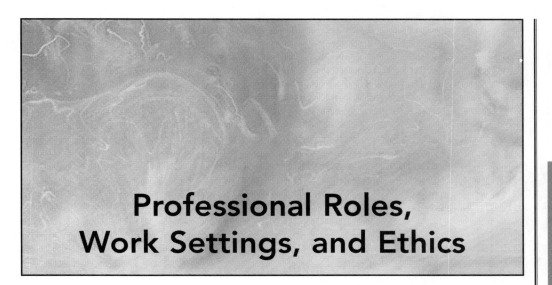

Professional Roles, Work Settings, and Ethics

Chapter 13

Learning Objectives

- Describe the responsibilities of speech-language pathologists and audiologists.

- Describe the roles of the American Speech-Language-Hearing Association.

- Describe at least seven of the roles of the speech-language pathologist and/or audiologist.

- Describe the process of becoming a speech-language pathologist or audiologist.

- Describe the role of a speech-language pathology assistant.

- List the primary requirements for obtaining a Certificate of Clinical Competence.

- Describe at least five of the work settings where speech-language pathologists and/or audiologists provide services.

- Describe the four primary principles in ASHA's Code of Ethics.

Chapter 13

Introduction

In Chapters 3 through 11, the focus was on children and adults who have communication disorders. This chapter discusses the professionals who have the primary responsibility for helping persons cope with these disorders: **speech-language pathologists (SLPs), speech-language pathology assistants (SLPAs), audiologists, and audiology assistants.** For a brief overview of these professionals, refer back to Chapter 2 on pages 30–31. ASHA's website also includes definitions of speech-language pathology (2005n) and audiology (2005c).

Speech-Language Pathology and Audiology Professionals

Although SLPs, audiologists, SLPAs, and audiologist assistants are committed to the same goal of promoting the welfare of people with communication disorders, their roles differ. Audiologists and SLPs are **independent professionals,** while SLPAs and audiology assistants work under the direct supervision of an SLP or audiologist.

Speech-Language Pathologists and Audiologists

SLPs and audiologists work in a variety of settings, each requiring a specific set of responsibilities. Very few SLPs and/or audiologists actually engage simultaneously in every one of the roles described here, but over the course of a career that includes the entire gamut of settings, one could function in a large number of the following roles.

Independent Professionals

As mentioned above, SLPs and audiologists are independent professionals. Other independent professionals in health-related fields are dentists, **psychiatrists**, and **optometrists.** Most nurses, **physical therapists,** and **occupational therapists** are not independent professionals because they are required by law to only accept referrals from physicians who prescribe what the nurses or therapists are to do.

Independent professionals assume full responsibility for what they do for a client or patient. The downside of this is that the professional can be sued for malpractice. Consequently, all independent professionals need professional liability (i.e., malpractice) insurance. Speech-language pathologists and audiologists in private practice purchase their own professional liability insurance. Those employed by a public school system, hospital, or other institution will almost always have the insurance furnished by their employer.

What does it mean to be a professional? Professionals have knowledge and expertise usually not possessed by those who buy their services. They are practitioners of occupations that require considerable formal training to perform at the level of competence consumers of their services expect. To learn more about the functioning of SLPs and audiologists as independent professionals and their risks for being sued for malpractice, see Silverman (1999a).

One of the main responsibilities of SLPs and audiologists as independent professionals is diagnosing and treating communication disorders in order to promote the welfare of people

Independent professional
A practitioner who is not required by law to have his or her activities regulated (i.e., controlled) by a member of another profession. Speech-language pathologists and audiologists (like physicians and dentists) are independent professionals. Speech-language pathology assistants (like nurses) are not.

Optometrist
A professional trained to provide care to improve vision with glasses, contact lenses, etc.

Introduction to Communication Sciences and Disorders

Code of Ethics of the American Speech-Language-Hearing Association
The ethical code to which all speech-language pathologists and audiologists are required to adhere. Failure to do so can result in one's certification and/or license to practice being suspended or revoked.

Clinician-investigator
A clinician who does therapy-outcome research which forms the basis for evidence-based practice. All speech-language pathologists and audiologists are required to collect some data on outcomes for purposes of accountability.

Objective attitude
A nonjudgmental attitude, such as viewing an impairment as a "challenge" rather than a "chain." This attitude assists a person who has an impairment to minimize the negative impact that the impairment has on his or her life.

with these disorders. They determine whether people referred to them have a communication disorder; determine the cause of a disorder; and develop and implement an intervention plan for reducing the disorder's severity. If it is not possible to determine the cause, as is the case with many language disorders, the SLP will usually develop an intervention plan that helps the person develop skills to succeed in school, compensate for the disorder, and/or function in his or her everyday life.

Clinician-Investigators

The **Code of Ethics of the American Speech-Language-Hearing Association** states that SLPs and audiologists "...shall evaluate services rendered to determine effectiveness" (ASHA, 2005a; p. 186). They must do therapy-outcome research, therefore, to function in a manner that is consistent with this code. This means they must function as **clinician-investigators** and assess the impact of their therapy programs on their clients. The information gleaned from such assessment enables professionals to improve their effectiveness as clinicians. It can, for example, enable them to identify intervention strategies that are not producing desired outcomes and that must, therefore, be modified or discarded.

Accountability is another reason clinicians need to assess the effectiveness of the services they render. Clinicians are required by their employers and by third-party payers (e.g., insurance companies) to document the impact they have on clients. They generate the data needed for documentation by doing therapy-outcome research—that is, by being investigators as well as clinicians. To learn more about the functioning of SLPs and audiologists as clinician-investigators, see Silverman (1998b). The topic of evidence-based practice is described in more detail in Chapter 16. You can find ASHA's code of ethics on their website (2005a).

Counselors

Speech-language pathologists and audiologists frequently function as counselors. They provide clients and their families with relevant information about communication disorders and how to cope with them. For example, they provide the families of people with aphasia with the information they need to cope with the behavioral changes that occur with brain damage.

Speech-language pathologists and audiologists also try to modify attitudes of clients and family members that could impede the rehabilitation process. An example of such an attitude would be the desire to conceal a hearing loss. If this attitude is not modified, it is likely to keep the client from wearing a hearing aid and benefiting from the device.

Furthermore, SLPs and audiologists help clients develop an **objective attitude** toward their disorder. This allows the person to minimize the negative impact of the disorder on his or her life—that is, to make it less handicapping. To learn more about the counseling role of SLPs and audiologists, see Crowe (1997) and Luterman (2002).

Educators

All SLPs and audiologists are called upon at some time to function as educators. They provide information to professionals in other fields and speak to professional and lay groups about people who have communication disorders. The majority of SLPs work in schools, so the role of educator is one they engage in daily. Most school-based SLPs work in classrooms, where they teach individuals, small groups, and entire classrooms of students. Many students majoring in audiology or speech-language pathology take a public speaking course to prepare themselves for meeting this responsibility.

Report Writers

Speech-language pathologists and audiologists are expected to prepare reports on their clients, which become a part of the client's clinical record. On request from the client and/or the client's family, these reports will be sent to professionals at other institutions or agencies. These reports are expected to include summaries of the findings of evaluations, progress notes, and discharge information.

Reports are one of the ways professionals judge each other's competence. Therefore, it is important that they be well written. Students majoring in speech-language pathology and audiology should develop their writing skills so they can write reports that are clear, informative, and free of grammatical and spelling errors. To learn more about the report writing responsibilities of SLPs and audiologists, see Pannbacker, Middleton, Vekovius, and Sanders (2001).

Team Members

Speech-language pathologists and audiologists often function as members of teams on which the professions represented are determined by the client's needs. Team members for a preschool child who is hypernasal because of a cleft palate, for example, may include an audiologist, an SLP, a plastic surgeon, a dentist, a psychiatrist, and a **social worker.** They will evaluate the client and jointly establish goals for the client.

School-based SLPs participate in a variety of teams. The school-based team responsible for writing the student's **Individualized Education Program (IEP)** will include the SLP for students who have communication disorders. In addition, many school-based SLPs provide service through teaching teams that include classroom teachers, special educators, an occupational therapist, a physical therapist, and the SLP.

Team members cooperate by each providing services aimed at the client's learning goals, including those related to communication. For example, when working with a child who has cerebral palsy, the SLP will encourage the child to use his or her hands in ways that the occupational therapist has recommended. Similarly, the occupational therapist will encourage the child to communicate in ways the SLP has determined is best for the child's developmental goals. Students majoring in speech-language pathology or audiology should become acquainted with the ways other health-care and education professionals can contribute to the treatment of children and adults who have communication impairments. To learn more about multidisciplinary teams for managing communication disorders, see Fawcus (2000) and Utley (1993).

Marketing Representatives

People with communication handicaps must be aware of services provided by audiologists and/or SLPs before they can be helped by the services. Raising awareness requires marketing. Most SLPs and audiologists engage in marketing of some form. For example, they give talks to lay and professional groups in which they describe aspects of their clinical service programs. School-based SLPs give presentations to parents, describing their work with students and how it contributes to academic success. To learn more about the marketing responsibilities of speech-language pathologists and audiologists, see Matthews (1993).

Individualized Education Program (IEP)
A program developed for each child who is eligible for special education, based on the child's unique needs, to provide the student with a free, appropriate, public education. The IEP contains a statement of the child's present level of performance, educational needs, and measurable goals and objectives. The IEP is reviewed at least annually.

Lobbying
In this context, attempting to encourage the passage of state or federal legislation that is likely to be helpful to persons who have communication disorders and to discourage the passage of legislation that is likely to be harmful to them.

Congressional Action Contact Network
A lobbying entity sponsored by the American Speech-Language-Hearing Association. A member of the association is assigned to each member of Congress to present its point of view on relevant upcoming bills.

Advocate
The role of helping clients deal with bureaucracy or other hurdles keeping them from receiving services.

Third-party payers
These include private insurance companies and governmental organizations (e.g., Medicare) that pay for client services.

Expert witness
Witnesses who give opinions in their areas of expertise at trials and hearings.

AuD
Doctor of Audiology degree.

Lobbyists and Advocates

ASHA's Code of Ethics states that SLPs and audiologists should hold paramount the welfare of persons served professionally (ASHA, 2005a). This refers to all persons who have communication disorders, not just those treated by clinicians.

The welfare of people with communication disorders is affected by both state and federal legislation. Such legislation can influence the availability of funding for needed services. It can influence, for example, whether a child with a severe communication impairment from a low-income family will be able to have the speech-generating communication device or the hearing aid that he or she needs.

One way SLPs and audiologists promote the welfare of people who have communication disorders is by **lobbying** for legislation favorable to client interests and against legislation that could be detrimental to clients. Most lobbying on the federal level is done through the **Congressional Action Contact Network.** A member of the American Speech-Language-Hearing Association is assigned to each senator and representative in the Congress. Whenever legislation is being considered that could affect people with communication disorders, they contact the members of Congress to whom they are assigned. Members provide legislators with evidence that supports the position they are advocating.

Speech-language pathologists and audiologists also promote the welfare of people with communication disorders by serving as **advocates** for them. Federal, state, and municipal administrative agencies (e.g., Medicare and local school districts), and other **third-party payers** sometimes deny people services or put them on waiting lists. They may not realize that the client is eligible to receive a service, or their funding may be inadequate to cover all of the services they are supposed to provide. A local school district, for example, may not provide an electronic communication device for a child with a severe communication disorder until the SLP helps provide necessary documentation. To learn more about how SLPs function as lobbyists and advocates, see Silverman (1999a).

Expert Witnesses

Speech-language pathologists and audiologists are occasionally asked to testify in trials as **expert witnesses.** They are hired by the attorney for the plaintiff or defendant in a lawsuit to provide opinions (backed by evidence) that will support or refute what has been testified to by the other side. An SLP may, for example, be asked to testify about the competency of a person with aphasia to continue to manage his or her financial affairs or to testify in a child custody case about which parent would be best able to provide for the child's therapy needs. To learn more about how SLPs function as expert witnesses, see Silverman (1999a).

Researchers

Some SLPs and audiologists spend more than half their time doing either pure or applied research. Their research may be funded by grants from governmental or private agencies. Most of them have a PhD or AuD degree and are on the faculty of a college or university.

Many practitioners in these fields who have master's or **AuD** degrees also do some research. Most of it tends to be both clinical and practical. They share their findings with other practitioners in their field by either publishing in professional publications or by presenting at professional meetings.

Supervisors

Many SLPs and audiologists function as supervisors, overseeing the activities of other SLPs, audiologists, or paraprofessionals (e.g., SLPAs). The facilities in which they supervise include school systems, hospitals, private practice, and rehabilitation centers. They also may supervise student clinicians at a college or university speech and hearing clinic. Any person who has earned a **Certificate of Clinical Competence (CCC)** from ASHA can supervise clinical practicum experiences in his or her area of certification (speech-language pathology or audiology). To learn more about how SLPs and audiologists function as clinical supervisors, see Farmer and Farmer (1989) and Leith, McNiece, and Fusilier (1989).

Administrators

Some SLPs and audiologists function as administrators as well as clinicians in clinical programs. The competencies required for administering a speech, language, and hearing clinical program are the same as those required for other administrative positions. To learn more about what is involved in administering a clinical program, see Cornett (1999); Hosford-Dunn, Dunn, and Harford (1995); Oyer (1987); and Rizzo Jr. and Trudeau (1994).

Authors

Many SLPs and audiologists author professional books, computer software, slide presentations, audiotapes, videotapes, diagnostic tests, or therapy kits for use by other clinicians. Also, some invent devices for diagnosing or treating communication disorders. Such activities are not limited to those with PhD or AuD degrees. To learn more about what is involved in authoring clinical intellectual property, see Silverman (1998a).

Consultants

Most SLPs and audiologists function at times as resource persons, or consultants. They consult with other SLPs about their clients, and they often consult and collaborate with teachers and other professionals to design and implement services.

It is important for SLPs and audiologists to fulfill each of the above roles. However, perhaps one of the most important characteristics of people in the profession is to be a person who genuinely wants to be helpful to others. A clinician who isn't a people person is unlikely to be successful, regardless of the amount of technical expertise he or she has. You can read about a client's experience with a clinician who was not caring in Study More 13.1 on page 226. To learn more about the human dimension to being an effective clinician, see Van Riper (1979).

Speech-Language Pathology Assistants (SLPAs)

Although **paraprofessionals** have been utilized in a number of health-care and education fields (e.g., physical therapy, nursing, teaching) for many years, their widespread utilization in the field of speech-language pathology is relatively recent. ASHA does not register (i.e., grant credentials to) SLPAs. However, they do have recommended guidelines for the supervision, use, and training of SLPAs. An SLPA should only perform tasks under the supervision of an ASHA certified SLP. ASHA recommends the following tasks to be delegated to SLPAs:

Certificate of Clinical Competence (CCC)
Clinical certification awarded by the American Speech-Language-Hearing Association once the person has met all the necessary academic and clinical requirements. The CCC-SLP is offered for speech-language pathology, and the CCC-A is offered for audiology.

Paraprofessionals
People who assist professionals in a particular field (e.g., speech-language pathology assistants).

Study More 13.1	A Client's Experiences with a Clinician Who Was Not Caring

This excerpt highlights the importance of a clinician exhibiting a genuine caring attitude. The author, who was a speech-language pathologist, had a stroke at the age of 29 that left her completely unable to communicate for almost one and one-half years.

I feel that the most important trait of a good clinician is a genuine, caring, patient attitude. If one has a lot of "textbook learning" and little empathy for the client, progress will be limited. One speech-language pathologist I had gave me the feeling that when she saw me she thought, "Well, here's Joy again. What shall I have her try today?" Needless to say, I made very little progress with this clinician. She was never really prepared for therapy, and I knew that she was just putting some things together on the spot to keep me "busy." I knew that her knowledge of my condition was severely limited, I think that a client without my background would have recognized this also. I did not get a feeling of professional or personal concern or even professional competency from this clinician. I needed a clinician who cared and was interested in me as a person, a clinician who could make me feel secure in her knowledge of my problem.

Another thing that has a big effect on the attitude of the client is enthusiasm. All speech-language pathologists need to be more enthused about their clients, to greet clients as if they were glad to see them, and to have a positive attitude about the clients. When I was depressed and the clinician was really not interested in me, I became even more depressed. It was wonderful when I would go to therapy and the clinician was cheerful and friendly. Knowing that the clinician cared would bring me out of my depression.

From "I'd Rather Tell a Story Than Be One," by J. G. Post and W. R. Leith, 1983, *ASHA, 25,* p. 27. © 1983 by the American Speech-Language-Hearing Association. Reprinted with permission.

Scope of practice
The services that practitioners in a field are recognized by licensing and certification boards and the courts as having the expertise to provide.

- Assisting the SLP with screening tests (without providing interpretation)

- Assisting the SLP with acquiring informal documentation

- Following the treatment plan developed by the SLP

- Documenting the client's performance (e.g., collecting data; tallying data; preparing charts, records, and graphs) and reporting this information to the SLP

- Assisting the SLP in assessing a client

- Assisting with clerical duties

- Providing support to the SLP in research, inservice training, and public relations programs

ASHA recommends that SLPAs receive an associate's degree from a training program for SLPAs. The two-year, 60-semester-hour program of study should include general education courses (20–40 semester hours) and courses intended to impart specific knowledge and skills required to be an SLPA (20–40 semester hours). The training program should include clinical observation and a minimum of one hundred clock hours of supervised field experience.

For more information on SLPAs, the ASHA webpage (2005f) defines the roles SLPAs play in providing services to people with communication disorders; how to become an SLPA; how SLPAs are supervised; and the training and fieldwork available for SLPAs. To learn more about the SLPAs **scope of practice**, see Thomas and Webster (1999).

Audiology Assistants

You may recall from Chapter 2 that the primary role of audiology assistants involves testing the hearing ability of people by means of various hearing tests. Using the results of those tests, along with information obtained from other sources, audiology assistants establish where the hearing impairment is located: in the middle ear, the inner ear, the nerve pathways, or the brain. In collaboration with a physician, audiology assistants can also adapt and adjust hearing aids. Audiology assistants working for hearing aid companies may fill other roles (e.g., repairs to hearing aids and earmolds; clerical duties; room and patient preparation; examination for abnormal ear conditions; taking of aural impressions and fitting of earmolds).

Some states require audiology assistants to obtain a license to practice. For instance, Texas's requirements for obtaining a license as an audiology assistant are:

- Baccalaureate degree with an emphasis in audiology

- 25 hours of clinical observation

- 25 hours of clinical assisting experience

- 24 semester hours in speech-language pathology and audiology with at least 18 in the area in which the applicant is applying

Becoming a Speech-Language Pathologist or Audiologist

In large part, the process of becoming an SLP or an audiologist consists of meeting the requirements for the Certificate of Clinical Competence (CCC-SLP or CCC-A). All employers accept the CCC-A as evidence of competency to function as an audiologist, and all employers except the public schools accept the CCC-SLP as evidence of competency to function as an SLP. Although most states require a license to practice as an SLP, the requirements for the license are usually the same as for the ASHA Certificate of Clinical Competence.

Each state department of public instruction has its own requirements for certifying SLPs as employable in its schools. Although an SLP who meets the requirements for one state will not necessarily meet those for other states, it is usually not difficult to meet them if you have met those for one state and ASHA's CCC-SLP.

If you are majoring in speech-language pathology, you would be wise to attempt to meet the requirements for both the ASHA Certificate of Clinical Competence (or state license) and the certificate required to work in the public schools of your state. It is advisable to do both even if you do not plan to work in a school setting. Having both credentials increases your possibilities for employment because it qualifies you to work as an SLP in either an educational or medical setting.

Most states license hearing aid dispensers. Audiologists who dispense hearing aids in these states must be licensed. Some states allow audiologists to dispense hearing aids with an audiology license alone (i.e., they do not require a separate hearing aid dispenser license).

Academic Degree Requirements

A master's degree is currently a prerequisite for obtaining the Certificate of Clinical Competence in Speech-Language Pathology or Audiology. The majority of people who hold these certificates now have master's degrees. The remainder have doctoral degrees, mostly the PhD or AuD. As pointed out earlier, the latter will replace the master's degree as a prerequisite for the CCC-A in the near future.

Although most states require a master's degree to be certified as employable in the public schools, a few will certify persons with only a bachelor's degree. However, the employment opportunities for SLPs who have only a bachelor's degree are limited and the salaries are low, making this a less attractive option.

Some SLPs and audiologists who are practitioners (as opposed to professors and/or researchers) have doctoral degrees. Many of them are directors of clinical programs or private practitioners. Most SLPs and audiologists who are directors of speech-language and/or hearing programs at Veteran's Administration hospitals, for example, have PhD degrees. Most people accumulate a few years of full-time clinical experience before beginning a doctoral program.

ASHA's Certificates of Clinical Competence

The formal training program for one of these certificates is usually six or seven years. A student enrolled in the program ordinarily earns both a bachelor's and a master's or AuD degree. The bachelor's portion usually takes four years to complete. A master's degree is then completed in two years or an AuD in three years. Some colleges and universities offer only the undergraduate (preprofessional) portion of the training program. All graduate coursework and graduate clinical practicum experience must have been initiated and completed at a college or university whose program is accredited by the Educational Standards Board of the American Speech-Language-Hearing Association in the area for which certification is sought—speech-language pathology or audiology.

It is possible for a person to earn both certificates. He or she is then qualified to treat anybody with a communication disorder. Meeting the requirements for both certificates usually involves earning two graduate degrees: one in speech-language pathology and one in audiology. The vast majority of members of ASHA are certified in only one of the two areas.

There are five requirements for obtaining one of these certificates: (1) successfully completing academic courses; (2) observing at least 25 hours of diagnostic and therapy sessions; (3) accumulating a minimum of 375 hours of supervised clinical practicum experience; (4) successfully completing a clinical fellowship year; and (5) passing a national examination. Also, the candidate must have a master's degree or an AuD from a program accredited by ASHA and be a member of ASHA or be willing to pay an annual certification maintenance fee to the association. An overview of these five requirements is presented in the next sections.

Academic Coursework Requirements

To be employed as an SLP or audiologist, it is necessary to have certain knowledge and skills. Because practitioners in both fields need some of the same information, some of the same courses are required for both ASHA certificates.

Before you can determine whether the speech and language abilities of an individual are within normal limits, you must be familiar with the speech and language skills of typically developing individuals. What kinds of information about normal hearing, speech, and language must SLPs and audiologists have? You have probably already surmised what is necessary by looking at the topics covered in this book. Several sections describe the normal structure and functioning of various mechanisms and processes, one of which, for example, is the normal anatomy and physiology of the speech and hearing mechanisms. To understand how people make sense of speech and how they are able to speak, you have to know how the parts of these mechanisms function. This information can be significant both diagnostically and therapeutically. Diagnostically, it enables clinicians to recognize possible organic causes for their clients' communication disorders. Therapeutically, it can enable them to predict whether it should be possible for a client to improve and, if so, how much.

For example, if an opening in a client's hard palate allowed air to flow into the nasal cavity, the clinician would know that the client will continue to be hypernasal until this opening is eliminated by surgery or by fitting a dental appliance into it. This information is acquired from the required course on the anatomy and physiology of the speech and hearing mechanism, as well as units of other courses that deal with components of this mechanism.

Another kind of information about normal hearing, speech, and language that a clinician must acquire pertains to the acoustical signals generated by the speech mechanism and interpreted by the ear. The signals result from the movements of the structures (e.g., the tongue) that make up the speech mechanism. When a person has a speech disorder, there is something abnormal about the acoustical signals being generated by his or her speech mechanism. Speech-language pathologists attempt to modify these acoustical signals—to make them more normal. Information about the acoustics of speech is acquired from courses on speech and hearing science, and phonetics.

Students must also acquire information about normal language development, which they need for both diagnosis and therapy. An SLP who does not know the typical development of grammatical rules will not know which ones to teach a three-year-old client who has a language disorder. Similarly, without information regarding children's development of metalinguistic abilities, the SLP will not be able to design appropriate intervention for children whose metalinguistic skills are not keeping pace with their peers. This kind of information is acquired from courses on normal language development.

Another kind of information that SLPs and audiologists must acquire pertains to the symptomatology, etiology, prognosis, diagnosis, and treatment of the various communication disorders. Students majoring in speech-language pathology or audiology are introduced to all types of communication disorders—not just to those that are treated by the professionals in their specific field. However, those majoring in audiology acquire information about hearing disorders in much greater depth than those majoring in speech-language pathology, and vice versa.

The clinical relationship is central to what audiologists and SLPs do. It is the structure within which they function clinically. They have to know how to manage the relationship proficiently in order to be maximally effective as clinicians, using the knowledge and skill they acquire in their clinical practicums.

Speech-language pathologists and audiologists must also know how behaviors are learned and unlearned. Students learn to utilize the various strategies that psychologists have developed for modifying behavior. They acquire the academic information needed for doing this from psychology courses and the skills for implementing the information in their clinical practicums.

The main responsibilities of most SLPs and audiologists are diagnosis and therapy. Students training to be clinicians acquire this information both from courses that focus directly

Introduction to Communication Sciences and Disorders

Scientific method
A logically organized and objective set of rules for investigating questions to maximize the likelihood of getting a correct answer.

on these topics (e.g., those dealing with diagnostic methods in speech-language pathology or hearing testing) and those that deal with specific communication disorders (e.g., aphasia or language-learning disabilities). They also acquire it from clinical practicums.

Both SLPs and audiologists need information about professional ethics and law as it affects clinical practice. They also need information about establishing and maintaining a clinical practice, record keeping, and marketing clinical services. Many training programs offer a course in which such information is presented (e.g., one on professional aspects of clinical practice in speech-language pathology and audiology).

All SLPs and audiologists function as consumers of research. They read professional journals in which research is reported, and utilize some of the journal information presented in their clinical practice. To know how to evaluate the findings of studies, they must become proficient in reading scientific reports and analyzing this information. They also have to know how to evaluate the impacts of their therapy programs on clients—that is, how to produce research. Most training programs offer a course from which students acquire the information needed for functioning as both a consumer and producer of clinical research.

While most SLPs and audiologists function more often as clinicians than as scientists, they nevertheless have to understand the **scientific method** because they utilize it for clinical decision making. All students majoring in speech-language pathology or audiology are required to take courses in biological/physical sciences and mathematics to facilitate the development of a scientific orientation.

Clinical Observation Requirement

All students majoring in speech-language pathology or audiology are required to observe a minimum of 25 hours of evaluation and/or therapy before beginning their clinical practicum experience. This is intended to increase their understanding of the dynamics of the clinical relationship.

Supervised Clinical Experience Requirements

All students majoring in speech-language pathology or audiology are required to accumulate a minimum of 375 hours of supervised clinical experience. At least 250 must be accumulated during the master's degree portion of the training program in the professional area in which certification is sought. In addition, these hours must be distributed in certain ways. A specified minimum number must be for evaluation and for treatment; for specific types of disorders; and for children and adults.

Students usually accumulate practicum hours in two types of settings. Almost all undergraduate practicum hours are likely to be accumulated in the clinical facilities of the college or university in which the student is enrolled. The remainder of the 375 hours are accumulated in community facilities that offer speech-language pathology and/or audiology services, such as public schools, hospitals, rehabilitation centers, and nursing homes.

The practicum experience at the college's or university's speech, language, and hearing clinic will be supervised by faculty who are certified by ASHA. Supervision at outside affiliations will be supervised by clinicians employed by these facilities who have volunteered to serve in this role. Any audiologist or speech-language pathologist can supervise practicum experience in the area in which he or she is certified by ASHA.

Clinical Fellowship Year Requirement

After a student has completed all the academic and practicum requirements for a Certificate of Clinical Competence and has received a graduate degree, he or she will begin a clinical fellowship year, which is similar to an internship. However, unlike some internships, the person receives a full salary. Any SLP or audiologist who is certified by ASHA in the student's professional area can serve as his or her clinical fellowship supervisor. This person may or may not be employed by the facility at which the intern is working. The supervisor interacts frequently during this year with the intern and submits a year-end evaluation of the intern's performance to ASHA.

The National Examination Requirement

The final requirement for attaining a Certificate of Clinical Competence is passing a national examination. The examinations are different for those seeking certification in speech-language pathology and in audiology. They are of the multiple-choice type and cover all aspects of clinical functioning. If candidates fail on the first try, they may take the test again.

Work Settings

Audiologists, SLPs, SLPAs, and audiologist assistants provide services in a variety of work settings. Several of these settings are discussed in the following paragraphs.

Schools

Public school systems historically have been one of the largest employers of SLPs. They are required by state and federal special education law to provide speech-language pathology services. Part of the local school district budget for these services comes from state and federal sources.

The clients served in this setting, of course, are school-age children and adolescents. Though the majority are of elementary-school age, federal law requires services to be provided to people from birth to 21 years. Children between the ages of birth to 3 are required by federal law to be offered therapy services if they are at risk for developing a communication disorder.

To qualify a child for special education services, a communication disorder must have a significant impact on a student's educational performance. Moore-Brown and Montgomery (2001) provide information on special education requirements related to speech-language pathology, and guidance on how children qualify for services.

The majority of children seen by SLPs in public schools have articulation or language disorders. The language services provided by SLPs in the schools address a wide variety of skills including phonological development, vocabulary development, story comprehension, and organizational skills. SLPs may also help older students with writing, oral presentations, and study skills.

Children are also seen for **fluency,** voice, and nasal resonance intervention. Speech-language pathologists, rather than audiologists, do the hearing habilitation in most school districts (except for that involving hearing aids).

Some school districts employ audiologists, who spend most of their time testing hearing and assisting children with hearing aids. Far fewer audiologists than SLPs are employed in public schools.

Some private schools have a full- or part-time SLP. If they do not employ one, their students may go to a nearby public school for therapy. To learn more about the scope of practice of SLPs in the public schools, see Blosser and Neidecker (2002); Dodge (2000); Moore-Brown and Montgomery (2001); and O'Connell (1997). ASHA (2005k) also provides a complete description of the scope of practice of SLPs, including public school settings, on their webpage.

Health-Care Settings

Hospitals, nursing homes, rehabilitation centers, and some HMOs offer speech-language pathology services. The SLP's caseload consists primarily of adults whose communication disorders are caused by brain damage—that is, **aphasia** and **dysarthria.** They also work with people who have lost the ability to swallow normally (i.e., **dysphagia**), which was described in Chapter 7 on pages 129–132. While assessing patients, SLPs may assist in or perform modified barium x-ray studies of their swallow (to learn more about dysphagia, see Groher, 1997).

Speech-language pathologists who work for HMOs, hospitals, and rehabilitation centers also treat some children. Some SLPs who are employed in hospitals, for example, work with medically fragile infants in neonatal intensive care units. One of their most important responsibilities when working with children is implementing feeding therapy programs. To learn more about such feeding programs, see Rossetti (2001).

Opportunities for audiologists are expanding in HMOs, hospitals, and rehabilitation centers. Increasing numbers of commercial health-care marketing groups, such as Blue Cross Blue Shield, provide audiology services and hearing aids (Gudmundsen, 1992). Also, the number of hospitals routinely screening newborns for hearing impairments is increasing (Marlowe, 1993).

Colleges and Universities

Learning institutions that have communication disorders training programs hire both audiologists and SLPs as instructors and as clinic supervisors. Instructors usually have a PhD degree, and clinic supervisors usually have a master's degree or AuD.

Businesses

Some corporations, particularly those in which employees are exposed to loud noise, employ audiologists. Audiologists who work for industry maintain hearing conservation programs, which include monitoring environmental noise levels, testing employees' hearing, and fitting employees with ear protectors.

A number of firms that publish books and other materials for SLPs, or manufacture devices for people who have communication disorders, employ SLPs. Some such firms are, in fact, owned by SLPs.

Schools for the Deaf

The primary responsibilities of audiologists in schools for the deaf are hearing testing and hearing aid maintenance. They also may become involved with hearing habilitation, including teaching speech. SLPs in schools for the deaf typically provide intervention in the areas of voice, articulation, **speechreading,** language comprehension, and language use.

Residential Facilities for People with Developmental Disabilities

Almost all of these residential facilities offer speech-language pathology services. Intervention focuses on functional communication skills (e.g., vocabulary needed to work at a sheltered workshop) and daily living skills. If a resident has severe developmental disabilities (and, hence, is incapable of acquiring sufficient speech to meet communication needs), services may include teaching gestural communication such as **American Sign Language (ASL)** or use of an augmentative/alternative communication device.

For-Profit Corporations that Sell Services to Other Institutions

These for-profit corporations employ large numbers of SLPs whose services are sold to hospitals, nursing homes, and other institutions. Some of these corporations service institutions in only a single city or a single state; others operate nationally. Many of them also sell the services of other health-care professionals (e.g., physical therapists, occupational therapists, and nurses).

Private Practice

The numbers of SLPs and audiologists who enter private practice either part- or full-time have increased dramatically during the past 30 years. A major factor in the increase in the field of audiology is because increasing numbers of audiologists are being licensed as hearing aid dispensers.

A number of SLPs in private practice specialize in treating English language learners (ELL). These are usually people who were born in non-English-speaking countries and who are working in the United States. Some corporations will pay for services to improve the intelligibility of their employees' speech.

Speech-language pathologists and audiologists usually rent offices in professional office buildings. They function professionally in the same manner as other independent practitioners who are in private practice.

One sign of the increased interest in private practice in audiology and speech-language pathology is the founding of a professional association for private practitioners—the **American Academy of Private Practice in Speech-Language Pathology and Audiology.** Spokespersons for this organization, as well as those for ASHA, predict that the private practice segment of the profession will continue to grow. To learn more about the private practice option, see Butler (1986), Coleman (2001), and Wood (1986).

American Academy of Private Practice in Speech-Language Pathology and Audiology An organization to which many of the speech-language pathologists and audiologists in private practice belong.

Ethics

Every profession is guided by a set of principles that ensure its members carry out their professional responsibilities with integrity, according to the highest standards of the profession. For SLPs and audiologists, this set of principles is codified in ASHA's Code of Ethics (2005a). It consists of four basic rules, which are paraphrased below.

1. Individuals must hold paramount the welfare of their clients and/or people who are participating in research studies. They must treat animals involved in their research in a humane manner. Services must be provided without discrimination and must maintain confidentiality regarding the client.

2. Individuals must achieve and maintain the highest level of professional competence. This includes providing service only in the areas of qualification, and routinely participating in continuing professional development activities.

3. Individuals must promote public understanding of their profession, support the development of services for unmet public needs, and provide accurate information in all their communications regarding the profession. Individuals must not misrepresent their qualifications, credentials, or services.

4. Individuals must respect all professions and maintain harmonious relationships with members of the professions with whom they work. Individuals must not engage in any dishonesty, fraud, deceit, or form of conduct that would reflect adversely on the profession.

ASHA's Code of Ethics is intended to provide specific standards to cover most situations encountered by SLPs and audiologists. It aims to protect and promote the welfare of the individuals and groups with whom SLPs and audiologists work and to educate members, students, and the public regarding ethical standards of the discipline. Members of ASHA believe that the Code of Ethics requires a lifelong personal commitment to act ethically; to encourage ethical behavior by colleagues, employees, supervisees, and students; and to consult with colleagues regarding ethical questions and issues.

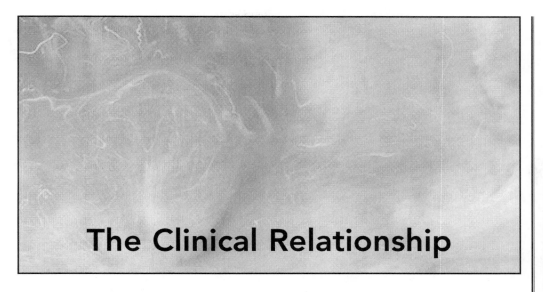

The Clinical Relationship

Chapter 14

Learning Objectives

- Identify the interactions comprising the clinical relationship.

- Describe the variables that influence a therapeutic relationship.

- Describe how a therapeutic relationship differs from other relationships.

- Identify the characteristics of a good therapeutic relationship.

- Discuss how the clinician's beliefs about the cause of a communication disorder affects a client's motivation and progress throughout the intervention process.

- Describe what a clinician must do to keep his or her own needs outside the therapeutic relationship.

- Describe how clinicians can best motivate clients and convey their belief that change is possible.

Introduction

The context within which clinical services are dispensed is a relationship involving the clinician, the **client,** and those close to the client (e.g., parents and other family members). This context may be one in which the clinician interacts with a number of members of the client's family (see Crais, 1992). The client is more likely to improve if these interactions are good ones, regardless of the disorder and the intervention strategy being used. Consequently, it is crucial that clinicians be aware of the variables that affect this relationship and, thereby, their ability to be helpful to their clients. This chapter discusses some of these variables in order to provide you with information that will make your interactions with clients more effective.

The term *client* is used in this chapter to designate the person the clinician is trying to help. Other terms may be used to designate this person, including patient or student. However, the term client was chosen both because of its wide utilization in medical and educational settings and because it implies that the person who ultimately is in charge is not the clinician, but either the person who sought the clinician's help or a member of his or her family.

What Is the Clinical Relationship?

The **clinical relationship** (i.e., therapeutic relationship) consists of more than the interaction between the clinician and the client. It also includes the relationship between the clinician and each of the client's significant others, and between the client and each of his or her significant others. The clinical relationship is illustrated in Figure 14.1 on page 238.

The most important of these interactions is usually the one between client and clinician. What these interactions entail is largely determined by the clinician's ability to treat the client as a person rather than as a disorder, or, as Oliver Sacks (1985) has put it, as a biography rather than a disease. The interactions between clinician and client (and/or significant others) may occur in several settings: in a **therapy room** in which the client and clinician sit facing each other; in the client's natural environment (e.g., home or classroom); on the Internet (e.g., via e-mail); or on the telephone. Doing therapy in the client's classroom rather than in a special therapy room is referred to as **collaborative/consultative service delivery** (Ferguson, 1991). This approach is particularly useful with children who have a language disorder (Masterson, 1993). For more information on classroom-based language intervention, see Miller (1989) and Moore-Brown and Montgomery (2001).

Another aspect of the clinical relationship is that between the clinician and the client's significant others. This includes the client's parents, spouse, partner, children, classroom teacher, other professionals, and **paraprofessionals.** In some instances, this relationship is more important for helping a client than that between the client and the clinician. For instance, when the SLP sees a preschool child whose parents are concerned that he or she is beginning to stutter, the SLP will need to develop a strong relationship with the child's family to provide maximally effective intervention (Zebrowski & Schum, 1993). Some clinicians manage the disorder in such children primarily by engaging in counseling the parents.

A third aspect of the clinical relationship is between a client and his or her significant others. Study More 14.1 on page 239 illustrates an example of how the relationship between spouses

Client
A person whom a clinician is trying to help. In some settings, this person is referred to as a patient or student.

Clinical relationship
The context within which clinical services are dispensed, involving the clinician, the client, and those close to the client. Also referred to as therapeutic relationship.

Therapy room
The office or other environment in which the clinician provides clinical services to the client.

Collaborative/ Consultative service delivery
Providing clinical services to a school-age child in his or her classroom, rather than a special therapy room.

Figure 14.1	Interactions in the Clinical Relationship

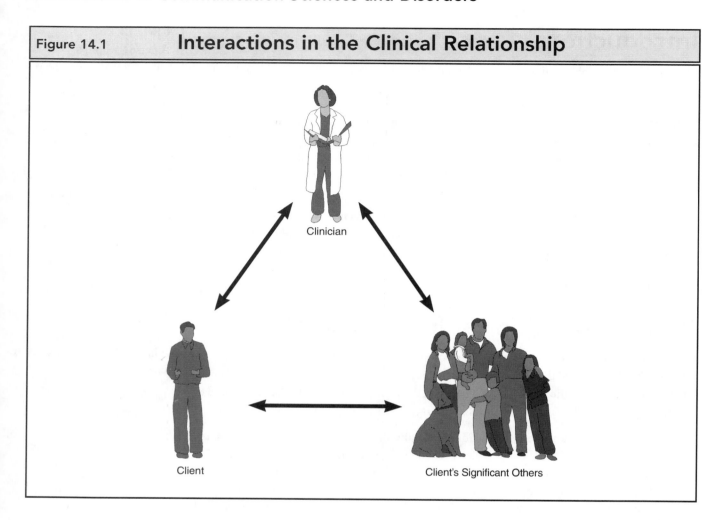

Clinician

Client

Client's Significant Others

can impact the success of intervention. This interaction can profoundly influence the likelihood that therapy will be successful. If, for example, those close to a client indicate that they are pleased with how he or she is changing, the client is more likely to continue trying to change than if they indicate dissatisfaction or concern with the client's progress.

Characteristics of a Good Therapeutic Relationship

One characteristic of a good therapeutic relationship is mutual respect. The client respects the clinician for his or her training and experience. The clinician respects the client and manifests this respect by not treating him or her as a "defective mouth" or a "defective ear," but as a person. Interacting with the client as a person, not as a stereotype, is particularly important if the client is from a culture different from the clinician's own (Anderson, 1992). Mutual respect also means the clinician does not refer to the client as his or her disorder (e.g., "the aphasic," "the LLD kid"), but rather as a person who has a particular condition (e.g., "the man with Wernicke's aphasia" or "the student with language-learning disabilities").

| Study More 14.1 | **Spousal Support and Improvement** |

One of the most common reasons for marital discord and divorce in our society is the husband, wife, or both no longer being willing to function like he, she, or they did previously. When this happens, the marital contract must be renegotiated if the relationship is to survive. Neither husbands nor wives tend to welcome changes in their marital roles and, consequently, will consciously or unconsciously resist their spouse changing in ways that may require them to do so.

A husband or wife who stutters may change in ways after improving (i.e., becoming more fluent and/or less willing to be handicapped by stuttering) that could affect his or her spouse, including the following:
- Relying less on the spouse for doing some of his or her communicating (e.g., making telephone calls)
- Becoming involved in new activities outside of the home that consume time previously spent with the spouse
- Becoming more assertive and less of a "people pleaser"

These have the potential to threaten a stutterer's spouse in a number of ways, some of which are indicated below.

Many stutterers rely on their spouse for doing some of their communicating (e.g., making telephone calls). If one of the roles that their spouse assumes and finds satisfying is being a "rescuer," a stutterer no longer needing someone to communicate for him or her (or needing this kind of assistance as often) can alter the spousal relationship. In fact, merely anticipating such an outcome can cause a spouse to consciously or unconsciously do things that will sabotage his or her partner's attempts to change.

When stutterers become less handicapped by stuttering, they tend to become more social and increase the number of activities in which they engage. As a consequence, they are likely to spend less time with their spouse. If a husband or wife has a strong need to be the "center" of their spouse's world, he or she may become threatened by his or her husband or wife becoming more social and consciously or unconsciously sabotage his or her attempts to improve.

Improvement can result in stutterers becoming more assertive and less willing to be "people pleasers." These changes would tend to make them less willing to be dominated by their spouse. If their spouse has been the dominant partner in the marriage and wishes to continue being so, he or she is likely to resist and possibly sabotage his or her husband's or wife's attempts to improve.

A marriage can survive the kinds of changes described here if the partners are willing to renegotiate their expectations for and roles in it. They are likely to need some professional help to do this. You may want to be proactive and routinely discuss with married stutterers and their wives how improvement could adversely affect their marriage and encourage them to seek marriage counseling as a preventative measure.

From *Second Thoughts about Stuttering: Musings of a Speech-Language Pathologist Who Has Stuttered for More Than Sixty Years* (pp. 5–6), by F. H. Silverman, 2000, Greendale, WI: CODI Publications. © 2000 by CODI Publications. Reprinted with permission.

While mutual respect is required for a good therapeutic relationship, mutual liking is not. It certainly is desirable for clinician and client to like each other as people, but it isn't essential. We all know people whom we respect a great deal professionally but would not enjoy spending time with socially. Maintaining objectivity and respecting the client as a person allows clinicians to provide services in a professional way whether or not they like the client. When clinicians want to be liked by a client, they can lose their objectivity and become less able to be helpful to the client.

In a good therapeutic relationship, the client can trust the clinician to treat what he or she is told as confidential. Clients must feel free to reveal things about themselves to the clinician that they do not want revealed to others.

In a good therapeutic relationship the participants are willing to be honest with each other. They do not tell the other what they want to hear if it is not the truth. Clients, for example, may tell their clinicians that they avoid speaking less often than they do because they want to please them. Or clinicians may not insist that their clients complete assignments regularly because they want to avoid upsetting them and possibly having them discontinue therapy. However, either action could adversely affect progress.

In a good therapeutic relationship the clinician has **empathy** for the client. If the client feels that the clinician does not really understand his or her reactions to the communication disorder, the client may not follow through on the clinician's recommendations.

Empathy
The ability to truly understand, at least a little, how another person feels about an event, experience, process, or idea.

239

Introduction to Communication Sciences and Disorders

Placebo effect
A change (usually a reduction) in the severity of an impairment or disorder elicited by a strong belief in the ability of something or someone to change its severity.

Learning style
The process(es) through which an individual (or cultural group) learns most efficiently.

Contract
A written or oral agreement that the parties agree to abide by voluntarily. The relationship between the client and clinician is a contractual one.

In a good therapeutic relationship the client and clinician successfully communicate with each other. Communication is the medium through which the clinician attempts to influence the client and the client attempts to make the clinician aware of his or her needs. With young children, it is also one of the media, through which language functioning can be enhanced (MacDonald & Carroll, 1992). However, communicating with children whose language development is impaired often requires using other media (e.g., play) to establish a relationship through which to communicate. In any case, the client is unlikely to be helped by the therapy experience if communication is poor.

In a good therapeutic relationship the client believes that the clinician values him or her as a person, believes the client's goals are paramount, and wants the client to reach his or her goals. It is crucial that the clinician communicate to the client in every way possible that this is the case. This communication is particularly important if the client does not have the same cultural background as the clinician (Anderson, 1992).

You are unlikely to be successful with a client you do not value as a person. Every clinician occasionally encounters a client with whom he or she cannot relate well. When such a situation occurs, the client should be referred to another clinician to satisfy the ASHA ethical requirement to hold paramount the welfare of the client.

In a good therapeutic relationship the clinician continually offers hope that the client can reach the goals he or she has set. Although clinicians cannot guarantee improvement, they can offer clients and their significant others hope that they can reach their goals. It is unethical for a clinician to accept a client for therapy or to continue treating a client if there is little likelihood of further improvement. A client who does not really believe that what the clinician is recommending will be effective is less likely to follow his or her recommendations, which would tend to reduce the effectiveness of the therapy program.

Another way hope affects the outcome of therapy is through the **placebo effect,** which is explained in Study More 14.2. For some disorders (e.g., aphasia, dysphagia, stuttering), this phenomenon appears to play a significant role in determining therapy outcome.

In a good therapeutic relationship the clinician gives the client the opportunity to experience success whenever possible. The most successful therapeutic programs are those designed to support clients in moving step-by-step from what they can do to things that are more difficult, eventually culminating in accomplishing things that initially might have seemed beyond the client's capabilities. If clients are asked to do things that are too difficult and that result in failure, clients are likely to terminate therapy rather than continue what, to them, is an unpleasant experience. Moreover, when clients set their own goals, they are more likely to want to reach them.

To maximize the opportunities for clients to experience success, clinicians must be sensitive to cultural differences in **learning style.** A strategy that tends to work well with white middle-class clients may not work with people from nonwhite cultures. To learn more about cultural differences in learning style, see Terrell and Hale (1992).

Successful therapeutic relationships are based on a **contract** between client and clinician. The contract (which may actually be written) specifies the obligations each agrees to assume in the relationship. The clinician promises to contribute his or her time and expertise, and the client promises to follow through on the clinician's recommendations for reaching his or her goals, which have been determined through collaboration between client and clinician. See

Study More 14.2 — The Placebo Effect

The traditional but unsatisfactory definition of the word placebo usually limits its meaning to inert or inactive drugs. In recent years the definition has been expanded...I would define it as any therapeutic procedure (or that component of any therapeutic procedure) which is given deliberately to have an effect, or unknowingly has an effect on a patient, symptom, syndrome, or disease, but which objectively without specific activity for the condition being treated...The placebo effect is defined as the changes produced by placebos.

The doctor's [clinician's] relationship to the patient [client] is basic to an understanding of the placebo effect. The interested doctor who imparts confidence, who is friendly and reassuring to patients, who performs a thorough examination, and who is not anxious, conflicted, or guilty about the patient or his treatment is more likely to elicit positive placebo reactions...Negative placebo reactions are more likely when the doctor is angry, rejecting, and contemptuous toward patients or seriously preoccupied with his own problems...Cures may occur when the patient per-

ceives the physician's strong needs for the patient to improve, and does so in order to gratify the doctor...

The doctor's attitude toward his treatment is an ingredient compounded into every prescription. Many studies have demonstrated that attitudes toward, faith and belief in, enthusiasms for, and bias about a particular treatment increase the effectiveness of placebos and of specific treatments.

[Faith is also basic to the placebo effect.] The importance of faith is reflected in the fact that one of the major, best educated, religious groups in the United States is able to deny the rational efficacy of any treatment or medicine, and to assign all treatment benefits to faith. When vague, but frequently mentioned, terms like warmth, trust, confidence, and faith in the doctor and in the treatment, the expectation and anticipation of relief, previous experience with doctors, knowledge and experience, and fame and popularity of a treatment, are coupled with the patient's magic expectation, we get back to the important elements in the doctor-patient relationship.

From "Factors Contributing to the Placebo Effect: Their Implications for Psychotherapy," by A. K. Shapiro, 1964, *American Journal of Psychotherapy, 18*(Supplement 1), pp. 73–88. © 1964 by the Association for the Advancement of Psychotherapy. Reprinted with permission.

Study More 14.3 on page 242 for further insights into the client's responsibilities in the rehabilitation process.

Finally, a good therapeutic relationship is one in which the clinician is willing to share experiences and feelings with the client if the clinician perceives this would benefit the client and encourage the client's reciprocal sharing. The use of life experience stories (described on pages 244–245) is one way for the clinician to share experiences and feelings with the client.

Sharing life experiences is one reason why **support groups** for persons who have a particular problem (e.g., Lost Chord clubs, the Learning Disabilities Association of America, or the National Stuttering Association) can be very helpful to those with similar experiences and communication needs. To learn more about the attributes of a good therapeutic relationship, see Study More 14.4 on page 243.

ASHA's website (2005i) contains a helpful article on the importance and ethics of maintaining confidentiality with colleagues (e.g., fellow SLPs). And the University of Michigan Health System website (2005) includes a worthwhile description of how to enhance your cultural communication skills. Although the focus in this material is on the physician-patient relationship, most of the content is relevant for SLPs and audiologists.

Support group
A group of people having a particular disability who support each other's attempts to cope with it. Members of such a group may communicate mainly face-to-face or online.

Variables That Influence a Clinical Relationship

Several variables affect the therapeutic relationship. A clinician's success at being helpful to a client is likely to be determined as much (or possibly even more) by the client as by the clinician's knowledge of therapeutic techniques. The clinician's beliefs, needs, and motivation also

	The Client as
Study More 14.3	Comanager in Rehabilitation

The effectiveness of rehabilitation, whether it involves physical, vocational, or emotional adjustment, depends largely upon the degree to which the client has made the plan his own. Barring special circumstances, this support on the part of the client in the long run is enhanced when he takes an active part in decision-making; it is often weakened when he feels that his life is being manipulated behind the scenes, even when it is by the experts who know best "where he is to go and how he is to get there."

The worker-client relationship tends to be an asymmetrical one in which the professional person has the higher status position. Just as in the case of doctor and patient, lawyer and client, or teacher and pupil the disabled person may easily feel in a dependent position in which it is hoped that the wisdom of the worker will guide him through his difficulties. But it is just such an atmosphere of a wise and powerful one, on the one hand, and a dependent, suppliant one on the other hand, that so easily can nourish the feelings of inadequacy and personal inferiority that true rehabilitation seeks to avoid. The inner strength and self-respect which we wish to build in the client grows in a relationship in which the disabled person feels that he has an important role in planning his life and that what he says and what he feels is respected... Even a disabled child needs to have a feeling that he knows what is happening to him and why,

that he has a choice in the decisions. How much more true this is of the person who has reached adulthood with all the independence of judgment and self-determination that this implies.

To repeat: Inner strength and self-respect grow in a relationship which the person feels that he has an important role in planning his life and that what he says and what he feels are regarded as important.

Motivation to make the plan work is the second important reason for stressing the participation of the adult in the evolving as well as the executing of the rehabilitation program... When the client feels that he had little to do with the plan in the first place, it is all too easy for him to dissipate his energies in minor complaints. He is less apt to be ready to make personal adjustments as required by new and sometimes disagreeable circumstances than when he has been a participant in mapping out the rehabilitation course...

A third consideration is the fact that our fund of knowledge is often not sufficiently exact to enable the counselor to know which course of action is best for the client. On these grounds alone it would seem desirable to allow for the views and intentions of the client.

From *Physical Disability—A Psychological Approach* (pp. 346–347), by B. A. Wright, 1960, New York: Harper and Row. © 1960 by Harper and Row. Reprinted with permission.

Evaluation
The initial step in the intervention process. Its purpose is to determine if the client has a communication disorder and, if so, to identify and describe the impairments, disabilities, and handicaps that it has caused or placed the client at risk for developing.

play an important role in the relationship. At bottom, though, the model (or combination of models) the clinician uses to provide service will influence the relationship. Dr. Carl Rogers, a renowned psychotherapist, describes the basic elements of a therapeutic relationship in Study More 14.5 on page 244.

The Medical Model

For a long time, the **medical model** was the approach most frequently used by speech-language pathologists (SLPs) and audiologists. Using the medical model, the clinician diagnoses the communication disorder and designs and directs the intervention process, which is focused on remediating the disorder. This approach grew out of an effort from the profession of communication disorders to incorporate scientifically supported approaches to the diagnosis and remediation of communication disorders. As Duchan explains it, the medical model involves "synthesizing what is going on at the biological, psychological and social levels. Such a synthesis is offered by the causal logic of the medical model" (Duchan, 2001b, ¶8).

One of a clinician's first tasks is establishing a therapeutic relationship with the client and/or with one or more significant others (e.g., a parent, spouse, partner, child, or classroom teacher). From the perspective of the medical model, the therapeutic relationship is different from other relationships in six ways. First, there is a predetermined time frame during which it can take place. An **evaluation** or therapy session is expected to begin and end at a prearranged

| Study More 14.4 | **The Clinician's Skill** |

Although the client's perception that he can trust the integrity of the therapist is basic, he also needs a clinician who can understand him deeply. Some of my clients have felt terribly alienated from society; most of them have felt helplessly alone far too often. It is always difficult to know another person, but I have found repeatedly that many of my mistakes were due to my insensitivity to the client's needs and feelings.

Clinicians must also learn how to arouse hope. It is a very powerful motivating force. The client cannot have much hope if the clinician has little. Somehow I've always been able to find enough favorable prognostic signs in the sorriest of my clients to believe that he can be helped, but you often have to hunt for these signs. You often have to blow hard on the embers before hope will flare.

All clinicians should also train themselves in the subtle skills that enable them to sense the hidden feelings of their clients. These are not to be found in textbooks or class-rooms. They must be mastered in the situations of intimate human encounter. Some of my students and clients have felt that I had an uncanny ability to read their thoughts—and at times I have indeed experienced something akin to clair-voyance—but only after I had observed and identified closely with the person long enough. I hate to give an example of this because it always sounds fraudulent. In any event, I do not feel that this ability is God- or devil-given. It is the result of very careful observation, uninhibited infer-ence making, and the calculation of probabilities. It comes through empathy.

Because the ability to understand another human being is so useful in therapy, I trained myself for many years to develop it in myself and in my students. I learned the skill of shadowing the speech of others, saying what they said at almost the same time they said it. First, I did this aloud when listening to speakers on the radio, then covertly when listening to others. I tried to match not only the words, but the tempo, voice inflections and pauses as well. One can also learn to "shadow" the gestures, postures, and move-ments of other people almost as actors do in learning a role.

I also worked hard to train myself in the psychothera-pist's art of reflecting—being able to express the real mean-ing of what your client is trying or wanting to say in your own words. I constantly tried to finish (covertly) the unfinished sentences that my client left hanging uncompleted so I might follow his chains of association. I endeavored to pre-dict his responses, to anticipate what he would do or say next. In short, I tried for the moment to be that other person. Oh, the failures that I had in this self-training—thousands of them—usually because I was out of tune, but the failures themselves led to more understanding. Of course, each new client presented a new problem in empathy, but grad-ually they became easier for me to read.

I do not wish to imply that my empathetic batting aver-age was ever very high; certainly it was never high enough to please me. Human beings are often hidden under many layers of veils and defenses. Moreover, they do not want these uncovered, lest they see themselves naked in the mir-ror of your eyes. (Because I respect these feelings I do my scanning as quietly and covertly as I can.) All I know is that when I have been completely unable to have any kind of close identification with a client, I have usually failed to help him, no matter what methods I used or how hard I tried.

From *A Career in Speech Pathology* (pp.107–108), by C. Van Riper, 1979, Englewood Cliffs, NJ: Prentice Hall. © 1979 by Prentice Hall. Reprinted with permission.

time on a prearranged day. The duration of the relationship is likely to be relatively short. In fact, the relationship may exist for only an hour or less (e.g., when an evaluation reveals that a child's speech or language development is within normal limits).

Second, the therapeutic relationship exists solely for accomplishing a specific task—eliminating or lessening the severity of the client's communication disorder. After the task is accomplished, or when further progress seems unlikely, the relationship is usually terminated.

Third, this relationship is not a symmetrical one—the parties play different roles. Metaphorically, the client usually plays the role of the person in need of care, and the clinician plays the role of care provider. For this reason, the client may develop a strong affection for the clinician. This situation can be helpful if handled appropriately by the clinician, because the client is more likely to do what the clinician recommends in order to please the clinician. On the other hand, the situation is less desirable if a clinician becomes overly emotionally attached to a client because the clinician is likely to lose some of the **objectivity** needed to be helpful to the client.

A fourth way the clinical relationship differs from others is that one party purchases the services of the other. The client either pays for the clinician's services or arranges for a third

Objectivity
Perceiving, documenting, and managing clients' impairments, disabilities, and handicaps without becoming emotionally involved and/or losing focus on the client's welfare.

Study More 14.5	Basic Elements of a Therapeutic Relationship

First is a warmth and responsiveness on the part of the counselor which makes rapport possible, and which gradually develops into a deeper emotional relationship. From the counselor's point of view, however, this is a definitely controlled relationship, an affectional bond with defined limits. It expresses itself in a genuine interest in the client and an acceptance of him as a person. The counselor frankly recognizes that he becomes to some extent emotionally involved in this relationship. He does not pretend to be superhuman and above the possibility of such involvement. He is sufficiently sensitive to the needs of the client, however, to control his own identification in order to serve best the person he is helping…

The second quality of a counseling relationship is its permissiveness in regard to expression of feeling. By the counselor's acceptance of his statements, by the complete lack of any moralistic or judgmental attitude, by the understanding attitude which pervades the counseling interview, the client comes to recognize that all feelings and attitudes may be expressed… In this respect the therapeutic relationship differs markedly from other relationships in ordinary life. It offers a place where the client may bring into the situation, as rapidly as his inhibitions will allow him, all the…unspoken attitudes which complicate his life.

While there is this complete freedom to express feelings, there are definite limits to action in the therapeutic interview, helping to give it a structure which the client can use in gaining insight into himself. These therapeutic limits are a third and an important aspect of the counseling situation. Take, for example, the matter of time. The client is free to keep an appointment or to break it, to come on time or to come late, to use the hour in idle talk in order to avoid his real problems, or to use it constructively. There is the limitation, however, that he is not free to control the counselor and gain more time, no matter by what subterfuge. Not infrequently the counselee waits until the last moments of the counseling hour to bring up some matter of vital importance, thus implicitly demanding more time. The small child is more direct about it and announces that he will stay two hours instead of one. The counselor is most wise, however, who holds to the essential time limits that have been set. The client can make much more effective use of a well-structured situation.

From *Counseling and Psychotherapy* (pp. 87–89), by C. R. Rogers, 1942, Boston, MA: Houghton Mifflin. © 1942 by Houghton Mifflin. Reprinted with permission.

Participation model
A clinical relationship characterized by client and clinician focusing on "what clients think about themselves, their abilities and accomplishments, their disabilities, and their future" (Duchan, 2003, ¶1).

party, such as a private or government insurance program (e.g., Medicare) or a school district, to make payment.

A fifth unique aspect of the therapeutic relationship is that only one party is expected to be concerned about the welfare of the other. The **Code of Ethics of the American Speech-Language-Hearing Association** obliges the clinician to hold paramount the welfare of persons served professionally (ASHA, 2005a). The client has no such obligation to the clinician.

A final unique aspect of this relationship is that only one party is obliged to treat as confidential what the other provides. ASHA's Code of Ethics (2005a) requires a clinician to treat as confidential all information that is received from a client or about a client from any source.

The Participation Model

As professionals in communication disorders have learned more about the nature of the clinical relationship and expanded the range of settings in which they interact with clients, clinicians (SLPs and audiologists alike) have developed an increasing awareness of other models that offer considerable insight into how we can best assist our clients in their daily lives (Duchan, 2001b). One model offered by Duchan is what she calls the **participation model,** in which the focus of the clinical relationship is not the communication disorder, but rather on who the client is as a person, how he or she experiences life, and what are his or her goals (Duchan, 2003). In this model, clients participate fully in the therapeutic process, select their intervention goals, plan the course of therapy, and evaluate their own progress in the context of their life outside the therapy setting.

The therapeutic relationship from the perspective of the participation model has four characteristics that distinguish it from other relationships. Clinicians using the participation model focus on: (1) what clients think about themselves; (2) clients' abilities and accomplishments; (3) clients' disabilities; and (4) clients' future (Duchan, 2003). The following are examples of participation models used by clinicians.

1. *Person-centered planning* allows the client to choose from among the many resources and tools offered by the clinician to determine the path he or she wishes to take during the intervention process.

2. *Client and clinician narratives* are used as a means for each to construct an ongoing life experience story that "charts" the therapeutic relationship. For the client, the story includes narrative regarding progress toward his or her goals. For the clinician, the story includes narrative regarding his or her participation in the client's story (Shields, 1997).

3. *Life inclusion intervention* emphasizes the therapeutic relationship as the care and support necessary for the client to be included in his or her community (Calculator & Jorgensen, 1994).

Duchan suggests that clinicians can best serve their clients by taking the best of both the medical and participation model. She advocates combining them in creative fashion to suit each client's unique needs and strengths.

The Clinician's Belief about the Cause of the Communication Disorder

The therapy program developed for a client should be based on the clinician's **hypotheses** about the cause(s) of the client's communication disorder, paired with the client's perceptions about the goals he or she believes would be best given his or her life experiences. These hypotheses are developed, in part, from the results of an initial evaluation, which is discussed in more detail in Chapter 15. A therapy program that is based on such hypotheses is more likely to be effective than one that is not.

These hypotheses also help the client and clinician develop realistic goals. The client's potential for improvement is likely to be partially determined by the etiology and severity of his or her communication disorder. If a child is unable to produce the /r/ phoneme correctly, the prognosis for improvement should be better if the reason is faulty learning rather than paralysis of the tongue.

Finally, the clinician's hypotheses can influence whether he or she will develop an intervention plan with the client or will refer the client to another practitioner. An SLP or audiologist is not the appropriate professional to treat some communication disorders. For instance, an adult who exhibits **hypernasality** because of **myasthenia gravis** should be treated by a neurologist because the **dysarthria** responsible for it often can be reduced by medication.

The Clinician's Needs

Clinicians have the same emotional needs as other people, including a need to be liked. However, clinicians must maintain their professional perspective and keep their own emotional

Hypotheses
In this context, preliminary explanations for clients' impairments, disabilities, and handicaps.

Positive reinforcement
A behavior modification technique to increase a desirable behavior with a reward. If a behavior is rewarded immediately after it occurs, it is said to have received response-contingent positive reinforcement.

Punishment
A technique for getting a behavior (e.g., interrupting) to occur less often by imposing something unpleasant on the client whenever the behavior appears.

Motivation
In this context, the willingness of the client to make the investments necessary to achieve therapy goals.

Goals
In this context, benefits the client hopes to derive from therapy.

needs out of the therapeutic process with their clients. This is not to say that clinicians must refrain from discussing feelings, fears, or perceptions. Rather, it means that the focus must remain on the clients and their communication needs and strengths.

Failure to act in a professional manner can impact negatively on the clinician's ability to help clients. For instance, they may hesitate recommending that clients do things that are not "fun," or they may not speak honestly to the client because they don't want to be disliked. Another possible professional pitfall is discussing one's personal problems with clients, which can lead to a role reversal in which clients function as clinicians and clinicians as clients.

Clinicians must constantly monitor their professional behavior, remembering that one of their primary goals is to promote the welfare of their clients. The therapeutic relationship must have at its center the client's communication needs and the steps that can be taken to assist them in their efforts to improve their communication abilities.

The Clinician's Approach to Modifying Behavior

The approach a clinician uses for modifying behavior can profoundly influence his or her interactions with clients. If a clinician usually modifies behavior by using **positive reinforcement,** his or her interactions with clients will tend to be different than if **punishment** is used. Responding positively to clients' behavior stems from the belief that people are inherently geared to improve, grow, and develop. Responding with punishment reflects a belief that "bad" behavior must be punished or it will continue to be exhibited. Most clinicians use positive reinforcement more often than punishment.

The Clinician's Ability to Motivate the Client

Clients are unlikely to change unless their **motivation** for change is strong. They will be unwilling to make the necessary investment unless they believe that doing it will be worth the sacrifice (i.e., will significantly improve the quality of their life). A clinician's ability to motivate a client is an important determiner of the benefit the client is likely to receive from therapy. One way a clinician can motivate clients is by helping them to identify **goals** that they are really interested in achieving. (See Miller, 1993b, for a description of some of the variables that influence people's motivation.)

A clinician can also motivate clients by making them aware of the progress they have made toward achieving their goals. Clients are more likely to continue investing in their therapy programs if they believe they are making real progress toward achieving such goals. A strategy that can be used for demonstrating that progress is occurring is described in Silverman (1980).

Helping the Client Believe Change Is Possible

Clients seeking therapy may not really believe they can change. They may, in fact, believe deep down that they cannot change. Clients who lack confidence in their ability to change are unlikely to do so. In addition, young children (and adolescents) often see no reason they should engage in activities that, from their perspective, lack relevance and meaning. In both these situations, the clinician must be able to communicate with the client in a way that results in the client understanding that the therapy activities lead to desired change.

Why might a client be certain he or she cannot change? One reason may be that previous therapy has been unsuccessful. The more often a client has experienced failure in a therapy experience, the more likely he or she will not believe change is possible. Similarly, children may have experienced therapy that was unpleasant or that took them away from what they perceive as more interesting. Or, like their adult counterparts, they may perceive previous therapy experiences as unsuccessful and be unwilling to participate further.

Here's an analogy that might help you understand how this situation might arise. Consider a change that you have tried to make at some time in your life (e.g., to lose weight by dieting). If your first diet was recommended by somebody you regarded as an authority on dieting, you probably began with a high degree of optimism. However, if your current diet is your fifth and you regarded the previous four as having been unsuccessful, you probably would not have begun this new diet with as much optimism as you did your first. You may, in fact, have begun it with the expectation (conscious or unconscious) that it would not work, and consequently you would be likely to go off it at the first indication that it was not working. Of course, going off your diet would result in your not losing weight, which, in turn, would reinforce your certainty that you are unable to lose weight by dieting.

When clients believe they cannot change, their clinician can play a major role in helping them change their mind. The best way is to help them change some aspect of their behavior so they can see they can change. While the aspect they change may not be a particularly important one, such a change can cause them to question their certainty that they cannot change—because they have just done it. If a client enters therapy with the certainty that it will not be effective, he or she is unlikely to change, regardless of the type and severity of the disorder, the skill of the clinician, or the management program used.

The clinician may have to engage in activities with which he or she knows the client will be successful, gradually introducing new tasks that are less familiar and more difficult. The key is to provide support throughout the therapeutic process so the client is taking small, successful steps rather than attempting a large one that could result in failure.

A clinician can cause a client to expect a therapy to be ineffective for another reason—by communicating a lack of confidence or competence. If the clinician communicates that he or she is bored, superior, or impatient, the client will surely get the message, regardless of what the clinician says. So, too, will the client if the clinician sincerely believes the client can make little or no progress, despite saying otherwise.

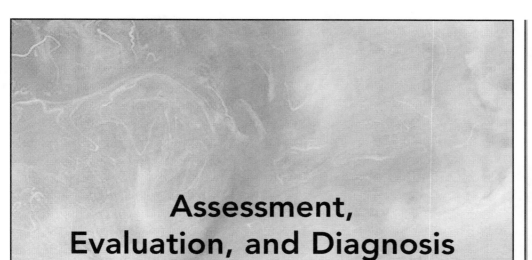

Assessment, Evaluation, and Diagnosis

Chapter 15

Learning Objectives

- Describe the clinical evaluation process.

- List the characteristics of appropriate, answerable questions.

- Describe three general approaches for making observations that answer evaluation questions.

- Describe how to ensure the validity of the data used to answer evaluation questions.

- Describe how to assess the reliability of the data used to answer evaluation questions.

- Describe the process of formulating and testing hypotheses.

- List six questions clinicians typically ask during an initial evaluation.

- List two questions typically asked during a reevaluation.

- Describe six types of standardized tests used during evaluation.

- Discuss how informal observations and interviewing informants contribute to the evaluation process.

Introduction

The **evaluation** process ordinarily both initiates and terminates intervention. It also occurs periodically throughout the course of intervention. This chapter describes how assessment and the decision-making process utilized for clinical evaluation lead to diagnosis (particularly **differential diagnosis),** which, in turn, leads to the design of appropriate intervention for individuals with communication disorders.

The Clinical Evaluation Process

The clinical evaluation process begins with the clinician asking certain **answerable questions** and making the observations necessary for answering them. From the answers to these questions, the clinician formulates and tests **hypotheses.** If these hypotheses seem invalid (i.e., not logical or reasonable) or if their validity is uncertain, the clinician reexamines the **observations** on which the hypotheses were based. Next, the clinician may ask and answer some additional questions based on the findings so far. Then, based upon what was learned from the answers to all these questions, the clinician reformulates and retests these hypotheses. The process is repeated until the clinician is satisfied that the hypotheses are sufficiently valid for planning intervention. This process is diagramed in Figure 15.1 on page 252 and is described in the following sections.

Asking Answerable Questions

The clinical evaluation process is initiated by asking appropriate, answerable questions. The term *answerable* in this context has a particular meaning. Questions are viewed as answerable if (1) they can be answered by making observations and (2) they specify the observations that have to be made to answer them. Consider the following question: "How well does my client, who has aphasia, understand speech?"

This question is answerable because it can be answered by making certain observations, and it specifies the observations that have to be made to answer it. In this case, the necessary observations would be those that provide information about the client's ability to understand speech. The following question, on the other hand, does not appear to be answerable based on how the term has been defined here: "How well will my client, who has aphasia, understand speech in two years?"

Although this question specifies the observations needed to answer it, there is no way to make them (unless one is a clairvoyant or has the ability to travel in time). However, the question can be addressed by making a prediction (i.e., prognosis) based on past experience—not the same thing as answering it, however. For further information about what constitutes an answerable question, see Study More 15.1 on page 253.

The specific questions a clinician will seek to answer during an evaluation are determined by the purpose of the evaluation. Some specific questions that may be asked include the following:

- Is the client's hearing for pure tones within normal limits?

- Why hasn't the client, who is 4 years old, begun to say words?

Differential diagnosis
A process for distinguishing between two or more conditions with similar characteristics by systematically comparing and contrasting their characteristics with clinical findings.

Answerable question
A question that can be answered by making observations and that indicates (directly or indirectly) the observations that have to be made to answer it.

Observations
The data used to answer the questions that an evaluation is intended to answer.

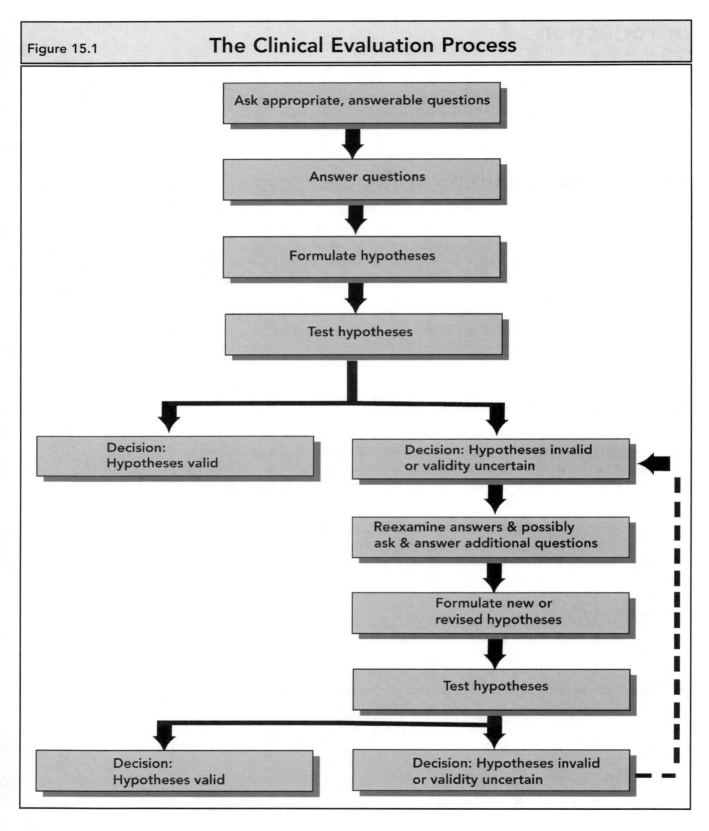

Figure 15.1

The Clinical Evaluation Process

Ask appropriate, answerable questions

Answer questions

Formulate hypotheses

Test hypotheses

Decision: Hypotheses valid

Decision: Hypotheses invalid or validity uncertain

Reexamine answers & possibly ask & answer additional questions

Formulate new or revised hypotheses

Test hypotheses

Decision: Hypotheses valid

Decision: Hypotheses invalid or validity uncertain

Study More 15.1 — The Ordeal of Asking Questions

"How much snush is there in ten tons of slerv?"

The lesson to be learned by staring at this "question" for a few moments is simple but fundamental: it is that the first principle of befuddlement lies in using words unclearly.

This being true, it follows that the surest way to get a clear answer is to ask a clear question. Only a fool who needs a psychiatrist—and possibly the psychiatrist he needs—could tell us what "snush" or "slerv" might mean in the above question. If for you these "words" are simply blanks, that is a good sign. If, on the other hand, you seriously wonder how much snush there really is in ten tons of slerv, your nearest of kin should be notified at once.

All this is, of course, too obvious to labor. One might not be quite as certain, however, as to what would be a sensible reaction to such a question as this: "What is the unpardonable sin?"

For most people it is quite likely that this question would create far more confusion than the previous one. The "snush" question would usually have little, if any effect; it would simply be dismissed as silly. This question as to what is the unpardonable sin, however, is more likely to be taken seriously. It seems to be about something real. It contains only standard English words, commonly used. It has a question mark at the end. It looks very much like hundreds of other questions that people ask—and seem to answer—every day. Most people might not feel sure they know the answer to it, but many would. Very few would doubt for a moment that there is a correct answer to the question, if only the man who knows it or the book that contains it might be found. It would be a rare and very wise person who would ask, "What does the question mean on the level of not-words, the level of observation and experience? That is, precisely what factual observations might I or anyone else make in order to answer it?"

If there is abroad in the land the one more great teacher mankind so desperately needs, surely he is telling us, among much else, that if the one who asks a question cannot indicate at least roughly how the factual observations needed to answer it are to be made, he has asked no question at all.

From *People in Quandaries* (pp. 52–53), by W. Johnson, 1946, New York: Harper & Brothers © 1946 by Harper & Brothers.

- Is the client more likely to understand a spoken or written message?

- Under what circumstances does the client avoid speaking?

- Does the client appear to fatigue easily?

- How concerned does the client appear to be about her syllable and word repetitions?

Plateau
A period during which the client makes no measurable progress toward achieving a therapy goal.

Although some of these questions are not all related directly to a client's speech, hearing, or language functions, the answers to them could directly affect how his or her case is managed and the type, length, and frequency of intervention sessions. If, for example, a client fatigues easily, the clinician might need to keep therapy sessions relatively short.

In addition to questions that are intended to define a client's communication disorder, others are asked after a period of therapy to determine how well a client is progressing. These include the following:

- How much reduction (if any) has there been in the severity of the client's stuttering?

- Does the client ask questions in class more frequently than before?

- Has the client learned to produce the /r/ sound correctly at the beginning of words?

- Have the client's parents accepted sign language being taught to their child?

- How well does the client understand speech with the hearing aid he or she is currently using?

- Has the client reached a **plateau,** or is improvement likely to occur with further therapy?

Chief complaint
The reason given by the client (or the person who requested the evaluation) indicating why the evaluation was requested.

Representative
Data that is consistent across situations (e.g., home, school, work).

How does a clinician decide which questions are appropriate for a particular evaluation? This decision is based partly on the client's **chief complaint.** However, certain questions are asked routinely, no matter what type of communication disorder the client has (e.g., Is the client's pure tone hearing within normal limits?).

The answers to both the routine and the specific questions are likely to suggest additional ones. Also, a clinician will routinely ask certain questions when assessing the impacts of intervention on a client. These questions will relate mostly to what the intervention was intended to accomplish and how the client responded throughout.

Answering Questions

After the initial set of questions has been selected, the clinician attempts to answer them. Because the answers are likely to suggest additional questions, the clinician will probably be formulating new questions while answering the original ones. Consequently, two of the tasks in the evaluation process (asking and answering questions) may be performed simultaneously.

How do clinicians answer questions? They make observations they hope will yield data that are **valid, reliable,** and **representative** of the client's functioning.

The validity of the data used to answer a question is determined by the appropriateness of the observations that yielded it for doing so. If a clinician makes observations that are appropriate for answering a question, the data yielded by them are likely to be adequately valid for the purpose. Suppose a clinician wanted to answer the question: "Does my client have a hearing loss?" Valid data for answering this question would be yielded by a **pure-tone** hearing test.

The reliability of the data used to answer a question is determined by the repeatability, or consistency of the observations that yielded it. If a clinician makes observations in a manner that can be repeated, the data yielded by them should be adequately reliable for the purpose. If an audiologist tests a client's hearing with a **pure-tone audiometer** that has not been **calibrated,** the reliability of the data yielded by the test will be uncertain. That is, the results might be different at a different time or with a different audiometer.

The representativeness of the data used to answer a question determines if the same answer will be given in other situations (e.g., home, school, work). If a clinician makes observations that are representative of those needed for answering a question, the data yielded by them should possess some generality. Suppose an SLP wanted to answer the following question: "How severe is a child's language disorder?" If the clinician observes the client at home as well as in school, the generality of the answer will be greater because the clinician will have gathered data from more than one context in which the child uses language.

Clinicians use three general approaches for making the observations needed to answer questions: (1) administering tests, (2) completing informal observations, and (3) interviewing informants.

Administering Tests

One approach that SLPs and audiologists utilize to generate the data they need to answer questions is to administer standardized tests. A wide variety of standardized test instruments is available for evaluating communication disorders. The following sections describes six basic types.

Audiometric Tests

The two most common audiometric tests are **pure-tone** audiometric testing and **tympanometry.** Pure-tone audiometric tests are used to assess the acuity sensitivity of a client's ears. They can detect disturbances in the functioning of the outer, middle, or inner portions of an ear, as well as the auditory nerve. Pure tones of various frequencies are presented at various loudness levels through earphones by an electronic instrument known as a **pure-tone audiometer.** (See Figure 11.1 on page 193.)

One type of pure-tone audiometric test is referred to as an **audiometric screening test**, which is used to determine whether a client's hearing acuity needs further testing. Pure tones of various frequencies are presented to one ear at a time (through earphones) at a loudness level that, though soft, can be heard by most people. Clients are told to raise their hand when they hear a tone. If they consistently respond when tones are presented and refrain from responding when no tones are presented, they pass the test. Otherwise, they fail the test and are usually given a complete audiometric assessment.

Tympanometry is the method used to detect disorders of the middle ear. Air pressure in the eustachian tube is varied to test the condition and mobility of the tympanic membrane. Tympanometry is typically used to check for these conditions:

- Fluid in the middle ear

- Perforated tympanic membrane

- Impacted cerumen

- Scarring of the tympanic membrane (usually from infection)

- Lack of contact between the ossicles

- A tumor in the middle ear

Language Tests for Children

Clinicians use tests to assess children's functioning across the areas of language development described in Chapter 4. Most language tests are standardized on a large number of children from across the United States who reflect the most current demographic statistics of the United States Census Bureau. Scores are collected from all types of children, which makes them representative of a wide range of children from all areas of the United States. In addition, valid and reliable tests can be used with confidence that they measure what they say they measure and that they will consistently measure the same thing, regardless of who administers the test or when it is administered.

Clinicians use language tests in order to determine whether a child has a general language disorder that crosses form, content, and use, or whether the child has a language disorder in one specific area. The most commonly used language tests assess children's abilities in the following areas:

- Vocabulary (comprehension and production)

- Syntax and morphology (comprehension and production)

Audiometric screening test
A brief pure-tone audiometric hearing test that is used to identify clients whose hearing may not be within normal limits. Those who fail it usually receive a complete hearing evaluation.

- Phonology

- Pragmatics

- Auditory processing

- Written language

If a child scores below average on a battery of language tests, one of the primary questions the clinician must ask is whether the scores reflect an actual language disorder or a language difference arising from English as the child's nonnative language. Children whose language abilities are different purely as a result of not knowing English well enough to score well, do not have a communication disorder. Most children in this situation are well able to learn language skills given appropriate support and instruction, while children with language disorders usually require intensive and specific intervention aimed at remediating their deficient language skills.

Language Tests for Adults

Adult language disorders usually stem from brain damage related to stroke, tumor, trauma, and/or **degenerative** disease. The language tests used with adults differ from those used with children in that adult instruments focus on how intact the person's language abilities are following the brain damage, while the tests used with children assess primarily developmental language abilities. Most standardized tests for adults with brain damage assess the following:

- Articulation

- Fluency

- Word-finding

- Repetition

- Grammar

- Auditory comprehension

- Reading

- Writing

- Visual-motor ability

- Spelling

In addition to **standardized assessments**, many SLPs use functional communication assessment tools, which are often less biased than standardized tests in evaluating clients from linguistically and/or culturally diverse backgrounds. Functional assessments usually assess the following:

- Telling time

- Using verbal and nonverbal contexts in communicating

- Role playing

- Observing social conventions (i.e., pragmatics)

- Understanding and using humor, metaphors, and absurdities

- Understanding and using number concepts

Articulation Tests

Articulation tests enable clinicians to both identify and inventory a client's articulation errors (i.e., sound omissions, substitutions, and distortions) at the beginning, middle, and end of words. (See Chapter 8 for information about disorders of articulation.) One type is the picture articulation test, which is used mostly with young children. The child is shown a series of drawings or photographs, as shown in Figure 15.2, and asked to name the objects depicted in them. Their names contain each English phoneme at least once at the beginning of a word (initial position), at the end of a word (final position), and in the middle of a word (medial position). The clinician indicates on a form whether the **target phoneme** was produced correctly and, if it was not, the type of error made. The resulting error inventory is used both for setting therapy goals and as a **baseline** for evaluating therapy effectiveness.

Tests of Motor Functioning

Motor functioning tests are used for assessing the functioning of the muscles used for respiration, phonation, and articulation. These tests provide the data necessary for determining

Articulation test
A test, usually consisting of a set of stimulus drawings or words, that is used to identify and inventory a client's articulation errors.

Target phoneme
The phoneme that a drawing or word in an articulation test is intended to elicit.

Figure 15.2	**Example Articulation Test Stimuli**

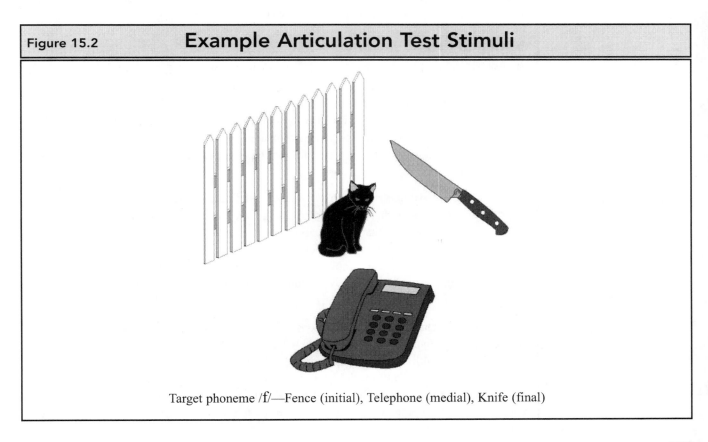

Target phoneme /f/—Fence (initial), Telephone (medial), Knife (final)

Diadochokinetic rate
The number of times in five seconds a client is able to repeat a specific consonant-vowel syllable. Used to test for neuromuscular disorders.

Aphasia test
A test used to identify language deficits that can result from damage to the cerebral cortex, particularly the left half.

whether the musculature is adequate to support the production of normal speech. A client who fails any of these tests may have a neuromuscular disorder.

One motor functioning test that is used with both children and adults is the determination of **diadochokinetic rates** for certain consonant-vowel syllables (e.g., the initial consonant and vowel in the word tub). The number of times the client is able to repeat the syllable in five seconds is compared to that of persons his or her age who are not neurologically impaired. Relatively low diadochokinetic rates (e.g., less than one repetition per second) suggest that the functioning of at least one articulator is not adequate to support the production of normal speech.

Tests of Attitude

Attitude tests can provide some insight into the nature of a client's attitude toward his or her communication disorder. Some contain statements similar to the following:

- A student with a communication disorder should not ask questions in class.

  Strongly Agree   Moderately Agree   Undecided   Moderately Disagree   Strongly Disagree

- A person should be embarrassed if he has a communication disorder.

  Strongly Agree   Moderately Agree   Undecided   Moderately Disagree   Strongly Disagree

The client responds to each statement by circling the words that best describe his or her reaction to it. If the responses are honest, they can provide considerable insight into the degree to which the client is handicapped by having the communication disorder.

Informal Observations

Gathering informal observations entails collecting the data needed to answer questions by observing relevant behaviors in natural contexts rather than by eliciting them in a testing context. For example, to identify and inventory a client's articulation errors, you could tape record a conversation with the client and later listen to the recording to abstract relevant information from it. Another example would be videotaping a child playing with his or her parent in order to determine mean length of utterance, different types of pragmatic intentions used, and types of words used in expressive language.

Informal observations have both advantages and disadvantages compared with administering standardized tests. Perhaps the main advantage of utilizing data samples that were gathered by informal observation is that they are more likely to reflect how a client typically communicates in his or her environment than when data samples are elicited by a test. Perhaps the main disadvantage of utilizing data samples that were generated by indirect observation rather than by testing is that this approach may be considerably more time consuming. This would, for example, tend to be the case for identifying and inventorying articulation errors.

On the other hand, for some questions, answering by informal observation is usually less time consuming than testing. An example would be the following: "Does a person with aphasia have a deficit in his ability to understand speech?" Having an informal conversation with the person would be likely to yield an answer as accurate as administering an **aphasia test.** However, the following question would probably be best answered through the use of a standardized test: "How impaired is the client's ability to understand speech?" Test data collected from a standardized instrument would be more likely than informal observation to yield an accurate estimate.

Data generated by informal observation are inherently neither more nor less objective (i.e., valid and reliable) than those generated by testing. However, depending on the question that is being addressed, data gathered through informal observation may be more or less valid and/or reliable than that generated by testing. The type of data that should be used to answer a question is the type most likely to yield an accurate answer.

Interviewing Informants

Clinicians interview **informants** (e.g., family members, teachers, other professionals) when they appear likely to have relevant information about the client. The type of data that can be collected from interviews ranges from developmental history and background of the communication disorder to current communication functioning in everyday life. Interviews can be performed live between clinician and interviewee or through interview checklists that are completed by the informant(s). As with informal observation data, the data collected by interviewing informants is neither more nor less valid and reliable than that generated by testing. Again, however, the data are only as useful as the questions asked in the interviewing process. For additional information about the relevance of such data for preschool children, see Study More 15.2.

All three of the above approaches (i.e., tests, observations, and interviews) may be utilized for making the observations needed to answer a question. Suppose an audiologist wanted to answer the question: "How well does a child's hearing aid compensate for his or her hearing loss?" To answer this question, the audiologist is likely to administer one or more hearing tests, informally observe how well the child seems to understand what is said while wearing the hearing aid, and question the child's parent about how well the child seems to understand what is said at home while wearing it.

All data yielded by such observations are unlikely to be given equal weight for answering questions. Some are likely to be regarded as having greater validity, reliability, and generality

Informants
In this context, people (including clients) who have information needed to answer a clinician's evaluation questions.

Study More 15.2	Reactive versus Proactive Approaches to Evaluation for Preschool Children

The relevance of getting input data from parents when evaluating preschool children is spelled out here.

Too often clinicians are reactive in their evaluations and also in recommendations to families. That is, clinicians respond in a predictable manner, carrying out assessment protocols that they usually use for all preschool children, identifying the problems and developing plans for the resolution of the problems. Although this process has worked in the past it frequently is less than ideal.

In contrast, a proactive approach to the evaluation and management of the preschool child encourages the parents' questions and considers the information provided by the parents as an integral part of both the assessment process and the intervention planning. Such an approach not only encourages input and questions from the family, but also uses the 'family perspective' to interpret and integrate assessment results. Dependence upon isolated instances of evaluation when designing an intervention plan, results in failure to recognize the dynamic nature of assessment and treatment. A proactive approach facilitates parental input at multiple levels and seeks parental involvement in problem identification and resolution. Active collaboration between professionals and families leads to mutually desired goals and likely success instead of failure to meet expectations.

From "Managing the Language and Learning Needs of the Communication-Impaired Preschool Child: A Proactive Approach," by P. A. Prelock, 1993, *Clinics in Communication Disorders, 3*(1), p. 2. © 1993 by Clinics in Communication Disorders. Reprinted with permission.

for the purpose than are others. The more valid and reliable the data used for answering a question, the more confidence a clinician can have in the accuracy of the answer.

Formulating Hypotheses

After the clinician's questions have been answered, the next task during an initial evaluation is to use the information obtained to formulate hypotheses about the etiology and severity of the client's communication disorder. If it is an ongoing evaluation, the next task would be to assess the impact that the therapy program had on the disorder. An example of such a hypothesis follows: "Based upon the information I currently have available, the most likely explanation for the problem that the client is having understanding speech is a conductive hearing loss."

The phrase "based upon the information I currently have available," suggests an important characteristic of such hypotheses: they always are viewed as tentative and subject to change as new information becomes available. New information may make it necessary to revise or abandon a hypothesis. Of course, it can also support a hypothesis.

An example of a hypothesis about the impact of a therapy program on a client follows: "Based upon the information I currently have available, the program has increased the severity of the client's stuttering."

Although few clinicians would welcome such an outcome, it is important to be aware when it happens so that the program can be modified to be more effective. Hypotheses concerning therapy outcome, like those concerning etiology, are always viewed as tentative and subject to change whenever new information becomes available.

Testing Hypotheses

After the hypothesis has been formulated, it is tested. The approach clinicians use depends on whether the hypothesis deals with etiology or therapy outcome.

Testing hypotheses about the etiology of a client's disorder involves determining whether the hypotheses allow the clinician to make accurate predictions about the disorder's symptoms and characteristics. That is, if a hypothesis about the etiology of a client's communication disorder is accurate, it should predict how the client's symptoms will vary under certain conditions. If, for example, an audiologist hypothesized that a client doesn't comprehend speech normally because of a conductive hearing loss caused by a bacterial infection, he or she would predict that antibiotics would improve the client's comprehension. If the client's comprehension improved under this condition (i.e., using antibiotics), the clinician's hypothesis would be supported. The clinician could also make other predictions about how the client's hearing would vary if the cause was a conductive hearing loss resulting from otitis media and check to see if the hearing varied in the predicted way(s).

A second type of prediction deals with the impact of intervention. If the hypothesis about the etiology of the disorder is accurate, it should allow the effect of intervention on the disorder to be predicted (assuming both that the disorder is treatable and other variables, such as a lack of motivation, are not impeding improvement).

The intervention program a clinician develops for a client should be based on the clinician's assumptions about the cause of the client's communication disorder. The alternative—using the same intervention for all people who have a particular disorder, regardless of its cause—is not acceptable because it is unlikely to be effective.

Testing hypotheses about therapy outcome involves determining what the available data indicate about differences (if any) between a client's current status and his or her status during the earlier evaluation period that serves as a baseline. Conclusions about program effectiveness are, in fact, hypotheses of this type, comparisons between baseline and periodic assessments of current status.

A clinician can reach one of three conclusions about the validity of a hypothesis. If the available data clearly supported it, the hypothesis would tentatively be regarded as valid. If the available data clearly appeared to refute it, the hypothesis would tentatively be regarded as invalid. And if the available data neither unequivocally supported nor refuted it, its validity would tentatively be regarded as uncertain.

Even when the clinician concludes that a hypothesis seems to be valid, the evaluation process does not stop. It is always possible that something may be learned in the future that is not consistent with the hypothesis. If this happens, the clinician will need to reconsider the conclusion that the hypothesis is valid.

If the clinician concludes that a hypothesis is invalid or that its validity is uncertain, the evaluation process continues in the manner shown in Figure 15.1 on page 252 and described in the next paragraph.

Reexamining Hypotheses

When a clinician judges a hypothesis to be invalid or of uncertain validity, he or she must reexamine the data on which it is based and decide whether the hypothesis is the only possible one that could be consistent with the data. The clinician must also decide whether additional data are needed to make this decision. If so, the clinician may formulate new questions and/or collect additional data relevant to ones that were already asked. This process of reexamining answers; asking and answering questions; and formulating and revising hypotheses will be repeated until the formulation of a hypothesis that appears to be valid is achieved.

Questions Clinicians Ask during an Initial Evaluation

The clinical evaluation process for an initial evaluation, which was summarized in the preceding paragraphs, begins with the asking of one or more answerable questions. This section clarifies what is meant by an answerable question by examining some of the more common questions SLPs and audiologists ask themselves and attempt to answer during an evaluation.

Normal limits
Statistically expected range within which a person's speech, hearing, and/or language abilities fall.

Developmental norms
Ages by which specific percentages of children in a given subpopulation have acquired particular abilities.

World Health Organization (WHO)
The agency of the United Nations that has healthcare as its primary focus.

Impairment
The failure to function normally. (In our context, the anomaly in hearing, speech, and/or language exhibited by the client.)

Disability
Something that an impairment prevents an individual from doing normally (e.g., a person who is deaf is highly unlikely to be able to communicate normally by telephone).

Handicap
Limitations that people impose on themselves because of their negative attitudes (e.g., shame, guilt, and/or embarrassment) toward their impairments and disabilities.

Are the Client's Speech, Language, and Hearing within Normal Limits?

This is the first question SLPs and audiologists seek to answer during an evaluation. They do not necessarily assume that people referred to them for an evaluation have a speech, language, or hearing disorder. Some of them will have speech, language, and hearing that are within **normal limits.** For example, a three-year-old whose parents are concerned that she isn't saying speech sounds correctly may be having difficulty producing the voiced and voiceless "th" sounds. Because many three-year-olds do not produce these sounds correctly, her ability to produce speech sounds (i.e., articulation) can be judged to be within normal limits.

To determine whether a client's speech, language, and hearing are within normal limits, relevant aspects are compared to accepted norms. For children, these would be **developmental norms.** Such norms specify the maximum age by which a child can exhibit a particular error (e.g., producing the /r/ sound incorrectly) and not be regarded as having a disorder.

Determining whether a particular aspect of behavior is within normal limits is somewhat arbitrary because it is determined by the percentage of the population labeled "abnormal." For instance, different states define "normal limits" differently, which affects the total number of children who qualify for special education services. Some states define "abnormal" more strictly than others, which means they have fewer special education students than states that define "abnormal" less strictly. Even though a clinician may determine that a child has a language disorder, whether the child qualifies for services through the school system depends on how the state defines "abnormal."

Unfortunately, there is no accepted standard for the percentage of children that it is appropriate to label "abnormal." Most clinicians use standardized assessments and/or procedures to help them make this decision. These instruments and/or procedures have been carefully standardized on a large population of people with similar speech, language, and/or hearing characteristics.

Is the Client at Risk for Developing a Disorder?

Although a client may not be judged to have a speech, language, or hearing disorder at the time of the evaluation, he or she may appear to be at greater than ordinary risk for developing one. When the clinician arrives at this conclusion, he or she has an ethical responsibility to do whatever possible to minimize the risk. If, for example, a client who works in a very noisy environment is given a hearing test and found to have hearing within normal limits, that client would, nevertheless, be at greater than ordinary risk for developing a noise-induced hearing loss. Consequently, some recommendations for hearing conservation would be warranted.

What Are the Characteristics of Impairment, Disability, and Handicap?

The **World Health Organization (WHO)** has suggested that, for purposes of rehabilitation, clients' disorders be viewed in three ways: (1) **impairments,** (2) **disabilities,** and (3) **handicaps.** If, for example, a client has a moderately severe sensorineural hearing loss, the hearing loss would be an impairment. If the hearing loss is severe enough to prevent the person from using a telephone, the inability to communicate in this way would be a disability. And if the person avoids parties and other social situations because of embarrassment about being hard-of-hearing, this avoidance of social situations would be a handicap.

If a client's communication behavior was judged not to be within normal limits, the clinician would attempt to describe the ways it deviated from normal, as well as any ways that it disabled and/or handicapped the client. The clinician would do this by making appropriate observations (i.e., by administering tests, observing the client informally, and/or interviewing informants). The resulting inventory of the client's communication impairments, disabilities, and handicaps would then be used to select goals for therapy.

Preventing or minimizing the development of disabilities and handicaps is usually easier than eliminating them or reducing their severity after they occur. Consequently, if an inventory of a client's communication impairments, disabilities, and handicaps indicates that the disorder is accompanied by disabilities and/or handicaps, a management goal should be to minimize the extent of the disabilities and/or handicaps. More important, perhaps, than waiting to determine whether the impairment has progressed to a disability and/or handicap would be for the clinician to provide proactive therapeutic intervention designed to prevent such a progression.

What Is the Cause of the Behaviors Constituting the Communication Disorder?

Once a client's communication impairments, disabilities, and/or handicaps have been identified, the next step is to formulate a tentative hypothesis for the cause of each in order to design appropriate and effective therapy. If, for example, a clinician assumed that a client is having difficulty understanding speech because of a hearing loss, intervention would be different from that designed for a client whose communication disorder was caused by receptive **aphasia.**

A clinician may have to perform a differential diagnosis before formulating a tentative hypothesis that describes the reason(s) a communication behavior deviates from normal. Making a differential diagnosis is a two-stage process. First, the clinician identifies all the possible reasons the communication behavior could deviate from normal in the ways it does. Second, the clinician systematically rules out as many of these reasons as possible. Ideally, this process will result in the elimination of all but one, which would be tentatively regarded as being the explanation for the behavior deviating from normal.

For a differential diagnosis to yield the "real" reason for a disorder or abnormal behavior, all possible reasons for it must be considered. If even one possibility is not considered, the diagnosis yielded by the process could be inaccurate.

To illustrate the differential diagnostic process, suppose that an adult client was reported to be having difficulty understanding speech. The following are some possible reasons that would have to be considered:

- Conductive hearing loss

- Sensorineural hearing loss

- Auditory nerve dysfunction

- Auditory agnosia

Educationally significant
Regarding eligibility for service in the schools, a speech, language, or hearing disorder that significantly interferes with a child's academic progress and cannot be adequately addressed through general education accommodations and modifications.

- Receptive aphasia

- Receptive language disorder

- Reduced auditory memory span

- Slow processing of auditory information

- Difficulty processing abstract information

- Feigning

- Severe depression

- Frequent petit mal seizures

- Frequent severe fatigue

- Schizophrenia

The information needed to rule some of these reasons in or out could be gleaned from testing; for others, it could be gathered from informal observation; and for still others it could be obtained from interviews with informants. There may, of course, be other reasons for a client not responding normally to speech sounds.

Is There Any Reason Why the Clinician Cannot or Should Not Provide Therapy?

Just because a client has a communication disorder does not necessarily mean that he or she is eligible to receive therapy. Eligibility is particularly likely to be a problem if someone other than the client or the client's family (i.e., a third party such as a school system or an insurance company) will be paying for it. To be eligible to receive therapy, the client may have to meet certain criteria, and the clinician will have to gather the data needed to document that the client meets the criteria (Ehren, 1993; Moore-Brown & Montgomery, 2001). In public schools, for example, children are eligible for services if their communication disorder is considered **educationally significant.** For a description of how data were gathered to document educational significance for a child who was being considered for discharge from therapy based on this criterion, see Gies-Zaborowski and Silverman, 1986.

The availability of funding is not the only legitimate reason for denying therapy to someone who has a communication disorder. Another is a lack of motivation. Almost all of the benefits that can be derived from therapy require a significant investment by the client and/or family. A prerequisite for clients making such an investment is motivation. Although a clinician should be able to generate the necessary motivation in a young child, in an older child or adult a clinician can usually do no more than reinforce the motivation the client already possesses. Consequently, an older child or adult must be intrinsically motivated to make the necessary investments of time, energy, and resources before beginning therapy. Otherwise, the client is unlikely to improve, and he or she may begin to develop uncertainty regarding progress. For further information about the development of such uncertainty, see Study More 15.3.

Study More 15.3	Unsuccessful Therapy Can Be Harmful

Stuttering therapy that is unsuccessful obviously does a little harm by wasting both the client's and clinician's time and somebody's money. Such harm, though regrettable, usually isn't serious enough to warrant discouraging a client from pursuing therapy. There is, however, a kind of harm that can result from unsuccessful stuttering therapy that is serious enough to warrant doing so—reinforcing the client's certainty that he or she can't change.

It is rarely justifiable to consider stuttering therapy successful unless the client changes in some way, at least a little. With a client who is an older child or adult, change is unlikely unless the client believes at a "gut level" that change is possible. If a client doesn't believe this or, worse yet, believes the opposite, a type of self-fulfilling prophecy is likely to be triggered that some psychologists refer to as a negative placebo effect.

Therapy that a client regards as having been unsuccessful can cause him or her to expect future therapy to be unsuccessful, thereby reducing the likelihood that future therapy will be successful. The more therapy experiences a client has had that he or she deems unsuccessful, the stronger the client's certainty of failure is likely to be.

A client will almost always have to make a substantial investment to benefit from therapy. The necessary investment will probably include an expenditure of time and energy between therapy sessions. And it may also require a willingness to be uncomfortable, including paying for services that aren't covered by insurance. Few clients will be willing to make such an investment if they don't anticipate (realistically or unrealistically) a substantial payoff from making it. That is, their motivation to make it will be determined, at least in part, by the size of the payoff they anticipate. Clients who don't anticipate a substantial payoff from

therapy are unlikely to invest much in it and, consequently, are unlikely to improve. All they are likely to take away from therapy is a strengthening of their certainty that they can't change.

Older children and adults who stutter should not be encouraged to pursue therapy if they appear to lack sufficient motivation to make the necessary investments. Encouraging them to do so will reduce the likelihood that they will benefit from therapy if at some future time they do have adequate motivation, because they will be entering therapy with an expectation of failure rather than of success. Consequently, they will have been harmed by the therapy experience.

The evaluation for older children and adults who stutter, for the reasons I have mentioned, should include an assessment of their motivation to invest in therapy...

And furthermore, for the reasons previously given, clients who stutter should be questioned about their previous therapy experiences. Specifically, it's important to determine whether they regard them as having been successful. If a client, rightly or wrongly, does not regard previous therapy as having been successful, the client is likely to be entering therapy without a strong expectation that it will be successful. His or her expectation, in fact, may be one of failure. Consequently, you're going to have to modify this certainty if the client is to have a reasonable chance of being successful. Perhaps the best way to do this is to begin with a behavior that you are almost certain the client has the ability to change and do whatever you can to facilitate his or her changing it. There is probably no better way to challenge a client's certainty that he or she can't change than to engineer it so that he or she does change. Nothing succeeds like success (nor, on the other hand, fails like failure)!

From *Second Thoughts About Stuttering: Musings of a Speech-Language Pathologist Who Has Stuttered for More Than Sixty Years* (pp. 51–53), by F. H. Silverman, 2000, Greendale, WI: CODI Publications © 2000 by CODI Publications. Reprinted with permission.

Questions Clinicians Ask during a Reevaluation

Clinicians **reevaluate** their clients periodically for a number of reasons, including the following:

- To meet **third-party payers'** (e.g., **Medicare**) and employers' requirements for accountability and documentation

- To check their tentative hypotheses about the causes of the behaviors they are attempting to modify and changing those hypotheses that need modification

- To assess their clients' progress toward meeting therapy goals

- To decide whether to recommend further therapy

- To fill requests for progress reports from other professionals and agencies (e.g., vocational rehabilitation, mental health services, educational systems)

Reevaluate
Conduct an evaluation after the initial diagnostic/assessment process.

Medicare
A federal health insurance program that partially pays for some of the services that speech-language pathologists and audiologists dispense to senior citizens.

Regardless of the setting in which SLPs or audiologists are employed, they will be required to document the outcome of intervention with clients. If clinicians are employed by a public school, they will be expected to document how well the goals and objectives specified in **Individualized Education Programs (IEPs)** have been met. If clinicians are employed in a medical setting, they will have to document client progress to receive funding from insurance programs for additional sessions.

To be maximally helpful to clients, clinicians use intervention strategies to modify communication behaviors based on what is hypothesized to have caused them. If clients change in the ways that would be expected if the hypotheses are valid, the change(s) would provide at least partial support for their validity. Unfortunately, if clients do not change in these ways, the reason could either be that the hypotheses are invalid or that some other factor (e.g., a lack of motivation to change) is impeding the clients' ability to change. Regardless, their lack of improvement would trigger a need for further evaluation.

Obviously, without periodic reevaluations it is not possible to gauge clients' progress toward achieving therapy goals. Neither would it be possible to make informed decisions about the likelihood of further therapy to be helpful.

Clinicians occasionally receive requests for progress reports on clients from other professionals and agencies. In order to provide these reports, clinicians typically conduct at least a partial reevaluation. The following paragraphs address several questions that would be asked routinely during a reevaluation.

Has There Been Any Change in the Severity of the Communication Disorder?

This is a routine question to ask at the termination of therapy, as well as at intervals during therapy, particularly if there were more than a few sessions. If the answer is "yes," the clinician would then ask, "In what way(s) has the client changed?" Answering these two questions involves comparing specific aspects of the client's communication behavior to what they were when therapy began.

How Likely Is the Client to Continue Improving If He or She Receives More Therapy?

This question is asked periodically throughout the period that a client is receiving therapy. The answer determines whether additional therapy will be recommended. Data used for answering it include information pertaining to the amount of improvement during the previous few sessions. If there has been a significant amount of improvement during this period, the prognosis for continued improvement tends to be better than if there has not been significant improvement. The **Code of Ethics of the American Speech-Language-Hearing Association** prohibits keeping clients in therapy beyond the point they are likely to benefit from it.

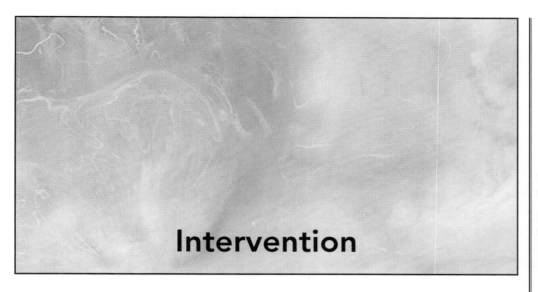

Intervention

Chapter 16

Learning Objectives

- Describe when intervention is not considered following an evaluation.

- Describe how to identify the behaviors that characterize a client's communication disorder.

- Discuss how to establish long-term goals and short-term objectives.

- List the factors that affect a clinician's choice regarding which intervention strategies to use.

- Describe two ways a clinician can document progress during intervention.

- Describe evidence-based practice and why it is important.

- Describe four reasons a clinician may terminate therapy with a client.

Chapter

16

Introduction

Once a client has been determined to have a speech, language, and/or hearing disorder and tentative **hypotheses** have been formulated about the etiology of at least some of the communication behaviors associated with the disorder, an intervention program is usually planned and implemented. Under some conditions, however, intervention is not considered. For example:

- The prognosis for improvement is extremely poor in spite of the client being adequately motivated to improve.

- The prognosis for improvement is good, but the client is not adequately motivated to make the investments necessary to improve.

- The client has the ability to remediate the disorder on his or her own.

- The client is being referred elsewhere for treatment, not necessarily to another SLP or audiologist. For example, a high school or college student might be referred to a debate coach as in Study More 16.1.

The intervention process described in this chapter is diagrammed in Figure 16.1 on page 270. This chapter provides an overview of the process that SLPs and audiologists utilize to accomplish each of these steps.

Study More 16.1	**Forensic Therapy**

A clinician sometimes can help a client achieve a goal by encouraging the client to become involved with some activity not ordinarily viewed as therapy. One such activity might be intercollegiate debating. This letter to the editor describes the experiences of three stutterers who participated in debates.

It has long been recognized that there are many educational benefits to be derived from competitive debating. In fact, it is usually justified upon this premise.

There is, however, a second area of benefit which, judging by the lack of literature in relation to it, seems to be largely unexplored. This neglected area is the "therapeutic" effect that debating can have upon the personality of the speech-defective debater.

I have discussed this at length with a number of coaches. The consensus was that few of them have ever had a "real" speech defective on their squad, nor have they seriously thought of encouraging one to go out for it. The question, therefore, seems to be: can an individual with a speech defect, everything else being equal, become an effective debater? It is my belief that he can. This conclusion is based primarily upon the experiences of three individuals, all stutterers. Admittedly, this is too small a group for any definite conclusions to be drawn. Nevertheless, the indications are quite encouraging.

One of the subjects is presently debating in high school, and the other two are debating in college. Though the former's stuttering tends to be quite severe in most situations, while debating she usually experiences no difficulty. This has had a positive effect upon her self-confidence which has carried over into all her activities. In this case the debate experience has definitely been of direct therapeutic value.

This same thing was true for the two college debaters. Both had definite feelings of inferiority because of their speech problem. However, after defeating several top-notch teams and accumulating some first-speaker ratings, their self-concepts became modified and more realistic. I can think of no other way that this change of attitude could have been brought about as rapidly.

If we accept the basic assumption that the primary justification for debating is to benefit the individual taking part (with the contest elements being secondary), then we must certainly agree that therapeutic benefits should be as acceptable as educational ones.

From "Forensic Therapy," by F. H. Silverman, 1960, *Quarterly Journal of Speech*, pp. 305–306. © 1960 by the Quarterly Journal of Speech. Reprinted with permission.

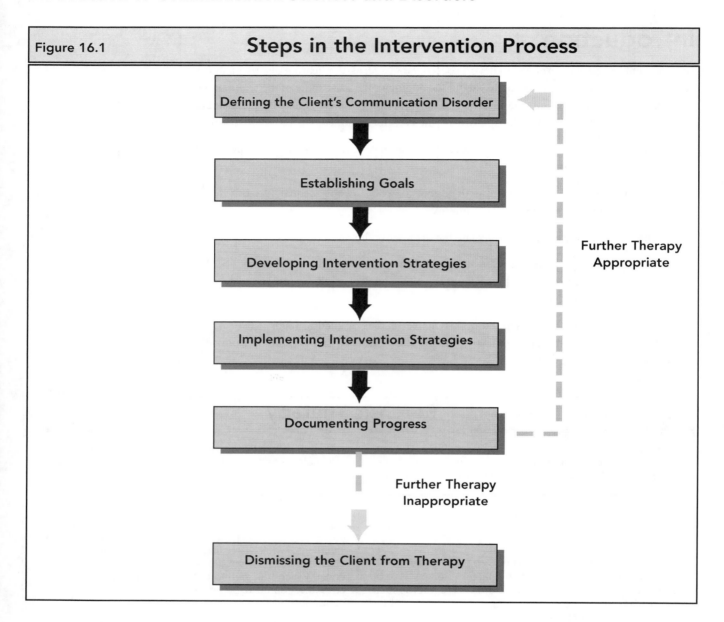

Figure 16.1 — Steps in the Intervention Process

Steps in the Intervention Process

Defining the Client's Communication Disorder

The first step in the intervention process is identifying the behaviors that characterize, or define, the client's communication disorder and formulating hypotheses about their cause. The term *behavior,* in this context, includes phenomena that most persons regard as attitudes and emotional states. We ascribe attitudes and emotional states to people by observing their behavior, both verbal and nonverbal.

There are several reasons why it is important to identify all behaviors related to a disorder and formulate a tentative hypothesis about why each occurs. First, these behaviors, if changed, can reduce the severity of the client's disorder. If, for example, a /w/ or /r/ sound substitution is one of the behaviors characterizing a client's communication disorder, one of the goals of therapy would likely be to teach the client to produce /r/ correctly.

Second, the hypothesis a clinician formulates about why an abnormal behavior occurs influences the choice of intervention strategies for modifying it. If, for example, the reason for a client's difficulty understanding speech is hypothesized to be a sensorineural hearing loss, the client will probably be fitted with a hearing aid. On the other hand, if it is hypothesized to be receptive **aphasia,** the client will probably be provided with a program of language stimulation appropriate for people with this disorder.

Third, identifying characteristics of a disorder provides a **baseline** for documenting therapy outcome(s). That is, to document changes in the severity of a client's disorder after a period of therapy, the status of the behaviors characterizing it at the beginning of therapy would be compared to those same behaviors after the period of therapy.

The behaviors that characterize a client's communication disorder may not consist solely of impairments in speech, hearing, or language. They may include psychological impairments that result in handicaps. An example of such a handicap would be avoiding certain situations because of a poor self-concept. It is important to identify these behaviors as well.

Establishing Intervention Goals

The next step in the intervention process is establishing **long-term** and **short-term goals**. These goals are derived in part from answering the question: "What is the purpose of intervention for this person's communication disorder?" Recall that, in Chapter 4, three purposes for intervention were discussed: changing the problem causing the disorder, changing the disorder, and teaching compensatory strategies. To set appropriate long-term goals and short-term objectives, the clinician must first identify which of these purposes is most likely to be achieved given the nature and severity of the disorder; the age of the client; previous intervention success and/or failures; and the client's communication needs in everyday life.

Both long-term and short-term goals are usually documented in written form. Study More 16.2 on page 272 describes the process used for documenting them in public schools in **Individualized Education Programs (IEPs).** The success of any intervention program is determined largely by the appropriateness of the goals and objectives to the client's specific disorder and communication needs.

Selecting goals affects therapy in at least two ways. First, it determines what is to be done to help the client. Second, it influences the client's level of motivation to invest in therapy. A client is likely to work harder to achieve some goals than to achieve others. Children, in particular, need to see how therapy goals are related directly to their everyday life.

The distinction between long-term goals and short-term goals is not absolute. A goal that is a first step or means to an end for one client may be the ultimate goal for another. For instance, for one client, the long-term goal might be to become aware of his or her communication disorder. For another client, the first short-term objective might be to become aware of his or her voice disorder, while the long-term goal might be to significantly change his or her use of voice at home and in school in order to eliminate vocal stress.

Study More 16.2	What Is an IEP?

An IEP is an educational program, specifically tailored to each individual child, taking into account his or her capabilities and limitations, and setting forth specific goals for the child's learning and personal growth.

The IEP is mandated by the federal law, most recently IDEA 2004 (Individuals with Disabilities Education Improvement Act 2004), governing special education. The IEP states the educational needs of the student, the goals and objectives directing the student's educational program, the student's educational programming and placement, and the evaluation and measurement criteria that were developed during the creation of the IEP.

Speech-language pathologists and audiologists who work in the schools use the IEP as a way to describe the goals and objectives that drive intervention for students with communication disorders. The following must be included in the IEP:

1. *Present Levels of Performance.* The IEP must provide a statement of the child's present levels of academic achievement and functional performance.

2. *Annual Goals.* The IEP must include a statement of measurable annual goals, including academic and functional goals. The IEPs of children who take alternate assessments must include a description of benchmarks or short-term objectives.

3. *Educational Progress.* This is a description of how the child's progress toward meeting the annual goals will be measured and when periodic reports on the progress the child is making toward meeting the annual goals will be provided (e.g., through the use of quarterly or other periodic reports, used with reportcards).

4. *Special Education and Related Services.* The child's IEP must include a statement of the special education and related services, and supplementary aids and services to be provided to the child. Services must be based on peer-reviewed research to the extent practicable. IEPs also include a statement of the program modifications or supports to be provided by school personnel.

5. *Accommodations and Alternate Assessments.* The child's IEP must include a statement of any individual appropriate accommodations that are necessary to measure the academic achievement and functional performance of the child on state and districtwide assessments. If the IEP Team determines that the child shall take an alternate assessment on a particular state or districtwide assessment of student achievement, a statement of why the child can't participate in the regular assessment and the alternate assessment that has been selected as appropriate for the child, must be stated.

6. *Transition.* The first IEP after the child is 16 (and updated annually) must include appropriate and measurable goals that address training, education, employment, and independent living skills (when appropriate) and the transition services necessary to assist the child in reaching these goals.

Source: United States Department of Education (2004)

Long-Term Goals

Long-term goals specify the outcomes the clinician is attempting to achieve through the intervention process. Attaining long-term goals should result in a meaningful reduction in the severity of the client's disorder. Some common long-term goals used by SLPs are:

1. *The client will produce speech that is at least 80 percent intelligible to most persons.* This is the type of long-term goal a clinician establishes when it is not feasible for a client to completely eliminate a communication impairment, but it is feasible for him or her to develop speech that can be understood by most persons. A clinician might set such a goal for a client whose speech musculature is not functioning normally because of a neuromuscular disorder (i.e., someone who has **dysarthria)** or for someone who is deaf or has had a **glossectomy.**

2. *The client will produce the /s/ phoneme correctly in all positions in words during nonstructured conversational speech at least 95 percent of the time.* This is the type of long-term goal clinicians establish when they believe it is feasible for a client to eliminate a speech disorder. A 100 percent success level is not expected because it might take years to achieve. In addition, it is reasonable to assume that if a client has

learned to produce /s/ correctly 95 percent of the time, he or she should be able to learn to produce it correctly 100 percent of the time without a need for further therapy. Consequently, it would almost always be safe to discharge a client who had achieved this level of success.

3. *The client will communicate functional, everyday communication needs.* This is the type of long-term goal clinicians establish for clients who have a severe communication impairment—people whose speech is inadequate (temporarily or permanently) for meeting at least some of their communication needs. Various strategies and devices are used with such clients to augment their ability to communicate (see Silverman, 1995).

4. *The client will use figurative language correctly in a written story.* This long-term goal is typical of the type school-based SLPs establish for students with language-learning disabilities. These students frequently have difficulty with the **metalinguistic** aspects of language, especially in writing.

A number of factors can influence a clinician's selection of long-term goals for a client. The following discusses some of the major factors.

The Severity of the Communication Disorder

Generally, the more severe the communication disorder, the more likely that long-term goals will focus on helping the client develop communication that is adequate for everyday functional needs. The less severe the communication disorder, the more likely that long-term goals will focus on speech, language, and/or hearing improvements that bring the client as close as possible to normal communication.

People with severe communication impairments either have no **intelligibility** or lack sufficient intelligible speech to meet their **functional communication needs.** Some of the conditions that result in severe communication impairments are **cognitive disabilities, autism, cerebral palsy, aphasia,** deafness, glossectomy, and laryngeal pathology (including **laryngectomy).** To learn more about people who have severe communication impairments, see Silverman (1995).

Clinicians who work with people with severe communication impairments have as their ultimate goal helping their clients develop the ability to communicate at a level adequate for meeting their daily, functional communication needs. To achieve this goal, clinicians will usually help their clients develop more intelligible speech (assuming this is possible), as well as provide them with communication strategies (which may include devices) to augment their ability to communicate. These strategies provided might include **American Sign Language (ASL), American Indian Hand Talk (Amer-Ind), Gestural Morse Code, communication boards,** and electronic communication devices. (For descriptions of these, see Silverman, 1995.) Augmenting a client's speech and other natural communication abilities by one or more of these strategies and/or devices can enable clients with sufficient cognitive abilities to meet their communication needs—or come closer to meeting them.

Functional communication needs
The basic communication abilities a person needs to function in everyday life (e.g., face-to-face or telephone conversations and writing).

American Indian Hand Talk (Amer-Ind)
A manual communication system adapted from one developed by Native Americans hundreds of years ago.

Gestural Morse Code
A communication system used by persons who have severe communication impairments in which words are spelled out letter-by-letter using gestures (e.g., blinking the eyes) for Morse Code dots and dashes.

Communication board
A sheet of cardboard or other material on which is printed the alphabet; commonly used words and phrases; and/or pictographic symbols. The user communicates by pointing to or otherwise indicating the symbols needed to transmit messages.

The Client's Communication Needs

Perhaps the greatest factor involved in designing long-term goals is the client's communication needs. The clinician first identifies these needs and then determines what the client has to do in order to develop, eliminate, or modify to meet their needs. Intervention consists of the clinician helping the client make the necessary changes in order to meet these needs.

To illustrate this point, suppose a clinician must develop long-term goals for an elementary-school-age girl who has normal intelligence, hearing, and vision, but who is unable to speak, write, or walk because of cerebral palsy. What are this child's communication needs? First, she should be able to converse with people face-to-face. A communication board as shown in Figure 16.2, or a laptop computer that has speech synthesizer circuitry built in might enable her to meet this communication need. Second, she must be able to do written work in the classroom. A laptop computer with a printer can enable her to do this if she has sufficient motor control to use the keyboard with any facility. Third, it would be desirable if she could communicate by telephone. This same laptop computer, if it has a built-in modem, can enable her to contact her state's **telecommunication relay service (TRS)** and have telephone services that are functionally equivalent to those available to other telephone users (see Silverman, 1999b to learn more). And, e-mailing is another option for communicating in an informal way with family and friends.

The Client's Prognosis for Improvement

The client's potential for change is an important component of the long-term goals that the clinician will establish. Obviously, the clinician will design goals the client is judged capable of achieving, because to do otherwise is to act unethically. If the client has difficulty achieving the goals, the clinician should reevaluate the goals to determine whether they are too difficult and need to be reformulated.

Available Resources

The resources available for treating a client can influence the long-term goals developed by a clinician. Such resources include available funding, administrative support, adequate physical facilities, access to appropriate materials, and continuing education opportunities.

Short-Term Goals (Objectives)

Short-term goals specify abilities clients must develop to achieve long-term goals. These abilities often have to be developed in a specific sequence, as illustrated in Figure 16.3 on page 276. The tasks specified in this figure almost always have to be carried out in the sequence indicated. A client, for example, would almost always have to be able to produce /s/ correctly in single words before doing so in sentences.

Developing Intervention Strategies

The development of intervention strategies arises directly from the long-term goals and short-term objectives the clinician has established for the client. There are several factors that affect clinicians' choices of which intervention strategies to use, including:

1. *The number of strategies that are appropriate for achieving a particular goal with which a clinician is familiar.* A clinician can select only from among the strategies he or she knows. If a clinician is familiar with only a single strategy for achieving a goal, the selection process will be easy. However, a clinician is more likely to be successful

Figure 16.2	An Example of a Communication Board

I CAN HEAR PERFECTLY	PLEASE REPEAT AS I TALK THIS IS HOW I TALK BY SPELLING OUT THE WORDS	WOULD YOU PLEASE CALL
A AN HE HER I IT ME MY HIM SHE THAT THE THESE THEY THIS WHOSE WHAT WHEN WHERE WHICH WHO WHY YOU WE YOUR	AM ARE ASK BE BEEN BRING CAN COME COULD DID DO DOES DON'T DRINK GET GIVE GO HAD HAS HAVE IS KEEP KNOW LET LIKE MAKE MAY PUT SAY SAID SEE SEEN SEND SHOULD TAKE TELL THINK THOUGHT WANT WAS WERE WILL WISH WON'T WOULD -ED -ER -EST -ING -LY -N'T -'S -TION	ABOUT ALL AND ALWAYS ALMOST AS AT BECAUSE BUT FOR FROM HOW IF IN OF ON OR TO UP WITH

A   B   C   D   E   F   G
  H   I   J   K   L   M
N   O   P   Qu   R   S   T
  U   V   W   X   Y   Z
1   2   3   4   5   6   7
  8   9   10   11   12   30
		AFTER AGAIN
		ANY EVEN
		EVERY HERE
		JUST MORE
		ONLY SO
		SOME SOON
		THERE VERY

SUN. MON. TUES. WED. THURS. FRI. SAT. BATHROOM	PLEASE THANK YOU GOING OUT MR. MRS. MISS. START OVER MOTHER DAD DOCTOR END OF WORD	$ ¢ 1/2 (SHHH!!)? Lynda Miller

in achieving a particular goal if he or she knows more than one strategy, because there are few (if any) that will work with all clients!

2. *The clinician's hypothesis about the primary cause(s) of the behavior to be changed.* The intervention strategy a clinician chooses is influenced by the assumptions he or she makes about the reason(s) the client continues to exhibit the target behavior. Its **maintaining cause** may be physiological, psychological, or a combination of the two. If the clinician's hypothesis is accurate, intervention is more likely to be successful than it would be if the hypothesis turns out to be inaccurate.

3. *The time and financial investments required.* Some intervention strategies require a greater time and/or financial investment than others. The more time a clinician must invest to implement an intervention strategy, the greater the cost to the client (or whoever is paying for the therapy). It may be possible, for example, for a clinician to reduce the time investment that is required to attain a particular goal and, consequently, the cost by conducting some sessions by telephone. For a description of how this approach was used in one clinic to reduce the number of face-to-face sessions needed to achieve a goal, see Study More 16.3 on page 277. Everything else being equal, a clinician will choose the strategy that requires the least time and financial investment.

Maintaining cause
Some factor that causes an impairment to persist.

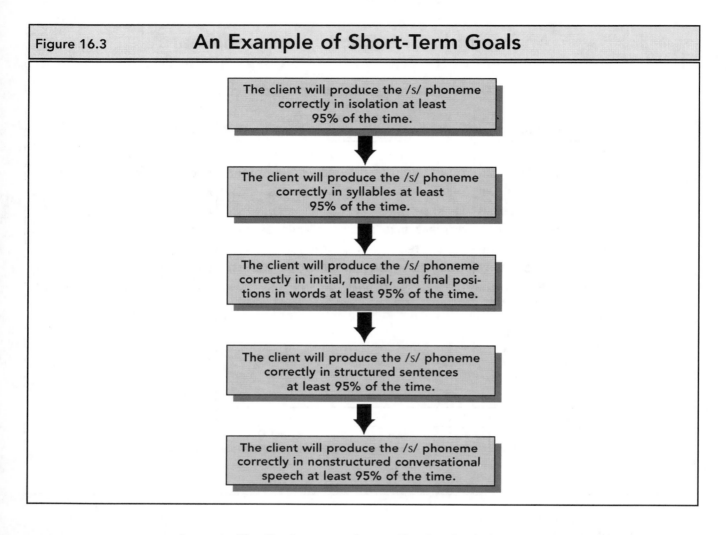

Figure 16.3   An Example of Short-Term Goals

The client will produce the /s/ phoneme correctly in isolation at least 95% of the time.

The client will produce the /s/ phoneme correctly in syllables at least 95% of the time.

The client will produce the /s/ phoneme correctly in initial, medial, and final positions in words at least 95% of the time.

The client will produce the /s/ phoneme correctly in structured sentences at least 95% of the time.

The client will produce the /s/ phoneme correctly in nonstructured conversational speech at least 95% of the time.

4. *The client's treatment history.* If a client has had previous therapy and believes that the approach used was effective, the clinician is likely to continue using it. On the other hand, if the client does not believe it was effective, the clinician is likely to use a different approach. A client's beliefs about the effectiveness of an intervention can reduce or enhance its effect. Clients tend to invest more time and energy in therapy when they anticipate success than when they anticipate failure.

5. *The client's intellectual level.* A client's level of cognitive functioning can influence the choice of an intervention strategy. It probably wouldn't be possible, for example, to use a communication board containing the alphabet and commonly used words as in Figure 16.2 on page 275 with people with significant cognitive deficits.

6. *Evidence-based practices.* **Evidence-based practice (EBP)** means integrating the clinician's individual clinical expertise with the best available external clinical evidence obtained from systematic research. The American Speech-Language-Hearing Association defines EBP as using current best research results to make clinical decisions about patient care. Based on the evidence from a comprehensive literature search and review of published research studies, the clinician develops interventions appropriate for each client.

Study More 16.3	Answering Machine Therapy

Sometimes a clinician can reduce the amount of time required for attaining a particular goal and the cost of doing so to the client by utilizing a telephone for some sessions. How this was done in one clinic is indicated here.

To increase parent involvement in the communication development of children in a local Head Start program, we explored the effectiveness of using a telephone answering machine call-in system to supplement the classroom enrichment activities that were part of the consultation program.

The system was first used in a pilot program with one classroom with 20 children. A telephone answering machine was installed in the Head Start office. Weekly language enrichment activities for parents to use with their children were provided by the speech-language pathologist and recorded by another member of the Head Start staff whom the parents knew well. A letter to the parents explained how to call in to hear the weekly language lesson. The letter also reinforced the parent's role in helping their children and encouraged extended family members to become involved in the language activities. Each week a different vocabulary enrichment activity was provided for the parents to coincide with classroom vocabulary lessons.

Source: Schubel & Erickson (1992)

Implementing Intervention Strategies

Speech-language pathologists and audiologists implement a wide range of intervention strategies. Much of learning to be an SLP or audiologist focuses on acquiring an understanding of these strategies. Table 16.1 provides examples that illustrate the link between intervention strategies and the goals they are intended to help clients attain.

Documenting Progress

A clinician cannot ethically continue providing intervention if the client does not demonstrate measurable progress toward the long-term goal established at the beginning of therapy. The clinician can modify the intervention strategies being used, refer the client to another

Table 16.1	Example Goals and Intervention Strategies

Goal	Intervention Strategy
The client will produce the /s/ phoneme correctly at the beginnings of single words at least 95 percent of the time.	The client will read aloud lists of words that begin with the /s/ phoneme. After the client says each word, the clinician will signal whether it was said correctly. The client will repeat the task until she is producing /s/ correctly at least 95 percent of the time in this context.
The client (who has a sensorineural hearing loss) will be fitted with a hearing aid that will enable him to understand at least 90 percent of words spoken in a quiet environment.	The client will be fitted with a hearing aid, and the percentage of the words on one or more special lists that he identifies correctly will be determined. The words will be presented over a loudspeaker in a sound-treated room. If the client doesn't appear to understand at least 90 percent of them, the process will be repeated with other hearing aids.
The client (who has a flaccid paralysis of the soft palate and is extremely hypernasal) will produce speech that is at least 90 percent intelligible.	The client will be fitted with a palatal lift prosthesis to reduce hypernasality and thus increase the intelligibility of his speech. First, a sample of the client's speech will be recorded with the prosthesis in place. Then, several listeners will transcribe the sample to determine whether it is at least 90 percent intelligible. This is an example of intervention for a communication disorder that requires the involvement of a clinician who is not an SLP or audiologist. In this case, the clinician involved probably would be a dentist who specializes in prostheses (i.e., a prosthodontist).

professional, or terminate therapy. In any case, the clinician must be able to show whether the client's communication behavior changed, and, if it did, how. The easiest way to show these changes is to document the client's communication behaviors during each therapy session. One way to document progress is to keep a running tally of the client's attempts to produce a target communication behavior, for example, the number of correct productions of the /s/ phoneme in initial position in words from a specified word list.

Another approach to documenting progress is to track the number of targeted communication behaviors used from session to session. For instance, the clinician working with a school-age child on developing the ability to tell a spontaneous story could track the story components the child included at the beginning of therapy, after four sessions, and again after eight sessions. If the intervention strategies used are appropriate, the number of story components the child includes will increase measurably.

Dismissing the Client from Therapy

The final step in the intervention process is dismissing the client from therapy and writing a summary report. Ideally, all the client's initial goals have been achieved and there doesn't appear to be a need for any new ones. However, several factors can result in terminating therapy before the client has reached his or her goals. Probably the most common is that the clinician determines the client is unlikely to make further progress toward the goals. Unless the client is likely to benefit from further therapy, the clinician is ethically bound to terminate the intervention process. This does not mean, however, that the clinician concludes that the client will never benefit from further intervention. To the contrary, often the clinician will arrange for periodic reevaluations to determine whether further therapy at that time would be beneficial to the client.

Another reason clients may be discharged before achieving their goals is that they want to change clinicians. Changing clinicians may result from the client moving away from the area or from the client having decided to enter the intervention process with a different clinician.

A third factor influencing discharging clients before they have achieved their goals is that they can no longer afford the clinic's fee. For instance, their insurance benefits for this type of therapy may have been exhausted, or their budget does not allow payment of further fees. In this situation, clients may seek therapy at a less-expensive facility, such as a university speech, language, and hearing clinic.

Finally, clients may be discharged before their goals are achieved simply because they want to be. They may no longer have time for therapy or be motivated to continue it, or they may feel capable of functioning as their own clinician. In fact, for some clients—particularly those whose communication impairments cannot be completely eliminated—assuming the responsibility for continued improvement may be one of the goals established when they began the therapeutic process. For these clients, terminating therapy with a clinician signals the achievement of their goal.

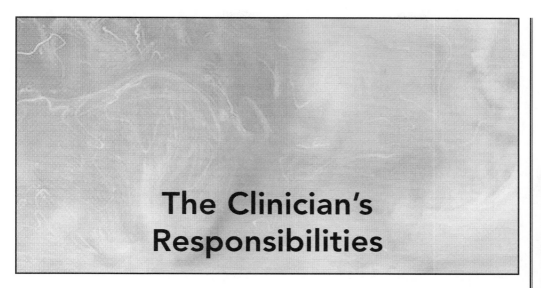

The Clinician's Responsibilities

Chapter 17

Learning Objectives

- Describe why speech-language pathologists and audiologists need to gather and disseminate information about the effectiveness of the clinical tools and techniques they use.

- Describe the clinician-investigator role and the benefits that speech-language pathologists and audiologists can derive from functioning in this role.

- List the six steps in the clinical research process.

- Describe why it is necessary to establish scientific justification for answering clinical questions through research.

- Demonstrate how the same data can be presented to imply greater or lesser improvement.

- Use 25 statistical terms to understand descriptions of clinical research in professional journals.

Introduction

Like most other health-care professionals, **speech-language pathologists (SLPs)** and **audiologists** rely considerably on the experience of others in their work. Most clinicians create few, if any, of the evaluation procedures and intervention strategies that they use. Instead, they acquire them by talking with colleagues; taking courses; reading books and professional journals; surfing the Internet; participating in continuing education activities; and attending professional meetings.

For clinical services to be maximally effective, clinicians need to share information about what works and what does not, described in the previous chapter as **evidence-based practice (EBP).** Because a publisher claims that a particular diagnostic test yields data that is **valid, reliable,** and **representative** does not necessarily mean that it does. However, publishers of **standardized assessments** almost always publish the statistical information necessary to determine whether their tests do possess adequate statistical power to be considered valid, reliable, and representative. Clinicians typically evaluate this information as part of deciding whether or not to use the test.

Similarly, because a particular intervention strategy is claimed by its creator to have been proven effective does not necessarily indicate that it really has. The amount of confidence a clinician can have in both these conclusions depends on who generated and interpreted the data. Unlike test instruments, which undergo rigorous statistical design and analysis, intervention programs are only recently being evaluated with the same rigor. Unfortunately, the desire of someone who creates an intervention process or program to have his or her creation be regarded as valid, reliable, and effective can bias both how he or she gathers data to evaluate it and how the data are interpreted. This phenomenon is referred to as **experimenter bias.** See Silverman, 1998b, to learn more about experimenter bias.

Consider this illustration of how experimenter bias can affect both the gathering of data to evaluate and interpret an intervention program. A hypothetical language program for school-age children has 23 participants enrolled in a summer program. The goal of the eight-week program is to increase the children's expressive language skills. At the beginning and end of the program, each child is interviewed by a clinician who records the conversation and then calculates the number of different sentence types used by each child. The results indicate that, at the beginning of the program, the children used mostly simple, active, declarative sentences. At the end of the program, the children's conversations contained several examples of compound sentences, interrogatives, and embedded phrases. From this information, the program director, who designed the program, concludes that the program is effective because the children's expressive language skills changed over the course of the intervention sessions.

Looking more closely at the data, however, reveals that there is no way to compare the children's sentences at the start of the program with their sentences at the program's conclusion. To measure and document actual change, the director would have needed to document changes through some sort of rigorous comparison of the children's expressive language skills at the beginning and end of the program. One way to do this would be to administer a well-documented test of expressive language skills to all children at the beginning and again at the end of the intervention program. Then the director could compare the pre- and post-program scores to see whether the changes, if any, reflect statistically significant differences.

Experimenter bias
Bias introduced by an experimenter's desire to have his or her findings be what is wanted.

Single-subject research
A research design in which questions are answered by data from individual subjects, rather than by data that are derived from the performances of groups of subjects.

Documentation
Regarding intervention, describing its impact on clients, using data that possess adequate levels of validity, reliability, and generality.

Unfortunately, for most therapies for speech, language, and hearing disorders, most (sometimes all) of the outcome data available were generated either by their creators or by people who are closely associated with them (e.g., their graduate students). Consequently, questions can legitimately be raised about the validity, reliability, and generality of data used to support statements about their effectiveness. How can the accuracy of such statements be assessed? Perhaps the best way is to encourage clinicians with no investment in the effectiveness of any given therapy to assess it.

The primary purpose of this chapter is to acquaint you with how clinicians gather and disseminate information about the effectiveness of clinical tools and techniques. It begins with a discussion of clinicians functioning as **clinician-investigators.** Then, the clinical research process is described, with particular emphasis on seven questions clinicians address when judging the effectiveness of any particular therapy.

The Clinician as Clinician-Investigator

SLPs and audiologists need to systematically evaluate and document their therapy in order to prevent experimenter bias. One way to systematically evaluate and document one's therapy is by functioning as a clinician-investigator. The research they do, usually **single-subject research,** results in the **documentation** necessary to show the effectiveness of particular therapy strategies and methodologies. It also serves an important function related to the ASHA **Code of Ethics,** which states that clinicians must evaluate the services they provide in order to determine their effectiveness.

Although there is considerable variation in the amount and type of therapy outcome research that individual SLPs and audiologists perform, they are all required to do some, regardless of whether they are employed in an educational, medical, or other setting. If they are employed in the public schools, they are required by their employer (usually the school district) to conduct research to document effectiveness because their employer needs the documentation to be eligible for reimbursement from the federal and/or state government for at least a part of their salary. If they are employed in a medical setting, they are required by their employer to document their practices because their employer needs the documentation to be paid for their services by private and governmental insurance entities (e.g., **Medicare**).

Another way people with communication impairments benefit from SLPs and audiologists functioning as clinician-investigators is that they receive higher quality services. Therapy service improves when SLPs and audiologists share information with their colleagues. An SLP, for example, may find that an intervention approach that is effective with one clinical population is also effective with another. An example is the gestural communication system known as **American Indian Hand Talk (Amer-Ind;** Skelly, Schinsky, Smith, Donaldson, & Griffin, 1975). Amer-Ind was developed at a Veteran's administration hospital for use with adults who are speechless because they have a neurological impairment or have had a **glossectomy.** An SLP who was working with children with **developmental disabilities** who had little or no speech wondered whether this system would facilitate their ability to communicate. She taught it to a group of 32 such children with encouraging results. She published a brief report of her experience (Duncan & Silverman, 1997), which was read by many SLPs in the United States, as well as in other countries. Many used it successfully with their clients who had severe speech disorders associated with developmental disabilities. By publishing this report, Duncan and Silverman helped a segment of the population with communication disorders receive a higher quality of service than they probably would have otherwise.

Clients also benefit when their clinicians routinely assess therapy outcomes because these clinicians are more likely to monitor more carefully the services they provide. Through this monitoring, clinicians are likely to identify and correct problems sooner, thereby increasing the potential that clients will benefit.

Finally, functioning as clinician-investigators makes it possible for clinicians to improve their effectiveness. By systematically evaluating the services they provide, they obtain information needed to identify both strategies that work for their clients and themselves and those that do not. One strategy may be more compatible with a clinician's personality and belief system than another. Clinicians' beliefs and subsequent expectations regarding the effectiveness of a particular therapy approach, for example, can directly affect likelihood of it helping their clients (Shapiro, 1964).

The Clinical Research Process

The clinical research process involves assessing and documenting therapy. This process is similar in many ways to the clinical evaluation process described in Chapter 15. Like the clinical evaluation process, the clinical research process involves asking **answerable questions** and making the observations needed to answer them. The clinical research process is diagrammed in Figure 17.1 on page 284.

Asking Relevant and Answerable Questions

The clinical research process starts with the clinician asking one or more answerable questions that have relevance for improving clinical effectiveness. Questions relevant to improving clinical effectiveness answer the "so what" and "who cares" questions regarding therapy. The most relevant questions carry the greatest **scientific justification** precisely because of their relevance. Questions regarding therapy outcome are examples of clinically relevant questions.

Many clinical research questions address the effectiveness of particular therapy strategies. The following questions are among those to which clinicians frequently seek answers when assessing the impact of such an approach (see Silverman, 1998b):

- *What is the impact of the approach on the communication behavior(s) that it is intended to modify?* The term *behavior* includes what are traditionally referred to as attitudes and feelings. We become aware of attitudes and feelings by observing behavior—that is, attitudes and feelings are explanations for behavior. Audiologists and SLPs are primarily concerned with impairment-, disability-, and handicap-related behaviors.

   In most cases, if the answer to this question is that an approach has no meaningful impact on the behavior it is intended to modify, answers would not be sought to any of the other questions listed below. However, occasionally one encounters a therapy approach that does not appear to do what it is intended to do but, nevertheless, has a very desirable **side effect.** Because such an approach might be considered worthy of further evaluation because of this side effect, answers would be sought to the other questions listed below.

Scientific justification
Providing answers to the "so what" and "who cares" questions for why it is important to carry out a particular clinical research project.

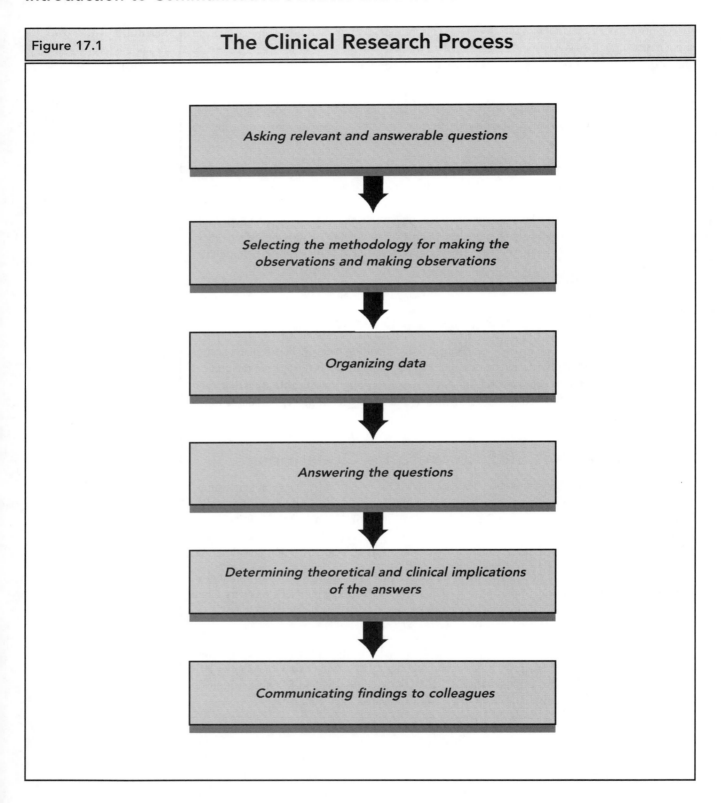

Figure 17.1 — The Clinical Research Process

Asking relevant and answerable questions

Selecting the methodology for making the observations and making observations

Organizing data

Answering the questions

Determining theoretical and clinical implications of the answers

Communicating findings to colleagues

- *What is the impact of the approach on other aspects of a client's communication?* An approach that has a desirable impact on behaviors that contribute to a client's communication disorder may have an undesirable impact on other aspects of the client's communication, including speaking rate; auditory acuity; speech rhythm and articulation; voice intensity and quality; language formulation; verbal output; spontaneity; and/or credibility as a communicator. If, for example, a person with a fluency disorder is taught to monitor his or her speech for moments of stuttering and voluntarily reduce their severity, this may result in a reduction in the stuttering severity but also reduce speaking rate, spontaneity, and inflection. If a client's communication behavior following intervention attracts more adverse attention than it did prior to intervention, the value of the approach would be questionable. On the other hand, the impact of an intervention approach on other aspects of a client's communication can be desirable. For example, approximately one-third of children and adults with severe speech disorders show a meaningful increase in verbal output after beginning to use an augmentative communication strategy or device (see Silverman, 1995).

- *What other effects is the approach having on the client?* That is, are there any side effects that are not directly related to communication? If so, are they desirable or not? Children with autism, for example, may often exhibit self-stimulating hand movements, which can lead to poor self-concept, reduced peer acceptance, disturbed biological rhythms, and increased anxiety. However, some children with autism exhibit fewer of these side effects after they have been taught a gestural communication system such as **American Sign Language** (see Silverman, 1995).

- *What is the client's attitude toward the approach and its effects on his or her communicative and other behavior?* A client's attitude toward an approach and its effects can reduce or enhance its effectiveness. If, for example, a client who has a hearing aid refuses to wear it, having the aid will not improve his or her ability to hear (unless, of course, the client's attitude can be changed through counseling). On the other hand, a client who has a strong belief that a particular therapy program will be of benefit is likely to invest the necessary time and energy in the program, which, in turn, will probably enhance its effectiveness.

- *What are the attitudes of a client's significant others toward the approach and its impact on the client's behavior?* Therapy is more likely to be successful if the clinician and the client's significant others believe it will be beneficial. For example, a clinician who lacks confidence in the effectiveness of an approach is likely to communicate this nonverbally to the client, reducing the odds that it will be effective. Similarly, if the client's family and friends have a positive attitude toward the therapy, the client will be more likely to respond positively.

- *What investment is required of the client and clinician?* Each type of therapy requires various types of investment, including financial; time and energy; and willingness to be uncomfortable. An approach may be effective but too expensive to be practical for many clients. For example, a highly sophisticated speech-generating communication device can cost more than $5,000, an amount that many persons with severe communication impairments cannot afford. Or an approach may be effective but cause clients to be so uncomfortable that few would be willing to make the necessary investment. One such approach is voluntary stuttering—fake stuttering—outside the therapy room (see

Quantitative data
Data that consist of numerical descriptions of various sorts of attributes.

Qualitative data
Information that is difficult to measure, count, or express in numerical terms (e.g., the nature of relationships among various groups).

Silverman, 1996). Many persons who stutter find this activity extremely noxious and refuse to do it.

- *What is the probability of relapse following termination of therapy?* People who have a communication disorder, particularly ones who stutter, often relapse to some degree after therapy is terminated. Although any client can suffer a relapse, the likelihood of relapse occurring when some approaches are used is unacceptably high. If the benefits yielded by a therapy are highly likely to wear off after a client is discharged, most clinicians would consider the therapy to be of questionable value. Consequently, it is important when evaluating a therapy to take the probability of relapse into consideration.

Selecting a Methodology and Making Observations

Once a research question has been formulated, the next task is to select a methodology for collecting the data needed and making observations. If the question is answerable, it will indicate (either directly or indirectly) both what and who to observe. For example, let's consider the question: "Does three months of daily sessions of a particular **aphasia** therapy improve the speech comprehension of people with **Wernicke's aphasia?**"

For this question, the what (which aspect of communication behavior to observe) is speech comprehension and the who (persons on whom observations are to be made) is clients with Wernicke's aphasia. The speech-comprehension levels of people with receptive aphasia after three months of the therapy would be compared to what they were at the beginning of the period (i.e., **baseline).** The method used to generate the data needed to answer the question would be to administer pre- and post-therapy tests of speech comprehension and then compare the scores. If the post-therapy scores were sufficiently higher to suggest there had been a meaningful improvement in speech comprehension, the investigator probably would conclude that the program had been effective. To draw this conclusion, however, the clinician must be certain that no other events occurred during the three-month period to account for the change in the clients' speech comprehension. For instance, if the clients with aphasia had received the therapy program within six months post-trauma, an alternative explanation for their improvement would be **spontaneous recovery.**

The data used to answer a question can be quantitative, qualitative, or a combination of the two. **Quantitative data** consist of numerical information, and **qualitative data** consist of observation, interviewing, and document review. Some questions can be answered more accurately by using quantitative data, others by using qualitative data, and still others by some combination of these two.

Organizing Data

After the data have been abstracted from the observations, the next task is to organize or summarize them in a way that makes it possible for them to be used for answering the question. The organizational structure used may be a table (see Table 17.1) or graphs (see Figure 17.2). Tables are appropriate for both qualitative data and quantitative data.

Table 17.1	Example Table	
Test Subject	**Pre-Therapy Score**	**Post-Therapy Score**
1	25	50
2	35	60
3	20	70
4	30	31
5	60	65
6	50	45
7	15	18
8	20	20
9	35	40
10	65	70
	35.5 = Mean	46.9 = Mean
Hypothetical pre- and post-therapy scores of 10 people with aphasia		

Figure 17.2	Example Graphs

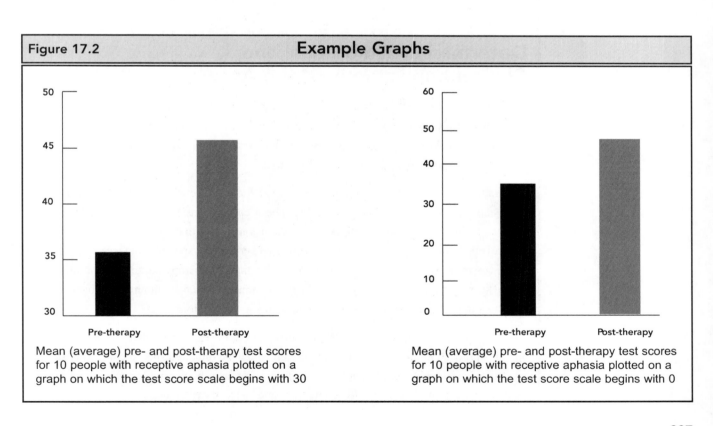

Mean (average) pre- and post-therapy test scores for 10 people with receptive aphasia plotted on a graph on which the test score scale begins with 30

Mean (average) pre- and post-therapy test scores for 10 people with receptive aphasia plotted on a graph on which the test score scale begins with 0

Statistical analyses
Numerical analyses for summarizing and otherwise treating quantitative data (e.g., to assess their validity and reliability) in order to answer research questions.

Note that Figure 17.2 on page 287 suggests a greater degree of improvement than do the scores in Table 17.1 even though both show the same data. The impression of improvement in the graph on the left in Figure 17.2 was enhanced by having the test score scale begin with 30 rather than 0. When the scale is begun with 0, as in the graph on the right, the amount of improvement appears to be less. These examples illustrate the importance of carefully examining the scales on graphs before interpreting them.

Quantitative data can also be summarized by performing various **statistical analyses** on them. For descriptions of those that are used most frequently in speech-language pathology and audiology research and the terminology associated with them, see Study More 17.1 and Silverman (1998b).

Answering the Questions

Once the data have been organized or summarized in a way that enables the questions to be answered, you are ready to answer them. Using the hypothetical example shown in Table 17.1 on page 287, one statistical analysis that could be used to show whether the differences between the pre- and post-therapy scores reflect real change is the t-test (see Study More 17.1). In our example, performing the t-test showed that the post-therapy scores are significantly higher than the pre-therapy scores. The clinician can conclude with confidence that the therapeutic intervention program used was effective for improving the speech comprehension of clients with Wernicke's aphasia.

Determining Theoretical and Clinical Implications of the Answer

Answering the research question naturally leads to two further considerations. First, what does the answer imply regarding the theoretical basis underlying the intervention program? Second, what does the answer imply about possible clinical implications for these clients (or others who may benefit from the same therapeutic approach)?

Using the example from Table 17.1 on page 287, once the clinician has determined that the intervention was effective in improving the speech comprehension of clients with Wernicke's aphasia, he or she considers what that information contributes to the theory underlying the theoretical approach. For instance, if the therapy involved pairing spoken sentences with the same sentences in print, the clinician could hypothesize that the therapy stimulated the brain with paired sensory stimuli, the theory being that stimulating the client's impaired language abilities increases the chances for improvement in speech comprehension.

One clinical implication that could be derived from the example is that this particular therapeutic approach might also work with children who have impaired speech comprehension. To test this idea, the clinician would use this implication as a beginning hypothesis for another clinical research study that would follow the same steps described here.

Study More 17.1 — Statistical Terms

You will need to know these 25 statistical terms to understand descriptions of clinical research in speech-language pathology and audiology publications. (For in-depth explanations of these and other statistical terms, see Silverman, 1998b.)

Analysis of variance—A statistical technique used mostly to assess the likelihood that observed differences between more than two means, medians, or other statistics are real ones (i.e., not merely the result of random sampling error). The scientific method requires such observed differences to be shown to be highly unlikely to result from random sampling error (i.e., chance) before they can be interpreted.

Confidence interval—An estimate of the value of a population statistic based on a sample of persons from the population (e.g., the percentage of persons in the United States who approve of the president's job performance estimated from the responses of a sample of 1,000 persons). The estimate is expressed as an interval within which it is 95 or 99 percent certain that the value falls (e.g., it is 95 percent certain the president's job approval rating is between 56 and 58 percent).

Correlation coefficient—A statistic that usually provides information about both the strength and direction of the relationship between two variables (e.g., height and weight). Correlation coefficients range in value from −1.0 to +1.0. The closer the value of the coefficient is to zero, the weaker the strength of the relationship. And the closer it is to either −1.0 or +1.0, the greater the strength of the relationship.

The minus or plus sign in front of a correlation coefficient indicates whether the relationship is a positive or negative one. If the relationship is a positive one, as the value of one variable increases, that of the other does also (e.g., height and weight are positively related). And if the relationship is a negative one, as the value of one variable increases, that of the other decreases (e.g., chronological age and number of articulation errors are negatively related for preschoolers).

Level of confidence—When you're doing a significance test, it is the level at which you want to be confident that an observed difference is real (i.e., not due to random sampling error) before concluding that it is real. The two levels of confidence that are used most often are 95 percent (0.05) and 99 percent (0.01). If you declare an observed difference between means to be a real one at the 0.05 (95 percent) level of confidence, there is a 5 percent chance that you will be wrong (i.e., that the observed difference really was due to random sampling error).

Linear relationship—Either a positive relationship in which both variables increase or decrease in value proportionally or a negative relationship in which the value of one variable increases as the value of the other decreases proportionally. If points for the two variables are plotted on a line graph (that is referred to as a scattergram—see A through C), the line of best fit to the points (i.e., the line from which they deviate the least) will be a straight line (rather than a curved line).

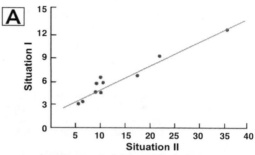

A scattergram depicting a relatively strong, positive, linear relationship between two variables.

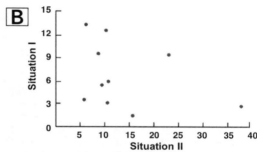

A scattergram depicting little or no relationship between two variables.

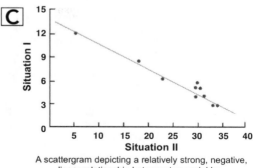

A scattergram depicting a relatively strong, negative, linear relationship between two variables.

Continued on next page

Study More 17.1—*Continued*	## Statistical Terms

Mean—A measure of "central tendency" that is the average of the numbers in a column or row. You add the numbers and then divide the total by how many numbers you added. The mean of the following numbers is five: 1, 10, 4.

Median—A measure of "central tendency" that is the number at the midpoint of a set of numbers when the numbers in the set are ordered from lowest to highest (or from highest to lowest). The median of the following set of five numbers is four: 1, 2, 4, 6, 30.

Mode—A measure of "central tendency" that is the most frequently occurring number in a set of numbers. The mode in the following set of ten numbers is five: 2, 3, 4, 4, 5, 5, 5, 5, 6, 8.

N—The abbreviation for the number of subjects or other entities (e.g., N = 10 subjects).

Negative relationship—If a relationship between two variables is a negative one, as the value of one increases, that of the other decreases (e.g., as children grow older, the number of articulation errors that they exhibit decreases).

Normal distribution—A symmetrical, bell-shaped curve in which certain relationships hold regarding its height at specified distances from its center (see following example).

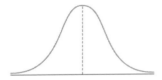

Percentile—The percentage of persons in a population who have a test score, or other numerical designation (e.g., height) that is less than a specified one. For example, having a test score at the 50th percentile means that half of the people who took the test had lower scores. The median, incidentally, is the 50th percentile.

Population—The group of persons to whom an investigator wants to be able to generalize. An example of such a population could be persons who have receptive aphasia and are more than one year post-trauma.

Positive relationship—If the relationship between two variables is a positive one, as the value of one increases, so does that of the other (e.g., increases in height tend to be accompanied by increases in weight).

Random error—A form of error present to some degree in all sampling and measurement processes. While such an error can make it difficult to detect relatively small differences and relatively weak relationships, it does not bias the data (i.e., cause incorrect conclusions to be reached about differences and relationships).

Random sample—A sample selected from a population by a random process (e.g., by using a table of random numbers). If a sample was not selected by a random process, the accuracy of conclusions about the population from which it came will be uncertain.

Range—A measure of "variability" that is the difference between the smallest number and the largest number (e.g., the subjects ranged in age from 5 years to 8 years). The larger the difference between the two numbers, the greater the variability.

Sample—A group of people or other entities that were selected from a population of such people or entities either randomly or by some other process.

Scattergram—A two-dimensional graphical display for visualizing the strength, nature (linear or curvilinear), and direction (positive or negative) of the relationship between two variables. It provides almost the same information about the strength and direction of a relationship as does a correlation coefficient.

Significance tests—Statistical techniques for assessing the likelihood that observed differences between means, medians, or other statistics are real ones (i.e., not merely the result of random sampling error). Two examples are analysis of variance and the t-test.

Standard deviation—A measure of the "variability" of the numbers in a row or column. The larger the standard deviation, the greater the variability. The standard deviation is less likely than the range to overestimate variability (because it isn't affected as much as is the range by a few extreme scores or other measures).

Statistically significant difference—A possible outcome of a significance test. Its usual interpretation is that it is 95 percent or more certain that the difference between means, medians, or other measures on which the test was performed was not due to chance. However, the difference in the population may not be as large as that observed, nor does it necessarily have any theoretical or practical implications. A difference between pre- and post-therapy measures may be statistically significant, but the amount of change it reflects may not be enough to yield any meaningful reduction in the severity of a client's impairments, disabilities, or handicaps.

Systematic error—A type of error present in a measurement process that biases the data (i.e., causes incorrect conclusions to be reached). For example, if a pure-tone audiometer is not calibrated properly, it may indicate hearing thresholds at one or more frequencies that are higher or lower than they should be.

T-test—A statistical technique for assessing the likelihood that the observed difference between two means, medians, or other statistics is a real one (i.e., not merely the result of random sampling error).

Variable—An entity than can assume more than one value. Two examples are chronological age and weight.

Communicating Findings to Colleagues

Clinician-researchers communicate their findings with colleagues in a variety of ways. They can be reported in clinical journals, such as the *American Journal of Speech-Language Pathology; American Journal of Audiology;* or *Language, Speech, and Hearing Services in Schools.* In addition, SLPs often submit their findings to journals published in related fields such as learning disabilities, exceptional children, and autism. Another means of reporting on the results of one's clinical research is to present a **platform presentation** or **poster presentation** at a professional meeting, such as the annual convention of ASHA or that of a state speech, language, and hearing association.

Platform presentation
An oral presentation of the findings of a research project at a professional association convention.

Poster presentation
A report of the findings of a research project at a professional association convention, printed on a poster and attached for an hour or so to a poster board. The presenter stands beside the poster to answer questions from colleagues.

Glossary

ABDUCT. To separate, or open.

ABLATIVE SURGERY. Surgical removal of all or part of a structure (e.g., the lips or mandible).

ABSTRACT-CONCRETE IMBALANCE. Having less than normal ability to categorize.

ACOUSTIC NEURITIS. Inflammation of the auditory nerve.

ACOUSTIC NEUROMA. A tumor that impedes the functioning of the auditory nerve by pressing on it.

ADDUCT. To bring together, or close. Also called approximation.

ADVOCATE. The role of helping clients deal with bureaucracy or other hurdles keeping them from receiving services.

AFFRICATE SOUND. Sound produced by narrowing an opening for air to pass in short bursts.

ALVEOLAR RIDGE. A ridged shelf in the upper jaw (i.e., maxilla) behind the upper teeth.

ALZHEIMER'S DISEASE. A brain disorder that often results in dementia.

AMERICAN ACADEMY OF PRIVATE PRACTICE IN SPEECH-LANGUAGE PATHOLOGY AND AUDIOLOGY. An organization to which many of the speech-language pathologists and audiologists in private practice belong.

AMERICAN INDIAN HAND TALK (AMER-IND). A manual communication system adapted from one developed by Native Americans hundreds of years ago.

AMERICAN SIGN LANGUAGE (ASL). The visual-gestural language used as a primary mode of communication by people with hearing loss. It is recognized as a natural language and is the native language of deaf people and deaf culture.

AMERICAN SPEECH-LANGUAGE-HEARING ASSOCIATION (ASHA). The primary national professional and scientific organization in the United States that regulates the training and practice of audiologists, speech-language pathologists, and speech-language pathology assistants.

AMUSICA. A disturbance in the recognition and processing of music, demonstrated by some persons who have damage to the right cerebral hemisphere.

AMYOTROPHIC LATERAL SCLEROSIS (ALS). A progressive, fatal neuromuscular disorder also known as Lou Gehrig's disease. Causes damage to nerve cells in the brain and spinal cord.

ANOMALY. An abnormality.

ANOMIC APHASIA. A disturbance in word finding. Persons with this problem have difficulty remembering the names of things. Also referred to as dysnomia.

ANOSOGNOSIA. Denial of illness, demonstrated by some persons who have damage to the right cerebral hemisphere.

ANOXIA. Oxygen deprivation, which frequently results in destruction of brain cells.

ANSWERABLE QUESTION. A question that can be answered by making observations and that indicates (directly or indirectly) the observations that have to be made to answer it.

ANTERIOR OPEN BITE. A type of dental malocclusion in which there is a relatively large space between the upper and lower incisors when the jaws are together.

APHASIA. A language disorder resulting from damage to the brain in which the person loses some ability to understand speech, formulate speech, read, write, calculate, or some combination of these abilities.

APHASIA TEST. A test used to identify language deficits that can result from damage to the cerebral cortex, particularly the left half.

APHONIA. The inability to phonate (i.e., produce voice).

APPIAN WAY. A road in ancient Rome that had cavelike apertures in the rocky outcrop on both sides, in which people who had mental handicaps, deformities, and communication impairments were caged to provide entertainment for travelers.

ARTICULATION TEST. A test, usually consisting of a set of stimulus drawings or words, that is used to identify and inventory a client's articulation errors.

ARTICULATORS. The structures within the oral cavity that move to change the configuration of the vocal tract (e.g., the tongue and velum).

ARYTENOID CARTILAGE. Two small cartilages in the larynx, the movements of which abduct and adduct the vocal folds.

ASPIRATION. Food or liquid entering the airway.

ASSISTIVE LISTENING DEVICE (ALD). A device that captures sound at its source (e.g., through a microphone) and delivers it directly to the listener (e.g., through earphones).

ATTENTION-DEFICIT/HYPERACTIVITY DISORDER (AD/HD). A neurobiological condition affecting an individual's ability to maintain attention.

AuD. Doctor of Audiology degree.

AUDIOGRAM. A graph for plotting the results of a hearing test that was administered with a pure-tone audiometer.

AUDIOLOGIST. An independent professional whose primary responsibility is helping persons who have a hearing disorder cope with it.

AUDIOLOGY ASSISTANT. A person working under the supervision of a licensed audiologist.

AUDIOMETER. An instrument used to measure hearing acuity.

AUDIOMETRIC. Used to measure hearing.

AUDIOMETRIC SCREENING TEST. A brief pure-tone audiometric hearing test that is used to identify clients whose hearing may not be within normal limits. Those who fail it usually receive a complete hearing evaluation.

AUDITORY AGNOSIA. A disorder of the central auditory nervous system in which the person has difficulty separating figure from background noise.

AUDITORY NERVE. A branch of the VIIIth cranial nerve that transmits electrochemical energy generated by the inner ear to the central auditory nervous system (CANS).

AUGMENTATIVE/ALTERNATIVE COMMUNICATION (AAC). Communication strategies and devices used to supplement or replace speech.

AURICLE. The largely cartilaginous, projecting portion of the outer ear. Also referred to as the pinna.

AUTISM. A neurologically based developmental disability with social, developmental, and physical symptoms. Usually described in terms of Autism Spectrum Disorder.

BABBLING. The sounds produced by babies at approximately 6 months of age when they begin to experiment with sounds and before they produce real words.

BALBUS. A surname given to some persons in ancient Greece and Rome who had a speech disorder.

BASAL GANGLIA. A group of nerve cells at the base of the brain that participate in regulating motor performance.

BASELINE. The reference point to which a client's current status is compared (e.g., the results of evaluation at the beginning of therapy) when measuring the degree of progress toward achieving a particular goal.

BASIC EPISODE. An early narrative form used by children; it consists of a problem, action taken by a character to solve the problem, and resolution of the problem.

BILABIAL SOUND. Sound produced with closure of the lips.

BILATERAL CONDUCTIVE HEARING LOSS. A conductive hearing loss in both ears.

BILINGUAL. Proficiency in (or developing proficiency in) two languages.

BIOFEEDBACK. A process in which a device (usually a computer-based one) is used to give clients feedback about whether they are making movements (e.g., producing speech sounds) correctly.

BOLUS. The rounded mass of food formed through chewing and saliva prior to swallowing.

BONE CONDUCTION. The conduction of sound to the inner ear through the bones of the skull.

BOUND MORPHEME. A morpheme that must be attached to a free morpheme or another bound morpheme.

BRAIN ABSCESSES. Walled-off cavities containing dead or dying white blood cells.

BROCA'S APHASIA. An impairment in the ability to produce speech voluntarily (i.e., moving the articulators in the manner required to produce words). Also known as motor aphasia, expressive aphasia, verbal apraxia, or disfluent aphasia.

CALIBRATED. Precisely adjusted in order to measure a particular function.

CATASTROPHIC REACTION. A reaction in which the person loses control and does something violent (e.g., throws something) when too many demands are made on him or her. Also referred to as challenging behavior.

CENTRAL AUDITORY NERVOUS SYSTEM (CANS). A group of sites within the central nervous system (brain) that process the electrical signals output by the auditory nerves. The CANS enables us to be aware of, and abstract information from, sounds in our environment.

CEREBELLAR ATAXIA. A neuromuscular disorder resulting from abnormal functioning of a part of the extrapyramidal system know as the cerebellum.

CEREBRAL ARTERIOSCLEROSIS. A thickening of the walls of cerebral arteries resulting in a slower rate of blood flow through them.

CEREBRAL CORTEX. The thin layer of nerve cells on the surface of the brain.

CEREBRAL LOCALIZATION OF FUNCTION. Dedication of nerve cells at specific locations in the cerebral cortex to performing specific functions.

CEREBRAL PALSY (CP). A neuromuscular disorder resulting from damage to the brain occurring prior to, during, or shortly after birth.

CERTIFICATE OF CLINICAL COMPETENCE (CCC). Clinical certification awarded by the American Speech-Language-Hearing Association once the person has met all the necessary academic and clinical requirements. The CCC-SLP is offered for speech-language pathology, and the CCC-A is offered for audiology.

CERUMEN. Ear wax.

CERUMEN IMPACTION. An overabundance of ear wax.

CERUMINOUS GLANDS. The glands that secrete cerumen.

CHIEF COMPLAINT. The reason given by the client (or the person who requested the evaluation) indicating why the evaluation was requested.

CHOLESTEATOMA. A type of tumor that can occur in the middle ear and cause a conductive hearing loss.

CILIA. Small hairs on the inner surface of the external auditory meatus.

CLEFT PALATE. A congenital disorder in which there is an opening in the hard palate, soft palate (velum), or both.

CLIENT. A person whom a clinician is trying to help. In some settings, this person is referred to as a patient or student.

CLINICAL RELATIONSHIP. The context within which clinical services are dispensed, involving the clinician, the client, and those close to the client. Also referred to as therapeutic relationship.

CLINICIAN-INVESTIGATOR. A clinician who does therapy-outcome research which forms the basis for evidence-based practice. All speech-language pathologists and audiologists are required to collect some data on outcomes for purposes of accountability.

CLUTTERING. A fluency disorder in which the person speaks very rapidly and hesitates a great deal because of doing so. Also referred to as tachyphemia.

COCHLEA. The structure in the inner ear responsible for hearing.

COCHLEAR IMPLANT. A surgically implanted inner ear prosthesis that can enable persons who are deaf to hear some sounds.

CODE OF ETHICS OF THE AMERICAN SPEECH-LANGUAGE-HEARING ASSOCIATION. The ethical code to which all speech-language pathologists and audiologists are required to adhere. Failure to do so can result in one's certification and/or license to practice being suspended or revoked.

CODE SWITCHING. Switching from one style of language usage to another, depending on context and the social situation.

COGNITIVE DISABILITY. A condition characterized by significantly below average intelligence and limitations in daily life functions; appears before the age of 18.

COLLABORATIVE/CONSULTATIVE SERVICE DELIVERY. Providing clinical services to a school-age child in his or her classroom, rather than a special therapy room.

COMMUNICATION. Any exchange of information between people using a common code, or symbol system, understood by those involved.

COMMUNICATION BOARD. A sheet of cardboard or other material on which is printed the alphabet; commonly used words and phrases; and/or pictographic symbols. The user communicates by pointing to or otherwise indicating the symbols needed to transmit messages.

COMORBID. The presence of coexisting or additional diseases with reference to an initial diagnosis.

CONDUCTIVE HEARING LOSS. A hearing loss caused by pathology in the outer or middle ear.

CONGENITAL. Present at birth.

CONGENITAL ATRESIA. A partial or complete absence or blockage of the external auditory meatus.

CONGRESSIONAL ACTION CONTACT NETWORK. A lobbying entity sponsored by the American Speech-Language-Hearing Association. A member of the Association is assigned to each member of Congress to present its point of view on relevant upcoming bills.

CONJUNCT. A device used to signal a logical relationship between sentences (e.g., *still, to conclude*).

CONSISTENCY EFFECT. The greater-than-chance tendency for stutterers to stutter on words that they stuttered on previously.

CONTINUANT. A phoneme that can be sustained.

CONTRACT. A written or oral agreement that the parties agree to abide by voluntarily. The relationship between the client and clinician is a contractual one.

CORPUS CALLOSUM. The structure that connects the right and left cerebral hemispheres.

CRICOID CARTILAGE. A cartilage that sits on top of the trachea and forms the base of the larynx.

CULTURAL SENSITIVITY. Awareness that cultures differ in their views of the world; knowing there is no one "right way" to view things.

CULTURE. The ways of thinking, talking, understanding, and relating to others that are characteristic of groups of people with a shared history (Paul, 2001, p. 165).

CYCLE. The time period required for a child to successively focus for two to six hours on each of his or her basic error patterns.

DECIBEL (dB). The unit of measurement for the loudness of sounds. The louder the sound, the larger the number.

DEGENERATIVE. Causing a gradual decline in quality, value, or strength.

DELAYED AUDITORY FEEDBACK (DAF). A procedure where you speak into a microphone and hear your voice through earphones, delayed by a fraction of a second.

DEMENTIA. A progressive disorder resulting from damage to the brain that impairs memory and cognitive functioning.

DEVELOPMENTAL APRAXIA OF SPEECH (DAS). A disturbance in the ability to voluntarily program the oral musculature to produce speech sounds resulting from damage to the central nervous system, usually either before, during, or immediately following birth. Also referred to as developmental verbal dyspraxia.

DEVELOPMENTAL DISABILITY. A diverse group of physical, cognitive, psychological, sensory, and speech-language impairments that arise any time before age 18.

DEVELOPMENTAL NORMS. Ages by which specific percentages of children in a given subpopulation have acquired particular abilities.

DIADOCHOKINETIC RATE. The number of times in five seconds a client is able to repeat a specific consonant-vowel syllable. Used to test for neuromuscular disorders.

DIAGNOSOGENIC THEORY. An anticipatory struggle theory for stuttering that states that the disorder is precipitated by parents (or others) diagnosing normal childhood syllable repetitions as stuttering and encouraging the child to avoid repeating them.

DIETICIAN. One who is trained in the science of food and nourishment.

DIFFERENTIAL DIAGNOSIS. A process for distinguishing between two or more conditions with similar characteristics by systematically comparing and contrasting their characteristics with clinical findings.

DISABILITY. Something that an impairment prevents an individual from doing normally (e.g., a person who is deaf is highly unlikely to be able to communicate normally by telephone).

DISCOURSE. The rule system governing how we combine phrases and sentences into larger units of meaning.

DISFLUENCY. Hesitations, repetitions, mispronunciations, and interjections in one's speech. They may be either normal or symptoms of stuttering or another fluency disorder. Also called moments of disfluency.

DOCUMENTATION. Regarding intervention, describing its impact on clients, using data that possess adequate levels of validity, reliability, and generality.

DRESSING APRAXIA. A deficit in which individuals may put on their clothes in a disorganized manner. For example, they might put their shirt on backwards.

DYSARTHRIA. A neuromuscular disorder that affects some or all of the vocal tract musculature.

DYSJUNCT. A device used to indicate the speaker's attitude toward the content of a sentence (e.g., *frankly, honestly*).

DYSLEXIA. Learning disabilities associated with reading.

DYSPHAGIA. Difficulty, discomfort, or pain when swallowing.

DYSRHYTHMIC PHONATIONS. Disturbances in the normal rhythms of words.

DYSTONIA. Abnormal muscle tone caused by involuntary muscle contractions.

ECHOLALIA. Repeating what others say without communicative intent.

EDUCATIONALLY SIGNIFICANT. Regarding eligibility for service in the schools, a speech, language, or hearing disorder that significantly interferes with a child's academic progress and cannot be adequately addressed through general education accommodations and modifications.

EFFICACY OF INTERVENTION. Demonstrating that changes in communication ability(ies) occurred that would not have occurred without intervention.

ELECTROLARYNX. A small battery-powered electrical device that can enable persons who have had a laryngectomy to produce a voice.

EMBOLUS. A blood clot that moves from its site of origin.

EMPATHY. The ability to truly understand, at least a little, how another person feels about an event, experience, process, or idea.

ENDOSCOPIC EXAMINATION. Insertion of an endoscope to observe the vocal folds.

ENDOTRACHEAL INTUBATION. Insertion of a flexible plastic tube through the mouth into the trachea to ensure the passage of air.

EPIGLOTTIS. A leaflike structure in the larynx that lowers during swallowing to prevent what is being swallowed from getting into the lungs.

ESOPHAGEAL SPEECH. A type of speech used by persons who have had a laryngectomy that requires air to be injected into the esophagus.

ESOPHAGUS. The tube that connects the oral cavity to the stomach.

EUSTACHIAN TUBE. A hollow structure that connects the middle ear to the back wall of the throat.

EVALUATION. The initial step in the intervention process. Its purpose is to determine if the client has a communication disorder and, if so, to identify and describe the impairments, disabilities, and handicaps that it has caused or placed the client at risk for developing.

EVIDENCE-BASED PRACTICE (EBP). Basing decisions about the care of individual clients on the best evidence available about what works. In EBP, clinicians integrate their clinical expertise and judgment with the best available external clinical evidence derived from systematic research.

EXCISED. To remove something surgically (e.g., a tumor).

EXECUTIVE FUNCTIONS. The many skills required to prepare for and execute complex behavior (e.g., plan, organize, multitask, use feedback).

EXHALATION. The process by which air is expelled from the lungs under pressure.

EXPECTANCY PHENOMENON. The ability of stutterers to predict moments of stuttering with greater-than-chance accuracy.

EXPERIMENTER BIAS. Bias introduced by an experimenter's desire to have his or her findings be what is wanted.

EXPERT WITNESS. Witnesses who give opinions in their areas of expertise at trials and hearings.

EXPOSITORY DISCOURSE. Discourse types other than narratives.

EXPRESSIVE. Relating to the skills of speaking and writing.

EXTERNAL AUDITORY MEATUS. The part of the outer ear that is also referred to as the ear canal.

EXTRAPYRAMIDAL SYSTEM. Groups of neurons within the central nervous system that are responsible for the refinement of movement patterns.

FIGURATIVE LANGUAGE. Nonliteral language or language forms that say one thing and mean another (e.g., idioms, polite forms, metaphors, parables, satires, aphorisms, and axioms).

FIRST TEMPORAL CONVOLUTION. A location in the temporal lobe of the left cerebral hemisphere that is referred to as Wernicke's area. A lesion in this area produces Wernicke's aphasia.

FLACCIDITY. Paralysis or weakness of muscle contraction resulting from damage to muscle fibers, myoneural junctions, or lower motor neurons.

FLUENCY. Effortless and smooth production of speech.

FREE MORPHEME. A morpheme that has meaning on its own.

FRICATIVE. A consonant sound produced by forcing air through a narrow opening.

FRONTAL LOBE. One of the four lobes of the cerebral cortex. The left frontal lobe facilitates cognitive functioning and motor speech.

FUNCTIONAL COMMUNICATION NEEDS. The basic communication abilities a person needs to function in everyday life (e.g., face-to-face or telephone conversations and writing).

FUNCTIONAL HEARING LOSS. A condition in which persons do not respond appropriately to speech or other sound and there does not appear to be an abnormality or lesion in their ears, auditory nerves, or CANS. Also referred to as psychogenic hearing loss, pseudohypacusis, and idiopathic sudden deafness.

GESTURAL MORSE CODE. A communication system used by persons who have severe communication impairments in which words are spelled out letter-by-letter using gestures (e.g., blinking the eyes) for Morse Code dots and dashes.

GLIDE SOUND. The two semivowels, /j/ as in *yes* and /w/ as in *well*.

GLOBAL APHASIA. Aphasia that causes severe impairment in all language areas.

GLOSSECTOMY. Surgical removal of a portion of the tongue. Such surgery is usually done to remove a malignant tumor from the tongue tissue.

GLOTTAL SOUND. Sound made with an open glottis.

GLOTTIS. The space between the vocal folds.

GOALS. In this context, benefits the client hopes to derive from therapy.

GRAND MAL SEIZURES. Seizures characterized by loss of consciousness.

GRAPHOPHONEMIC AWARENESS. The ability to associate letters of the alphabet with speech sounds.

HANDICAP. Limitations that people impose on themselves because of their negative attitudes (e.g., shame, guilt, and/or embarrassment) toward their impairments and disabilities.

HARD PALATE. The anterior portion of the roof of the mouth.

HEARING. The perception of sound.

HEARING AID. A portable amplifier that can improve the ability of some persons who have a hearing loss to understand speech.

HEMATOMA. Blood that has formed as a result of a broken blood vessel.

HEMIANOPIA. A visual field disturbance in which there is a loss of vision in either the right or left halves of the visual field in each eye.

HEMIPLEGIA. A neuromuscular disorder that affects only one side of the body.

HEMORRHAGE. A loss of a large amount of blood in a short time.

HEMORRHAGIC STROKE. When a cerebral artery bursts and blood can no longer flow through it to the areas of the brain it nourishes.

HERTZ (Hz). The unit of measurement for the pitch of sounds. The higher the pitch, the larger the number.

HUNTINGTON'S DISEASE. A genetic disease resulting in gradual loss of brain cells. Both neurological functioning and intelligence are affected. Also referred to as Huntington's chorea.

HYOID BONE. A complex of bones at the base of the tongue and above the thyroid cartilage that supports the tongue and its muscles.

HYPERNASALITY. A disorder in which air flows through the nasal cavity while producing sounds for which it should not.

HYPONASALITY. A disorder in which air does not flow through the nasal cavity while producing sounds for which it should.

HYPOTHESES. In this context, preliminary explanations for clients' impairments, disabilities, and handicaps.

IDEOGRAPHIC. A set of written characters that symbolize ideas without indicating the pronunciation of the words represented.

IDIOMS. An expression with both a literal and nonliteral (i.e., figurative) meaning, the latter understood by a particular group of people to have its own unique meaning (e.g., *to kick the bucket* meaning *to die*).

IDIOSYNCRATIC. Unique, one-of-a-kind, or distinctive.

IMPAIRMENT. The failure to function normally. (In our context, the anomaly in hearing, speech, and/or language exhibited by the client.)

INCISORS. The four front teeth in each jaw (i.e., the two front and two lateral incisors).

INCUS. The second of the three tiny bones in the middle ear.

INDEPENDENT PROFESSIONAL. A practitioner who is not required by law to have his or her activities regulated (i.e., controlled) by a member of another profession. Speech-language pathologists and audiologists (like physicians and dentists) are independent professionals. Speech-language pathology assistants (like nurses) are not.

INDIRECT LARYNGOSCOPY. A procedure for viewing the top surface and edges of the vocal folds through a laryngeal mirror.

INDIVIDUALIZED EDUCATION PROGRAM (IEP). A program developed for each child who is eligible for special education, based on the child's unique needs, to provide the student with a free, appropriate, public education. The IEP contains a statement of the child's present level of performance, educational needs, and measurable goals and objectives. The IEP is reviewed at least annually.

INFORMANTS. In this context, people (including clients) who have information needed to answer a clinician's evaluation questions.

INHALATION. The process by which air from the environment is drawn into the lungs.

INTELLIGIBILITY. How understandable a speaker is to a listener.

INTELLIGIBLE. Understandable.

INTERJECTIONS. Sounds, syllables, words, and/or phrases added between words.

INTERVENTION STRATEGY. The approach used to try to achieve an intervention goal (i.e., to be helpful to the client).

JOINT ATTENDING. An infant and adult attend to the same external object or process.

JOINT REFERENCING. An infant and adult jointly attend to an external object which the adult talks about.

LABIO-DENTAL SOUND. Sound produced with the upper teeth placed on the lower lip.

LANGUAGE. The code used for communicating ideas with others.

LANGUAGE CONTENT. Semantics.

LANGUAGE DIFFERENCE. Variation of language used by a group of individuals with shared regional, social, or cultural/ethnic factors.

LANGUAGE DISORDER. Impaired comprehension and/or expression of language form, content, and/or use.

LANGUAGE FORM. Phonology, syntax, and morphology.

LANGUAGE USE. Pragmatics.

LARYNGEAL TONE. The buzzing sound produced by phonation.

LARYNGECTOMY. The surgical removal of all or part of the larynx.

LARYNGOSCOPIC VIEW. The view of the top surface of the vocal folds through a round laryngeal mirror. It is the view of the larynx yielded by indirect laryngoscopy.

LARYNX. The structure that contains the vocal folds (i.e., the mechanism that produces voice). The larynx also functions as a valve which prevents food and liquids from getting into the lungs.

LEARNING STYLE. The process(es) through which an individual (or cultural group) learns most efficiently.

LEFT CEREBRAL HEMISPHERE. The left half of the brian. Damage may impair the ability to comprehend and/or use language.

LEFT NEGLECT. Lack of attention to environmental stimuli on the left. Also referred to as hemi-attention.

LICENSE. A permit issued by a governmental entity (usually a state) to practice a profession.

LINGUA-ALVEOLAR SOUND. Sound produced with the tongue against the alveolar ridge.

LINGUA-DENTAL SOUND. Sound produced with the tongue between the upper and lower teeth.

LINGUAL FRENUM. A fold of membrane that extends from the floor of the mouth at the midline to the underside of the tongue.

LINGUISTICS. The study of the structure and development of a particular language and its relationship to other languages.

LIPREADING. An older term for speechreading. Using visual facial information to augment hearing for understanding speech.

LIQUID SOUND. Sound produced by air passing along one or both sides of the tongue.

LISPING. Either a substitution of the voiceless /θ/ sound for /s/ (e.g., *th*ip for *s*ip) or a distortion of /s/ in which the airstream is directed at the side rather than the front teeth. The former is referred to as a frontal lisp and the latter as a lateral lisp.

LOBBYING. In this context, attempting to encourage the passage of state and federal legislation that is likely to be helpful to persons who have communication disorders and to discourage the passage of legislation that is likely to be harmful to them.

Locked-in syndrome. Severe motoric impairment in which the only muscles that usually aren't paralyzed are those of the eyes. The person may be able to learn to communicate by Morse code by blinking the eyes.

Logopedics. The study of speech disorders.

Long-term goals. Statements that specify the measurable outcomes that the clinician is attempting to achieve through the intervention process.

Loudness recruitment. An abnormally rapid growth of loudness with an increase in intensity.

Lower motor neurons. The structures within the motor system that come into most direct contact with muscle fibers. They conduct electrical signals to muscles.

Lungs. The two lungs are the main component of the respiratory system. They are the source of the air for vibrating the vocal folds to produce voice.

Maintaining cause. Some factor that causes an impairment to persist.

Malleus. The first of the three tiny bones in the middle ear.

Mandible. Lower jaw.

Manual communication system. A communication system that uses gestures, body language, and facial expressions in place of the voice to mediate a message.

Maxilla. Upper jaw.

Medical model. Abnormal behavior (e.g., stuttering) is viewed as a symptom of some underlying disorder. Treatment focuses on what is assumed to be the underlying disorder rather than on the abnormal behavior (i.e., symptom).

Medicare. A federal health insurance program that partially pays for some of the services that speech-language pathologists and audiologists dispense to senior citizens.

Memory wallet. A small loose-leaf binder containing photographs and words on index cards (e.g., names and photographs of family members and friends) that a person with Alzheimer's disease or dementia has difficulty remembering.

Ménière's disease. A disease of the vestibular system (part of the inner ear) that has a sensorineural hearing loss as one of its components.

Metacognitive ability. The ability to think and talk about thinking.

Metalinguistic ability. The ability to think and talk about language.

Metaphor. A figure of speech that involves an implicit comparison between two things (e.g., *He's a brick*).

Metapragmatic ability. The ability to think and talk about how language is used.

Morpheme. The smallest grammatical unit that carries meaning.

Morphological disorder. Difficulties understanding and/or producing morphemes, the smallest units of meaning.

MORPHOLOGY. The rule system governing the smallest units of meaning in language.

MOTHERESE. The language used by adults communicating with infants in which they use altered pitch, loudness, and intonation patterns to talk about what is going on in the immediate environment.

MOTIVATION. In this context, the willingness of the client to make the investments necessary to achieve therapy goals.

MOTOR SYSTEM. The parts of the peripheral and central nervous systems that regulate the contraction of muscle fibers.

MULTIPLE SCLEROSIS (MS). A neurological disorder that can affect the functioning of the auditory nerves and other structures within the brain that support motor and sensory abilities. Typical symptoms are weakness, incoordination, paresthesias, speech disturbances, and visual complaints.

MUSCULAR DYSTROPHY. A neuromuscular disorder of genetic origin in which muscle weakness results from muscle abnormality, rather than myoneural junction or nerve abnormality.

MUTUAL ATTENDING. An infant and an adult attend to each other.

MYASTHENIA GRAVIS. A neuromuscular disorder characterized by muscle weakness.

MYOFUNCTIONAL THERAPY. Therapy intended to eliminate tongue thrusting.

MYONEURAL JUNCTIONS. The space between the tips of lower motor neurons and muscle fibers that contain a chemical for conducting electrical signals.

NARRATIVE DISCOURSE. Telling actions, feelings, or thoughts of fictional or nonfictional characters.

NASAL CAVITY. The interior of the nose.

NASAL SOUND. Sound produced with air flowing through the nose.

NASALITY. Nasal resonance.

NASOGASTRIC TUBE. A flexible plastic tube running from the nose, through the esophagus, and into the stomach. It is used to either drain the stomach or to deliver medications and/or nutrients.

NATIONAL STUDENT SPEECH LANGUAGE HEARING ASSOCIATION (NSSLHA). The preprofessional membership association for students interested in the study of communication sciences and disorders.

NEGLECT DYSLEXIA. A tendency to frequently misread the beginnings of words. It is demonstrated by some persons who have damage to the right cerebral hemisphere.

NEOPLASMS. Tumors (i.e., abnormal masses of tissue) either malignant or benign.

NEUROFIBRILLARY TANGLES. Brain abnormality in persons who have Alzheimer's disease.

NEUROGENIC ACQUIRED STUTTERING. A fluency disorder, usually acquired during adulthood, that is caused by damage to the central nervous system (e.g., a stroke or head trauma).

NONSTANDARDIZED ASSESSMENTS. Instruments or procedures for which norms have not been collected and which may include procedures that are not standardized or specified completely.

NORMAL LIMITS. Statistically expected range within which a person's speech, hearing, and/or language abilities fall.

OBJECTIVE ATTITUDE. A nonjudgmental attitude such as viewing an impairment as a "challenge" rather than a "chain." This attitude assists a person who has an impairment to minimize the negative impact that the impairment has on his or her life.

OBJECTIVITY. Perceiving, documenting, and managing clients' impairments, disabilities, and handicaps without becoming emotionally involved and/or losing focus on the client's welfare.

OBSERVATIONS. The data used to answer the questions that an evaluation is intended to answer.

OBTURATOR. A prosthetic device used to close an opening in the body.

OCCIPITAL LOBE. One of the four lobes of the cerebral cortex. The left occipital lobe facilitates visual functioning.

OCCLUDE. To create a blockage.

OCCUPATIONAL THERAPIST. A professional who helps people improve basic motor functions to perform daily living and work tasks.

ONCOLOGIST. A physician who specializes in the treatment of cancer.

OPTOMETRIST. A professional trained to provide care to improve vision with glasses, contact lenses, etc.

ORAL CAVITY. The mouth.

ORAL METHOD. The method used to teach individuals with hearing impairments to communicate through speech.

ORALITY. Oral resonance.

OSSICULAR CHAIN. The three tiny bones in the middle ear.

OSSICULAR DISCONTINUITY. One of the three tiny bones that form the ossicular chain in the middle ear breaks or somehow becomes disconnected from the other two. The result is a conductive hearing loss.

OTITIS MEDIA. An inflammation in the middle ear that can cause a conductive hearing loss.

OTOLARYNGOLOGIST. A physician who specializes in treatment of disease of the ear, larynx, and upper respiratory tract.

OTOSCLEROSIS. A disease in which the stapes (the third bone in the ossicular chain) becomes fixated in the oval window, thereby causing a conductive hearing loss.

OVAL WINDOW. The membrane that separates the middle ear from the inner ear.

PALATAL SOUND. Sound produced with the tongue against the hard palate.

PARAPHASIA. Producing unintended syllables, words, or phrases during speech.

PARAPROFESSIONALS. People who assist professionals in a particular field (e.g., speech-language pathology assistants).

PARIETAL LOBE. One of the four lobes of the cerebral cortex. The left parietal lobe facilitates one's ability to repeat.

PARKINSON'S DISEASE. A neuromuscular disorder resulting from abnormal functioning of the extrapyramidal system.

PARTICIPATION MODEL. A clinical relationship characterized by client and clinician focusing on "what clients think about themselves, their abilities and accomplishments, their disabilities, and their future" (Duchan, 2003, ¶1).

PART-WORD REPETITIONS. Repetitions of sounds and syllables in words.

PEDIATRICIAN. A physician who specializes in the care of infants and children.

PERINATAL. An event occurring during the birth process.

PERSEVERATION. Continuing to repeat a behavior to an exceptional degree (e.g., saying a word or phrase over and over).

PERVASIVE DEVELOPMENTAL DISORDER (PDD). A set of five syndromes including autistic disorder, Asperger syndrome, childhood disintegrative disorder, Rett's syndrome, and pervasive developmental disorder (not otherwise specified).

PETIT MAL SEIZURES. Seizures characterized by frequent, momentary loss of contact with the environment.

PHARYNGEAL CAVITY. The throat. Also referred to as the pharynx.

PHONATION. Voice produced by vibration of the vocal folds.

PHONEME COLLAPSE. The production of one sound by the child for several different adult target sounds, or the deletion of several adult target sounds in a given position (e.g., /t/ substituted for /f, p, h, θ, n/.

PHONEMES. Speech sounds.

PHONETICS. The study and classification of the sounds made in a spoken language.

PHONIATRICS. The study of voice disorders.

PHONOLOGICAL AWARENESS. Understanding elements of words, such as syllables; initial, medial, and final sounds; sound sequencing; rhyming; and syllabication.

PHONOLOGICAL DISORDER. A language disorder in which sound substitutions and omissions result from a lack of awareness of the phonemes that words contain, rather than errors programming the articulators to produce desired phonemes (as is the case with an articulation disorder).

PHONOLOGICAL PROCESSES. Ways children below the age of 3.5 years sometimes simplify their production of words.

PHONOLOGY. The rule system governing how we combine sounds.

PHRASE REPETITIONS. Repetitions of units of two or more words.

PHYSICAL THERAPIST. A professional who helps those suffering from disease or injury restore function, improve mobility, relieve pain, and prevent or limit permanent physical disabilities.

PICTOGRAPHIC. Symbols that somewhat resemble the units of experience they represent.

PLACEBO EFFECT. A change (usually a reduction) in the severity of an impairment or disorder elicited by a strong belief in the ability of something or someone to change its severity.

PLATEAU. A period during which the client makes no measurable progress toward achieving a therapy goal.

PLATFORM PRESENTATION. An oral presentation of the findings of a research project at a professional association convention.

PLOSIVE. A consonant sound that cannot be sustained.

POLIO. A viral disease that damages lower motor neurons and causes flaccidity. Function of the velum is frequently affected.

POSITIVE REINFORCEMENT. A behavior modification technique to increase desirable behaviors with a reward. If a behavior is rewarded immediately after it occurs, it is said to have received response-contingent positive reinforcement.

POSTER PRESENTATION. A report of the findings of a research project at a professional association convention printed on a poster and attached for an hour or so to a poster board. The presenter stands beside the poster to answer questions from colleagues.

POSTLINGUAL DEAFNESS. Hearing loss acquired after age 5.

POSTNATAL. An event occurring just after birth.

PRAGMATIC DISORDER. Difficulties understanding how to use language in different ways for a variety of intentions, situations, and listeners.

PRAGMATICS. The rule system governing how language is used.

PREDISPOSING CAUSE. A psychological or organic factor that makes some persons more "at risk" than others for developing a disorder.

PRELINGUAL DEAFNESS. Hearing loss acquired before the onset of language development.

PRENATAL. An event occurring prior to birth.

PRESBYCUSIS. Sensorineural hearing loss resulting—directly or indirectly (e.g., long-term exposure to noise)—from the effect of the aging process on the inner ear.

PROSODY. Variations in stress, pitch, and rhythms of speech that carry meaning.

PROSOPAGNOSIA. Failure to recognize familiar faces, such as that of one's spouse.

PROSTHESIS. An artificial body part.

PROSTHODONTIST. A person who specializes in the part of dentistry pertaining to replacement of missing teeth and tissues with artificial substitutes.

PROVERBS, ADAGES, AND MAXIMS. Short, witty, popular sayings that impart wisdom.

PSYCHIATRIST. A physician who specializes in the diagnosis, treatment, and prevention of mental and emotional disorders.

PSYCHOANALYSIS. A system of psychotherapy developed in the late 1800s by Sigmund Freud.

PSYCHOGENIC ACQUIRED STUTTERING. A fluency disorder, usually acquired during adulthood, that is caused by an acute or chronic psychological disturbance.

PSYCHOLOGICAL OVERLAY. When psychological factors influence the severity of an organic impairment.

PUNISHMENT. A technique for getting a behavior (e.g., interrupting) to occur less often by imposing something unpleasant on the client whenever the behavior appears.

PURE TONE. A sound in which particles of air vibrate at a single frequency.

PURE TONE AUDIOMETER. An instrument for measuring hearing using pure tones.

PYRAMIDAL SYSTEM. The system responsible for controlling voluntary motor movements.

QUALITATIVE DATA. Information that is difficult to measure, count, or express in numerical terms (e.g., the nature of relationships among various groups).

QUANTITATIVE DATA. Data that consist of numerical descriptions of various sorts of attributes.

RECEPTIVE. Relating to the skills of listening and reading.

REEVALUATE. Conduct an evaluation after the initial diagnostic/assessment process.

RELIABLE. Consistently gives the same result on successive trials.

REPRESENTATIVE. Data that is consistent across situations (e.g., home, school, work).

RESONATE. Intensification of sound produced by vibrations interacting with the tissues of the vocal tract.

RESPIRATORY SYSTEM. The organs that generate the raw material (i.e., air) for vibrating the vocal folds to produce voice.

RESPIRATORY THERAPIST. A professional who evaluates, treats, and cares for individuals with breathing or other cardiopulmonary disorders.

REVISION-INCOMPLETE PHRASES. Disfluencies in which the speaker begins an utterance but does not complete it.

RIGHT HEMIPLEGIA. Weakness or paralysis of the right side of the body due to damage to the left cerebral hemisphere.

SCIENTIFIC JUSTIFICATION. Providing answers to the "so what" and "who cares" questions for why it is important to carry out a particular clinical research project.

SCIENTIFIC METHOD. A logically organized and objective set of rules for investigating questions to maximize the likelihood of getting a correct answer.

SCOPE OF PRACTICE. The services that practitioners in a field are recognized by licensing and certification boards and the courts as having the expertise to provide.

SECONDARY BEHAVIORS. Behaviors that accompany moments of stuttering, particularly those of adults (e.g., using interjections or eye blinking). Also referred to as secondaries.

SELF-IMAGE. The manner in which a person views himself or herself.

SEMANTIC DISORDER. Difficulty understanding and/or assigning meaning to words.

SEMANTICS. The rule system governing how words are used.

SEMICIRCULAR CANALS. The structures in the inner ear responsible for the detection of rotation.

SENSORINEURAL HEARING LOSS. A hearing loss caused by pathology in the inner ear.

SEVERE COMMUNICATION IMPAIRMENT. The inability to speak intelligibly enough to meet communication needs. Augmentative communication strategies and devices can enable these clients to meet their communication needs.

SHORT-TERM GOALS. These are "stepping stones" to achieving long-term goals . They often have to be accomplished in a specific order. Also referred to as short-term objectives.

SIDE EFFECT. Something an intervention strategy changes other than what it's intended to change. A side effect can be physiological, psychological, desirable, or undesirable.

SIGNING EXACT ENGLISH (SEE). A manual communication system based on spoken English.

SIMILE. A figure of speech that involves an explicit comparison between two things with the use of *like* (e.g., *He's like a big cat).*

SINE WAVE. The waveform for a pure tone.

SINGLE-SUBJECT RESEARCH. A research design in which questions are answered by data from individual subjects, rather than by data that are derived from the performances of groups of subjects.

SOCIAL WORKER. A professional who helps individuals function their best in their environments; help deal with relationships, and help solve personal and family problems.

SOUND DISTORTION. An articulation error in which a phoneme that does not occur in a language is substituted for one that does.

SOUND OMISSION. An articulation error in which a phoneme is omitted from words.

SOUND SUBSTITUTION. An articulation error in which one phoneme that occurs in a language is substituted for another that occurs in that language.

SPASMODIC DYSPHONIA. A voice disorder in which the voice, at times, sounds tense or strained.

SPASTICITY. A condition in which certain muscles are continuously contracted. It is the result of a lesion in the pyramidal and extrapyramidal systems.

SPECIFIC LANGUAGE IMPAIRMENT (SLI). Difficulties with language (i.e., communication) in the absence of another problem such as cognitive disability, hearing loss, or emotional disorder (NIDCD, 2005). Also referred to as language learning disability (LLD).

SPEECH. The production of phonemes by the vocal tract.

SPEECH-LANGUAGE PATHOLOGIST (SLP). An independent professional whose primary responsibility is helping persons who have speech and/or language disorders cope with them as impairments, disabilities, and handicaps.

SPEECH-LANGUAGE PATHOLOGY ASSISTANT (SLPA). A paraprofessional who helps people who have speech and/or language disorders cope with them under the supervision of a speech-language pathologist.

SPEECHREADING. Using visual information to augment hearing for understanding speech. Less accurately called "lipreading."

SPONTANEOUS RECOVERY. The tendency for aphasic impairments to decrease in severity during the first six months posttrauma.

STANDARDIZED ASSESSMENTS. Tests that are based on the scores of a large number of people with the same characteristics as the person being tested.

STAPES. The third of three tiny bones in the middle ear.

STARTERS. A device that stutterers use to avoid stuttering. They inject sounds, syllables, words, or phrases they believe they can say without stuttering before words on which they expect to stutter.

STATISTICAL ANALYSES. Numerical analyses for summarizing and otherwise treating quantitative data (e.g., to assess their validity and reliability) in order to answer research questions.

STROKE. Occurs when a cerebral artery is blocked and the area of the brain it nourishes is damaged or destroyed. Also referred to as cerebrovascular accident, or CVA.

STUTTERING. A fluency disorder that usually begins in early childhood.

SUPPORT GROUP. A group of people having a particular disability who support each other's attempts to cope with it. Members of such a group may communicate mainly face-to-face or online.

SUPRAMARGINAL GYRUS. A brain structure above Wernicke's area that carries out some language functions.

SYLLABARY. A set of written symbols that represent syllables.

SYNTACTIC DISORDER. Difficulties understanding sentence structures and/or combining words into phrases and sentences.

SYNTAX. The rule system governing the use of the grammatical structures of language.

TARGET PHONEME. The phoneme that a drawing or word in an articulation test is intended to elicit.

TELECOMMUNICATION RELAY SERVICES (TRS). Organizations that provide telephone services to persons who do not hear or speak well enough to use a standard telephone. They were mandated by the Americans with Disabilities Act of 1990.

TEMPORAL LOBE. One of the four lobes of the cerebral cortex. The left temporal lobe facilitates speech comprehension.

TEMPORARY THRESHOLD SHIFT. A temporary hearing loss after being exposed to loud noise that affects the functioning of the inner ear.

TENSE PAUSES. Pauses filled with barely audible heavy breathing or muscle tightening. Also referred to as blocks.

TEXT TELEPHONE (TTY): A device used by deaf persons to communicate over telephone lines. Both messages and responses are keyboarded. Also referred to as telecommunication device for the deaf (TDD).

THERAPY ROOM. The office or other environment in which the clinician provides clinical services to the client.

THIRD FRONTAL CONVOLUTION. A location in the frontal lobe of the left cerebral hemisphere that is referred to as Broca's area.

THIRD-PARTY PAYERS. These include private insurance companies and governmental organizations (e.g., Medicare) that pay for client services.

THRESHOLD. The lowest intensity level (in decibels) that a person hears for a frequency.

THROMBOEMBOLIC STROKE. Occurs when a piece breaks off a blood clot that formed outside the brain, and the clot is carried to a cerebral artery and blocks it.

THROMBOTIC STROKE. Occurs when a blood clot forms in and blocks a cerebral artery.

THYROARYTENOID MUSCLE. The muscle in each vocal fold.

THYROID CARTILAGE. A part of the larynx; the bulge in the neck referred to as the Adam's apple.

TINNITUS. A constant or almost constant ringing, whistling, or roaring sound that appears to the person experiencing it to be located in one or both ears or somewhere in the head.

TONGUE THRUST. Thrusting the tongue against the incisors (i.e., front teeth) while speaking and swallowing.

TONGUE TIED. Having a lingual frenum that extends too near the tip of the tongue and, consequently, restricts the ability of the tongue tip to move.

TRACHEA. A hollow tube-like structure below the larynx through which air flows to the lungs.

TRACHEO-ESOPHAGEAL SPEECH. A type of speech used by persons who have had a laryngectomy in which air passes from the lungs into the esophagus through a small opening in the wall that separates the trachea from the esophagus.

TRACHEOSTOMY. Opening the trachea surgically in order to allow air into the lungs.

TRANSDUCE. Convert energy from one form into another. The inner ear transduces sound-induced vibration into a form of electrochemical energy.

TRAUMA. Damage that is usually accidental to the nervous system or other bodily structures .

TRAUMATIC BRAIN INJURY (TBI). Injury to the brain that results from an accident (e.g., a traffic accident involving a motorcycle). TBI is the most common cause of brain damage in children and young adults.

TYMPANIC MEMBRANE. The eardrum.

TYMPANOMETER. An instrument used to measure the mobility of the eardrum (i.e., tympanic membrane) at different levels of air pressure.

TYMPANOMETRY. The measurement of the energy of a sound signal reflected by the tympanic membrane at different levels of air pressure.

UNFILLED PAUSES. Long pauses between words without tension.

UNILATERAL CONDUCTIVE HEARING LOSS. A conductive hearing loss in only one ear.

UNINTELLIGIBLE. Speech with so many errors it is difficult or impossible to understand.

UNITS OF EXPERIENCE. The objects and events to which words refer.

UPPER MOTOR NEURONS. Motor neurons in the central nervous system that control the lower motor neurons in the peripheral nervous system.

VALID. Measures what is says it measures.

VELAR SOUND. Sound produced with the tongue against the velum.

VELOPHARYNGEAL CLOSURE. Elevation of the velum to contact the posterior and lateral walls of the pharynx, thereby closing off the opening between the oral and the nasal cavities.

VELOPHARYNGEAL PORT. The soft palate and nasopharyngeal wall.

VELUM. The posterior portion of the roof of the mouth. Also referred to as soft palate.

VENTILATOR-DEPENDENCE. Dependency on a mechanical device (ventilator/respirator) in order to breathe.

VENTRICULAR FOLDS. A pair of soft, flaccid folds above the true vocal folds that contain little muscle fiber. Also referred to as false vocal cords.

VERBAL APRAXIA. A disturbance in the ability to voluntarily program the oral musculature to produce speech sounds, resulting from damage to the central nervous system. There is no weakness, paralysis, or incoordination of the oral musculature while it is being used for vegetative purposes (i.e., eating and drinking), as there is with dysarthria.

VESTIBULE. The structure in the inner ear responsible for the detection of linear acceleration and gravity.

VISUAL FIELD DISTURBANCE. Blindness in a portion of the visual field.

VOCAL FOLDS. Two mucous-covered muscles that stretch horizontally across the larynx; they vibrate to produce sound.

VOCAL TRACT. The mechanism that molds the "buzz" generated by the vocal folds into speech sounds. It consists of the pharyngeal, oral, and nasal cavities.

VOICED SOUND. Sounds produced when air particles entering the vocal tract are set into vibration by the vocal folds (e.g., /z/ and /v/).

VOICELESS SOUNDS. Sounds produced when air particles entering the vocal tract are not set into vibration by the vocal folds (e.g., /s/ and /f/).

WAVEFORM. The manner in which particles of air that are perceived as sound vibrate. There is a unique vibration pattern for each speech sound.

WERNICKE'S APHASIA. A disorder of the central auditory nervous system in which the person loses some ability to relate heard words to units of experience. It is also referred to as receptive aphasia and fluent aphasia.

WORD-FINDING PROBLEMS. Difficulty retrieving specific words accompanied by pauses, repetitions, starting over, and use of generic terms such as *thing* or *stuff*. Also referred to as word-retrieval problems.

WORD REPETITIONS. Repetitions of entire words. In most cases they are single syllable ones.

WORLD HEALTH ORGANIZATION (WHO). The agency of the United Nations that has health-care as its primary focus.

References

Alsarraf, R., Jung, C. J., Perkins, J., et. al. (1998). Otitis media health status evaluation: A pilot study for the investigation of cost-effective outcomes of recurrent acute otitis media treatment. *Annals of Otology, Rhinology and Laryngology, 107*(2), 120–128.

American Community Survey. (2002). *Ranking tables.* Retrieved February 7, 2005, from http://www.census.gov/acs/www/Products/Ranking/Ranking3.htm

American Psychiatric Association. (2000). *Diagnostic and statistical manual of mental disorders IV–TR* (4th ed., text revision). Arlington, VA: Author.

American Speech-Language-Hearing Association. (1996). *Intervention with multicultural populations.* Retrieved October 4, 2005, from http://www.asha.org/about/leadership-projects/multicultural/readings/reading_4.html

American Speech-Language-Hearing Association. (2003). *Cultural differences in communication and learning styles,* ¶3. Retrieved March 2, 2005, from http://www.asha.org/about/leadership-projects/multicultural/readings/reading_2.html

American Speech-Language-Hearing Association. (2004a). *2004 schools survey: Caseload characteristics.* Retrieved March 1, 2005, from http://www.asha.org/NR/rdonlyres/22D66325-4CE6-460D-8D61-9E0388219EC3/0/SchoolsSurveycaseloads.pdf

American Speech-Language-Hearing Association. (2004b). *Communication difference versus language disorder.* Retrieved March 2, 2005, from http://www.asha.org/about/leadership-projects/multicultural/issues/diff.htm, ¶1.

American Speech-Language-Hearing Association. (2005a). *ASHA's online reference library. Volume I. Code of ethics,* p. 186. Retrieved March 31, 2005, from http://www.asha.org/about/ethics/

American Speech-Language-Hearing Association. (2005b). *Attention deficit hyperactivity disorder.* Retrieved March 1, 2005, from http://www.asha.org/public/speech/disorders/ADHD.html

American Speech-Language-Hearing Association. (2005c). *Audiology.* Retrieved March 31, 2005, from http://www.asha.org/students/professions/overview/audiology.htm

American Speech-Language-Hearing Association. (2005d). *Audiology in culturally and linguistically diverse populations.* Retrieved February 8, 2005, from http://www.asha.org/about/leadership-projects/multicultural/issues/audcld.htm

American Speech-Language-Hearing Association. (2005e). *Childhood apraxia of speech.* Retrieved April 28, 2005, from http://www.asha.org/public/speech/disorders/childhood-apraxia.html

American Speech-Language-Hearing Association. (2005f). *Frequently asked questions. Speech-language pathology assistants.* Retrieved April 7, 2005, from http://www.asha.org/about/membership-certification/faq_slpasst.html

American Speech-Language-Hearing Association. (2005g). *Introduction to augmentative and alternative communication*. Retrieved April 28, 2005, from http://www.asha.org/public/ speech/disorders/Augmentative-and-Alternative.html

American Speech-Language-Hearing Association. (2005h). *Language-based learning disabilities*. Retrieved March 1, 2005, from http://www.asha.org/public/speech/disorders/ Language-Based-Learning-Disabilities.html

American Speech-Language-Hearing Association. (2005i). *Loose lips: Confidentiality in relationships with colleagues*. Retrieved April 11, 2005, from http://www.asha.org/ Templates/about/aEthicsTemplate.aspx?NRMODE=Published&NRORIGINALURL=%2f about%2fethics%2floose_lips%2ehtm&NRNODEGUID=%7bFBF78C4A-2AB8-412D-AC67-0A77D6789463%7d&NRCACHEHINT=Guest&guest=true

American Speech-Language-Hearing Association. (2005j). *Orofacial myofunctional disorders*. Retrieved April 28, 2005, from http://www.asha.org/public/speech/disorders/ Orofacial-Myofunctional-Disorders.html

American Speech-Language-Hearing Association. (2005k). *Scope of practice in speech-language pathology*. Retrieved April 7, 2005, from http://www.asha.org/NR/rdonlyres/ 4FDEE27B-BAF5-4D06-AC4D-8D1F311C1B06/0/19446_1.pdf

American Speech-Language-Hearing Association. (2005l). *Self-assessment for cultural competency*. Retrieved February 8, 2005, from http://www.asha.org/Templates/about/ aLeadershipTemplate.aspx?NRMODE=Published NRORIGINALURL=%2fabout%2fleadership-projects%2fmulticultural%2fself%2ehtm&NRNODEGUID=%7b733431C8-2677-44B0-B4AD-53B756C5E05D%7d&NRCACHEHINT=Guest&guest=true

American Speech-Language-Hearing Association. (2005m). *Speech, language, and swallowing*. Retrieved March 31, 2005, from http://www.asha.org/public/speech/

American Speech-Language-Hearing Association. (2005n). *Speech-language disorders and the speech-language pathologist*. Retrieved February 24, 2005, from http://www.asha.org/ students/professions/overview/sld.html

American Speech-Language-Hearing Association. (2005o). *Speech-language pathology in culturally and linguistically diverse populations*. Retrieved February 8, 2005, from http://www.asha.org/about/leadership-projects/multicultural/issues/SLPCLD.htm

American Speech-Language-Hearing Association (2006). *Communication facts: Special populations: Autism–2006 edition*. Retrieved March 1, 2005, from http://www.asha.org/members/research/reports/autism

American Speech-Language-Hearing Association Ad Hoc Committee on Service Delivery in the Schools. (1993). Definitions of communication disorders and variations. *ASHA*, *35*(Suppl. 10), 40–41.

Anderson, N. B. (1992). Understanding cultural diversity. *American Journal of Speech-Language Pathology, 1*(1), 9–10.

Arizona Behavioral Health Associates. (2005). *What is biofeedback?* Retrieved March 28, 2005, from http://www.psychotherapy.com/bio.html

Arnold, G. E. (1965). Cluttering: Tachyphemia. In R. Luchsinger & G. E. Arnold (Eds.), *Voice-speech-language* (pp. 598–618). Belmont, CA: Wadsworth.

ASLinfo.com. (2005). *Deaf time-line: 1000 B.C.–1816.* Retrieved March 30, 2005, from http://www.aslinfo.com/trivia.cfm

Bates, E. (1976). *Language and context: The acquisition of pragmatics.* New York: Academic Press.

Battle, D. E. (Ed.). (1993). *Communication disorders in multicultural populations.* Stoneham, MA: Andover Medical.

Battle, D. E., & Anderson, N. (1998). Culturally diverse families and the development of language. In D. E. Battle (Ed.), *Communication disorders and language disorders.* New York: Macmillan.

Bauby, J. (1998). *The driving bell and the butterfly.* New York, NY: Vintage Books.

Bellenir, K. (Ed.). (2003). *Alzheimer's disease sourcebook* (3rd ed.). Detroit, MI: Omnigraphics.

Benton, A. L. (1964). Contributions to aphasia before Broca. *Cortex, 1,* 314–327.

Benton, A. L. (1981). Aphasia: Historical perspectives. In M. T. Sarno. (Ed.), *Acquired aphasia.* New York, NY: Academic Press.

Benton, A. L., & Joynt, R. J. (1960). Early descriptions of aphasia. *Archives of Neurology, 3,* 199–226.

Bernthal, J. E., & Bankson, N.W. (1998). *Articulation and phonological disorders* (4th ed.). Boston, MA: Allyn and Bacon.

Bhatnagar, S. C. (2002). *Neuroscience for the study of communicative disorders* (2nd ed.). Philadelphia: Lippincott.

Bleile, J. M., & Wallach, H. (1992). A sociolinguistic investigation of the speech of African American preschoolers. *American Journal of Speech-Language Pathology, 1*(2), 54–62.

Bloodstein, O. (1993). *Stuttering: The search for a cause and cure.* Boston, MA: Allyn and Bacon.

Bloom, C., & Cooperman, D. K. (1999). *Synergistic stuttering therapy: A holistic approach.* Boston, MA: Butterworth-Heinemann.

Bloom, E. D., Singer, M. L., & Hamaker, R. C. (1998). *Tracheoesophageal voice restoration following total laryngectomy.* San Diego, CA: Singular.

Bloom, L., Rocissano, L., & Hood, L. (1976). Adult-child discourse: Developmental interaction between information processing and linguistic knowledge. *Cognitive Psychology, 8,* 521–552.

Blosser, J., & Neidecker, E. A. (2002). *School programs in speech-language pathology: Organization and service delivery* (4th ed.). Boston, MA: Allyn and Bacon.

Boone, D. R., & McFarlane, S. C. (2000). *The voice and voice therapy* (6th ed.). Boston, MA: Allyn and Bacon.

Borden, G. J., Harris, K. S., & Raphael, L. J. (1994). *Speech science primer* (3rd ed.). Baltimore, MD: Williams & Wilkins.

Bourgeois, M. S. (1992). Evaluating memory wallets in conversations with persons with dementia. *Journal of Speech and Hearing Research, 35,* 1344–1357.

Bruner, J. (1975). The ontogenesis of speech acts. *Journal of Child Language, 2,* 1–9.

Buteau, C. L., & Hodson, B. W. (1989). *Phonological remediation targets: Words and primary pictures for highly unintelligible children.* Austin, TX: Pro-Ed.

Butler, K. G. (Ed.). (1986). *Prospering in private practice: A handbook for speech-language pathology and audiology.* Rockville, MD: Aspen Publishers.

Calculator, S., & Jorgensen, C. (1994). *Including students with severe disabilities in schools.* San Diego: Singular.

Campbell, L. R. (1993). Integrity of home linguistic varieties: Black English vernacular. *American Journal of Speech-Language Pathology, 2*(1), 11–12.

Canalis, R. F., & Lambert, P. R. (2000). *The ear: Comprehensive otology.* Philadelphia, PA: Lippincott.

Carroll, L. (2001). *Jabberwocky and other poems.* Mineola, NY: Dover.

Caruso, A. J., & E. Strand. (1999). *Clinical management of motor speech disorders in children.* New York: Thieme.

Casby, M. W. (1992). An intervention approach for naming problems in children. *American Journal of Speech-Language Pathology, 1*(3), 35–42.

Casper, J. K., & Colton, R. H. (1998). *Clinical manual for laryngectomy and head/neck cancer rehabilitation* (2nd ed.). San Diego, CA: Singular.

Chapey, R. (Ed.). (2001). *Language intervention strategies in aphasia and related neurogenic communication disorders* (4th ed.). Philadelphia, PA: Lippincott.

Chermak, G. D., & Musiek, F. E. (1992). Managing central auditory processing disorders in children and youth. *American Journal of Audiology, 1*(3), 61–65.

Cirrin, F. M., & Magnusson, D. L. (1992). Determining the need for speech-language intervention services for infants and toddlers. *Clinics in Communication Disorders, 2*(3), 1–12.

Clover Park School District. (2005). *About CPSD.* Retrieved March 2, 2005, from http://cpsd.cloverpark.k12.wa.us/aboutus/aboutus.asp

Coleman, A. M. (2001). *On your own: A resource manual for starting a successful private practice as a solo practitioner in speech-language pathology.* Austin, TX: Pro-Ed.

Community Unit School District. (2004). *District and community profile.* Retrieved March 2, 2005, from http://www.cusd200.org/programs/technology/Section%203.pdf

Cooper, E. B., & Cooper, C. S. (1992). A fluency disorders prevention program for preschoolers and children in the primary grades. *American Journal of Speech-Language Pathology, 1*(1), 28–31.

Cornett, B. S. (1999). *Clinical practice management for speech-language pathologists.* Gaithersburg, MD: Aspen Publishers.

Crais, E. R. (1992). Moving from "parent involvement" to family-centered services. *American Journal of Speech-Language Pathology, 1*(1), 5–8.

Creech, R., & Viggiano, J. (1981). Consumers speak out on the life of the non-speaker. *ASHA, 23*(8), 550–551.

Crowe, T. A. (Ed.). (1997). *Applications of counseling in speech-language pathology and audiology.* Baltimore, MD: Williams & Wilkins.

Cunningham, M., & Cox, E. O. (2003). Hearing assessment in infants and children: Recommendations beyond neonatal screening. *Pediatrics, 111,* 436–440.

Dallas Independent School District. (2003). *DISD at a glance.* Retrieved March 2, 2005, from http://www.dallasnews.com/s/dws/spe/2004/dallas/graphics/12_disd.pdf

Daly, D. A. (1986). The clutterer. In K. O. St. Louis (Ed.), *The atypical stutterer.* Orlando, FL: Academic Press.

Daly, D. A. (1993). Cluttering: The orphan of speech-language pathology. *American Journal of Speech-Language Pathology, 2*(2), 6–8

Darley, F. L., Aronson, A. E., & Brown, J. R. (1975). *Motor speech disorders.* Philadelphia: Saunders.

Davis, G. A. (1993). *A survey of adult aphasia and related language disorders* (2nd ed.). Englewood Cliffs, NJ: Prentice Hall.

Deem, J. F., & Miller, L. (2000). *Manual of voice therapy* (2nd ed.). Austin, TX: Pro-Ed.

Dhooge, I. J. (2003). Risk factors for the development of otitis media. *Current Allergy and Asthma Reports, 3,* 321–325.

Dikeman, K. J., & Kazandijan, M. S. (2004, October 19). Managing adults with tracheostomies and ventilator dependence: Current concepts. *The ASHA Leader,* pp. 6–7, 19–20.

Dodge, E. P. (Ed.). (2000). *The survival guide for school-based speech-language pathologists.* San Diego, CA: Singular.

Duchan, J. F. (2001a). *Getting here: A short history of speech pathology in America.* Retrieved March 30, 2005, from http://www.acsu.buffalo.edu/~duchan/history.html

Duchan, J. F. (2001b, May 12). *Learning leveling and leveling learning: Graduation speech.* Department of Communicative Disorders and Sciences, University of Buffalo. Retrieved October 30, 2005, from http://www.acsu.buffalo.edu/~duchan/leveling.html

Duchan. J. F. (2003, November). *Identity based therapies*. Paper presented at the American Speech-Language-Hearing Association. Retrieved October 3, 2005, from http://www.acsu. buffalo.edu/~duchan/identity_based_therapies.html

Duncan, J. L., & Silverman, F. H. (1997). Impacts of learning American Indian Sign Language on mentally retarded children. *Perceptual and Motor Skills, 44,* 1138.

Durand, V. M. (1993). Functional communication training for challenging behaviors. *Clinics in Communication Disorders, 3*(2), 59–70.

Ehren, T. C. (1993). Tests: A significant difference? *American Journal of Speech-Language Pathology, 2*(1), 17–19.

Eisenberg, M. G., Glueckauf, R. L., & Zaretsky, H. H. (Eds.). (1999). *Medical aspects of disability: A handbook for the rehabilitation professional.* New York: Springer.

Eldridge, M. (1968). *A history of the treatment of speech disorders.* Edinburgh, Scotland: Livingstone.

Fact Monster. (2005). *Embolus.* Retrieved March 28, 2005, from http://www.factmonster. com/ce6/sci/A0817238.html

Farmer, S. S., & Farmer, J. L. (1989). *Supervision in communication disorders.* Columbus, OH: Merrill.

Fawcus, R. (Ed.). (2000). *Stroke rehabilitation: A collaborative approach.* Malden, MA: Blackwell Science.

Felsenfeld, S., Broen, P. A., & McGue, M. (1992). A 28-year follow-up study of adults with a history of moderate phonological disorder: Linguistic and personality results. *Journal of Speech and Hearing Research, 35,* 1114–1125.

Ferguson, M. L. (1991). Collaborative/consultative service delivery: An introduction. *Language, Speech, and Hearing Services in Schools, 22,* 147.

Ferrand, C. T. (2001). *Speech science: An integrated approach to theory and clinical practice.* Boston, MA: Allyn and Bacon.

Garliner, D. (Ed.). (1976). *Myofunctional therapy.* Philadelphia: Saunders.

Geffner, D. (2005). *Attention-deficit/hyperactivity disorder: What professionals need to know.* Eau Claire, WI: Thinking Publications.

Gies-Zaborowski, J., & Silverman, F. H. (1986). Documenting the impact of a mild dysarthria on peer perception. *Language, Speech, and Hearing Services in Schools, 17,* 143.

Gillam, R. G., & Bedore, L. M. (2000). Communication across the lifespan. In R. B. Gillam, T. P. Marquardt, & F. N. Martin. (Eds.), *Communication Sciences and Disorders: From Science to Clinical Practice* (pp. 25–61). San Diego, CA: Singular.

Gleason, J. B. (2001). *The development of language* (5th ed.). Boston, MA: Allyn and Bacon.

Glickstein, J. K., & Neustadt, G. K. (1993). Speech-language interventions in Alzheimer's disease: A functional communication approach. *Clinics in Communication Disorders, 3*(1), 15–30.

Goldstein, K. (1948). *Language and language disturbances, aphasic symptom complexes and their significance for medicine and theory of language.* New York: Grune & Stratton.

Gordon, P. A., & Luper, H. L. (1992a). The early identification of beginning stuttering I: Protocols. *American Journal of Speech-Language Pathology, 1*(3), 48–53.

Gordon, P. A., & Luper, H. L. (1992b). The early identification of beginning stuttering II: Problems. *American Journal of Speech-Language Pathology, 1*(3), 49–55.

Gould, G. M., & Pyle, W. L. (1937). *Abnormalities and curiosities of medicine.* New York: Sydenham.

Grandin, T. (1995). *Thinking in pictures: And other reports from my life with autism.* New York: Doubleday.

Groher, M. E. (1997). *Dysphagia: Diagnosis and management* (3rd ed.). Boston, MA: Butterworth-Heinemann.

Gudmundsen, G. (1992). Expanding opportunities for audiologists in hear-care delivery. *American Journal of Audiology, 1*(1), 21.

Gudykunst, W. B. (1998). *Bridging differences, effective intergroup communication* (3rd ed.). London: Sage.

Gustason, G. (1983). *Teaching and learning Signing Exact English.* Los Alamitos, CA: Modern Signs Press.

Hahn, E. F. (1956). *Stuttering: Significant theories and therapies* (2nd ed.). Stanford, CA: Stanford University Press.

Hall, E. T. (1966). *The hidden dimension.* Garden City, NY: Doubleday.

Hall, K. D. (2001). *Pediatric dysphagia resource guide.* San Diego, CA: Singular.

Hall, P. K. (1992). At the center of the controversy: Developmental apraxia. *American Journal of Speech-Language Pathology, 1*(3), 23–25.

Halper, A. S., Cherney, L. R., & Burns, M. S. (1996). *Clinical management of right hemisphere dysfunction* (2nd ed.). Gaithersburg, MD: Aspen

Halvorson, J. (1999). *Abandoned: Now stutter my orphan.* Hager City, WI: Halvorson Farms of Wisconsin.

Hanson, M. L., & Barrett, R. H. (1988). *Fundamentals of orofacial myology.* Springfield, IL: Charles C. Thomas.

Hargrove, P. M., & Katz, K. B. (1992). Achieving cultural sensitivity: A process, not a product. *Clinics in Communication Disorders, 2*(3), 13–22.

Hodson, B. W. (1997). *Perspectives in applied phonology.* Gaithersburg, MD: Aspen Publishers.

Hodson, B. W., & Paden, E. P. (1991). *Targeting intelligible speech: A phonological approach to remediation* (2nd ed.). Austin, TX: Pro-Ed.

Hosford-Dunn, H., Dunn, D. R., & Harford, E .R. (1995). *Audiology business and practice management*. San Diego, CA: Singular.

Hulit, L. M., & Howard, M. R. (1997). *Born to talk: An introduction to speech and language development*. Boston: Allyn and Bacon.

Hulit, L. M., & Howard, M. R. (2006). *Born to talk: An introduction to speech and language development* (4th ed.). Boston: Allyn and Bacon.

Hull, R. H. (Ed.). (2001). *Aural rehabilitation: Serving children and adults* (4th ed.). San Diego, CA: Singular.

Individuals with Disabilities Education Improvement Act of 2004. (IDEA), 20 U.S.C. § 1400 *et seq*. (2004).

Johnson, W. (1946). *People in quandaries*. New York: Harper & Brothers.

Johnson, W., & Associates. (1959). *The onset of stuttering*. Minneapolis, MN: University of Minnesota Press.

Johnston, J. (2006). *Thinking about child language: Research to practice*. Eau Claire, WI: Thinking Publications.

JSOnline (2005). *Stuttering research no secret to scholars*. Retrieved March 21, 2005, from http://www.jsonline.com/news/metro/jun01/stut16061501a.asp

Kaufman, N. J., & Larson, V. Lord (2005). *Asperger syndrome: Strategies for solving the social puzzle*. Eau Claire, WI: Thinking Publications.

Kemper, A. R., & Downs, S. M. (2000). A cost-effectiveness analysis of newborn hearing screening strategies. *Archives of Pediatric and Adolescent Medicine, 154,* 484–488.

Klingbeil, G. M. (1939a). The historical background of the modern speech clinic: Aphasia. *Journal of Speech Disorders, 4,* 26–284.

Klingbeil, G. M. (1939b). The historical background of the modern speech clinic: Stuttering and stammering. *Journal of Speech Disorders, 4,* 115–132.

Kuster, J. (2005a). *Other related fluency disorders: Cluttering*. Retrieved March 22, 2005, from http://www.mnsu.edu/comdis/kuster/related.html

Kuster, J. (2005b). *Other related fluency disorders: Neurogenic stuttering*. Retrieved March 22, 2005, from http://www.mnsu.edu/comdis/kuster/related.html

Kuster, J. (2005c). *Stuttering homepage*. Retrieved March 21, 2005, from http://www.mnsu.edu/comdis/kuster/stutter.html

LaFond, D., Joanette, Y., Ponzio, J., Degiovani, R., & Sarno, M. T. (1993). *Living with aphasia: Psychosocial issues*. San Diego, CA: Singular.

Larson, V. L., & McKinley, N. L. (2003). *Communication solutions for older students: Assessment and intervention strategies*. Eau Claire, WI: Thinking Publications.

Lass, N. J., Ruscello, D. M., Schmitt, J. F., Pannbacker, M. D., Orlando, M. B., Dean, K. A., Ruziska, J. C, & Bradshaw, K. H. (1992). Teachers' perceptions of stutterers. *Language, Speech, and Hearing Services in Schools, 23,* 78–81.

Leinhard, J. H. (2005). No. 327: *Ambroise Paré.* Retrieved March 30, 2005, from http://www.uh.edu/engines/epi327.htm

Leith, W. R., McNiece, E. M., & Fusilier, B. B. (1989). *Handbook of supervision: A cognitive behavioral approach.* Boston, MA: Little, Brown.

Leonard, R., Goodrich, S., McMenamin, P., & Donald, P. (1992). Differentiation of speakers with glossectomies by acoustic and perceptual measures. *American Journal of Speech-Language Pathology, 1*(4), 56–63.

Lewis, B. (1992). Genetics in speech disorders. *Clinics in Communication Disorders, 2*(4), 48–58.

Life Captured (Producer). (n.d.). *Cry of the cat* [Video recording]. North Sydney, Australia.

Lubinski, R. (Ed.). (1995). *Dementia and communication.* San Diego, CA: Singular.

Luterman, D. (1995). *In the shadows: Living and coping with a loved one's chronic illness.* Bedford, MA: Jade Press.

Luterman, D. (2002). *Counseling persons with communication disorders and their families* (4th ed.). Boston, MA: Little Brown.

MacDonald, J. D., & Carroll, J. Y. (1992). Communicating with young children: An ecological model for clinicians, parents, and collaborative professionals. *American Journal of Speech-Language Pathology, 1*(4), 39–48.

Mace, N. L., & Rabins, P. V. (1999). *The 36-hour day: A family guide to caring for person with Alzheimer disease, related dementing illnesses, and memory loss* (3rd ed.). Baltimore, MD: Johns Hopkins University Press.

Maestas, A. G., & Erickson, J. G. (1992). Mexican immigrant mothers' beliefs about disabilities. *American Journal of Speech-Language Pathology, 1*(4), 5–10.

Marlowe, J. A. (1993). Screening all newborns for hearing impairment in a community hospital. *American Journal of Audiology, 2*(1), 22–25.

Martin, F. N. (2000). *Introduction to audiology* (7th ed.). Boston, MA: Allyn and Bacon.

Masterson, J. J. (1993). Classroom-based phonological intervention. *American Journal of Speech-Language Pathology, 2*(1), 5–9.

Mathieson, L. (2001). *Greene and Mathieson's the voice and its disorders* (6th ed.). Philadelphia, PA: Whurr Publishers.

Matsuki, C. (1989). The clinical study of functional deafness [Japanese]. *Nippon Jibiinkoka Gakkai Kaiho, 92*(9), 1371–1380.

Matthews, C. B. (1993). *Marketing speech-language pathology and audiology services.* San Diego, CA: Singular.

Merriam-Webster Online Dictionary. (2005). *Homepage.* Retrieved March 30, 2005, from http://www.merriam-webster.com

Meyers, F. L., & St. Louis, K. O. (1992). *Cluttering: A clinical perspective.* Kibworth, England: Far Communications.

Meyers, P. S. (1999). *Right hemisphere damage: Disorders of communication and cognition.* San Diego, CA: Singular.

Miller, L. (1989). Classroom-based language intervention. *Language, Speech, and Hearing Services in Schools, 20,* 153–169.

Miller, L. (1993a). Testing and the creation of disorder. *American Journal of Speech-Language Pathology, 2*(1), 13–16.

Miller, L. (1993b). *What we call smart: A new narrative for intelligence and learning.* San Diego, CA: Singular Publishing Group.

Moore-Brown, B., & Montgomery, J. (2001). *Making a difference for America's children: Speech-language pathologist in public schools.* Eau Claire, WI: Thinking Publications.

Murry, T., & Carrau, R. L. (2001). *Clinical manual for swallowing disorders.* San Diego, CA: Singular.

Nadeau, S. E., Gonzales-Rothi, L. J., & Crosson, B. (Eds.). (2000). *Aphasia and language: Theory to practice.* New York: Guilford Press.

National Center on Birth Defects and Developmental Disabilities, Centers for Disease Control and Prevention. (2002, December 17). *Developmental disabilities.* Retrieved August 26, 2003, from http://www.cdc.gov/ncbddd/dd/default.htm

National Center on Birth Defects and Developmental Disabilities, Centers for Disease Control and Prevention. (2003, July 7). *The genetics of infant hearing loss.* Retrieved August 31, 2003, from http://www.cdc.gov/ncbddd/ehdi/genetics.htm

National Information Center for Children and Youth with Disabilities. (2004, January). *Deafness and hearing loss* (Pub. No. FS3). Washington, DC: Author.

National Institute on Deafness and Other Communication Disorders. (2002a, July). *Otitis media* (ear infection) (NIH Pub. No. 974216). Bethesda, MD: Author.

National Institute on Deafness and Other Communication Disorders. (2002b, December 12). *Statistics and human communication.* Retrieved August 31, 2003, from http://www.nidcd.nih.gov/health/statistics/

National Institute on Deafness and Other Communication Disorders (2005a). *Cochlear implants.* Retrieved March 29, 2005, from http://www.nidcd.nih.gov/health/hearing/coch.asp

National Institute on Deafness and Other Communication Disorders (2005b). *Dysphagia.* Retrieved April 7, 2005, from http://www.nidcd.nih.gov/health/voice/dysph.asp

National Institute on Deafness and Other Communication Disorders. (2005c). *Ear infections: Facts for parents about otitis media.* Retrieved March 25, 2005, from http://www.nidcd.nih.gov/health/hearing/otitismedia.asp

National Institute on Deafness and Other Communication Disorders (2005d). *Facts about telecommunication relay services and national 711*. Retrieved March 30, 2005, from http://www.nidcd.nih.gov/health/hearing/telecomm.asp

National Institute on Deafness and Other Communication Disorders. (2005e). *Glossary*. Retrieved February 9, 2005, from http://www.nidcd.nih.gov/health/glossary/glossary.asp

National Institute on Deafness and Other Communication Disorders (2005f). *The noise in your ears: Facts about tinnitus*. Retrieved March 21, 2005, from http://www.nidcd.nih.gov/health/hearing/noiseinear.asp

National Institute on Deafness and Other Communication Disorders. (2005g). *Otitis media (ear infection)*. Retrieved March 25, 2005, from http://www.nidcd.nih.gov/health/hearing/otitism.asp

National Institute on Deafness and Other Communication Disorders. (2005h). *Otosclerosis*. Retrieved February 25, 2005, from http://www.nidcd.nih.gov/health/hearing/otosclerosis.asp

National Institute on Deafness and Other Communication Disorders (2005i). *Presbycusis*. Retrieved March 28, 2005, from http://www.nidcd.nih.gov/health/hearing/presbycusis.asp

National Institute on Neurological Disorders and Stroke. (2003). *Autism fact sheet*. Retrieved March 1, 2005, from http://www.ninds.nih.gov/health_and_medical/pubs/autism.htm

National Institute on Neurological Disorders and Stroke. (2005a). *NINDS multiple sclerosis information page*. Retrieved March 28, 2005, from http://www.ninds.nih.gov/disorders/multiple_sclerosis/multiple_sclerosis.htm

National Institute on Neurological Disorders and Stroke. (2005b). *NINDS muscular dystrophy information page*. Retrieved April 27, 2005, from http://www.ninds.nih.gov/disorders/md/md.htm

National Institute on Neurological Disorders and Stroke. (2005c). *NINDS myasthenia gravis information page*. Retrieved April 27, 2005, from http://www.ninds.nih.gov/disorders/myasthenia_gravis/myasthenia_gravis.htm

National Institute on Neurological Disorders and Stroke. (2005d). *NINDS Parkinson's disease information page*. Retrieved April 27, 2005, from http://www.ninds.nih.gov/disorders/parkinsons_disease/parkinsons_disease.htm

National Student Speech Language Hearing Association. (2004). *Homepage*. Retrieved May 15, 2005, from http://www.nsslha.org/nsslha/

National Stuttering Association. (2005). *Homepage*. Retrieved March 21, 2005, from http://www.nsastutter.org/

Nippold, M. A., Ward-Lonergan, J. M., & Fanning, J. L. (2005). Persuasive writing in children, adolescents, and adults: A study of syntactic, semantic, and pragmatic development. *Language, Speech and Hearing Services in Schools, 36,* 125–138.

O'Connell, P. F. (Ed.). (1997). *Speech, language, and hearing programs in schools: A guide for students and practitioners.* Gaithersburg, MD: Aspen Publishers.

O'Hare, W. P. (2001). *The child population: First data from the 2000 census.* Retrieved February 7, 2005, from http://www.aecf.org/kidscount/trends_children.pdf

Olswang, L. & Bain, B. (1991). Intervention issues for toddlers with specific language impairments. *Topics in Language Disorders, 11,* 69–86.

O'Neill, Y. V. (1980). *Speech and speech disorders in western thought before 1600.* Westport, CT: Greenwood Press.

Onslow, M. (1992). Identification of early stuttering: Issues and suggested strategies. *American Journal of Speech-Language Pathology, 1*(4), 21–27.

Osberger, M. J., Maso, M., & Sam, L. K. (1993). Speech intelligibility of children with cochlear implants, tactical aids, or hearing aids. *Journal of Speech and Hearing Research, 36,* 186–203.

Owens, R. E., Jr. (2001). *Language development: An introduction* (5th ed.). Needham Heights, MA: Allyn and Bacon.

Oyer, H. J. (1987). *Administration of programs in speech-language pathology and audiology.* Englewood Cliffs, NJ: Prentice-Hall.

Paden, E. (1970). *A history of the American Speech and Hearing Association 1925 to 1958.* Washington, DC: American Speech and Hearing Association.

Pannbacker, M., Middleton, G., Vekovius, G. T., & Sanders, K. L. (2001). *Report writing for speech language pathologists and audiologists* (2nd ed.). Austin, TX: Pro-Ed.

Patterson, K., & Wilson, B. (1990). A ROSE is a ROSE or a NOSE: A deficit in initial letter identification. *Cognitive Psychology, 7,* 447–478.

Paul, R. (2001). *Language disorders from infancy through adolescence: Assessment and intervention* (2nd ed.). St. Louis: Mosby.

Pedrey, C. (1950). Letter to the editor. *Journal of Speech and Hearing Disorders, 15,* 266–269.

Penman, R., Cross, T., Milgrom-Friedman, J., & Meares, R. (1983). Mothers' speech to prelingual infants: A pragmatic analysis. *Journal of Child Language, 10,* 17–34.

Perkins, W. H. (1992). Fluency controls and automatic fluency. *American Journal of Speech-Language Pathology, 1*(2), 9–10.

Pichora-Fuller, M. K., & Benguerel, A. (1991). The design of CAST (computer-aided speechreading training). *Journal of Speech and Hearing Research, 34,* 202–212.

Polloway, E., Miller, L., & Smith, T. E. C. (2004). *Language instruction for students with disabilities* (3rd ed.). Denver: Love.

Post, J. G., & Leith, W. R. (1983). I'd rather tell a story than be one. *ASHA, 25,* 23–26.

Prelock, P. A. (1993). Managing the language and learning needs of the communication-impaired preschool child: A proactive approach. *Clinics in Communication Disorders, 3*(1), 1–14.

Registry of Interpreters for the Deaf. (2005). *Homepage.* Retrieved March 29, 2005, from http://www.rid.org/

Rizzo, Jr., S. R., & Trudeau, M. D. (Eds.). (1994). *Clinical administration in audiology and speech-language pathology.* San Diego, CA: Singular.

Robbins, S. D. (1948). Chapter 10. In E. Froeschels (Ed.), *Twentieth century speech correction.* New York: Philosophical Library.

Robin, D. A. (1992). Developmental apraxia of speech: Just another motor problem. *American Journal of Speech-Language Pathology, 1*(3), 19–22.

Rogers, C. R. (1942). *Counseling & psychotherapy.* Boston, MA: Houghton Mifflin.

Roseberry-McKibbin, C. (1997). Understanding Filipino families: A foundation for effective service delivery. *American Journal of Speech-Language Pathology, 6*(3), 5–14.

Roseberry-McKibbin, C., & Hegde, M. N. (2000). *Advanced review of speech-language pathology.* Austin, TX: Pro-Ed.

Rossetti, L. M. (2001). *Communication intervention: Birth to three* (2nd ed.). San Diego, CA: Singular.

Roth, C. R., Aronson, A. E., & Davis, Jr., L. J. (1989). Clinical studies in psychogenic stuttering of adult onset. *Journal of Speech and Hearing Disorders, 5*(4), 634–646.

Ruscello, D. M., St. Louis, K. O., & Mason, N. (1991). School-age children with phonological disorders: Coexistence with other speech/language disorders. *Journal of Speech and Hearing Research, 34,* 236–242.

Sacks, O. (1985). *The man who mistook his wife for a hat.* New York: Touchstone.

Salvi, R. J. (1993). 4000 Hz noise damage. *American Journal of Audiology, 2*(1), 21.

Sander, E. (1972). When are speech sounds learned? *Journal of Speech and Hearing Disorders, 37,* 62.

Sandlin, R. E. (Ed.). (1991). *Textbook of hearing aid amplification* (2nd ed.). San Diego, CA: Singular.

Sarno, M. T. (1981). *Acquired aphasia.* San Diego, CA: Academic Press.

Sarno, M. T. (1998). *Acquired aphasia* (3rd ed.). San Diego, CA: Academic Press.

Schubel, R. J., & Erickson, J. G. (1992). Model program for increasing parent involvement through telephone technology. *Language, Speech, and Hearing Services in Schools, 23,* 125–129.

Schuster, L. I., Ruscello, D. M., & Smith, K. D. (1992). Evoking /r/ using visual feedback. *American Journal of Speech-Language Pathology, 1*(3), 29–34.

Shallice, T. (1987). Impairments of semantic processing: Multiple dissociations. In M. Coltheart, G. Sartori, & R. Job (Eds.), *The cognitive neuropsychology of language* (pp. 111–127). London: Erlbaum.

Shapiro, A. K. (1964). Factors contributing to the placebo effect: Their implications for psychotherapy. *American Journal of Psychotherapy, 18*(Suppl. 1), 73–88.

Shields, C. (1997). *Behind objective description: Special education and the reality of lived experience.* Unpublished doctoral thesis, University of Toronto.

Silverman, F. H. (1960). Forensic therapy. *Quarterly Journal of Speech,* 305–306.

Silverman, F. H. (1980). The Stuttering Problem Profile: A task that assists both client and clinician in defining therapy goals. *Journal of Speech and Hearing Disorders, 45,* 119–123.

Silverman, F. H. (1988a). Impact of a t-shirt message on stutterer stereotypes. *Journal of Fluency Disorders, 13,* 279–281.

Silverman, F. H. (1988b). The monster study. *Journal of Fluency Disorders, 13,* 225–231.

Silverman, F. H. (1990). Are professors likely to report having "beliefs" about the intelligence and competence of students who stutter? *Journal of Fluency Disorders, 15,* 319–321.

Silverman, F. H. (1995). *Communication for the speechless* (3rd ed.). Boston, MA: Allyn and Bacon.

Silverman, F. H. (1996). *Stuttering and other fluency disorders* (2nd ed.). Boston, MA: Allyn and Bacon.

Silverman, F. H. (1998a). *Authoring books and materials for students, academics, and professionals.* Westport, CT: Praeger.

Silverman, F. H. (1998b). *Research design and evaluation in speech-language pathology and audiology* (4th ed.). Boston, MA: Allyn and Bacon.

Silverman, F. H. (1999a). *Professional issues in speech-language pathology and audiology.* Boston, MA: Allyn and Bacon.

Silverman, F. H. (1999b). *The telecommunication relay service (TRS) handbook.* Newport, RI: Aegis Publishing Group.

Silverman, F. H. (2000). *Second thoughts about stuttering: Musings of a speech-language pathologist who has stuttered for more than sixty years.* Greendale, WI: CODI Publications.

Silverman, F. H. (2004). *Introduction to speech, language, and hearing disorders* (3rd ed.). Cincinnati, OH: Atomic Dog Publishing.

Silverman, F. H., & Flack, S. M. (1992). Attitudes of teenagers toward peers who have a single articulation error. *Language, Speech, and Hearing Services in Schools, 23,* 187.

Silverman, F. H., Gazzolo, M., & Peterson, Y. (1990). Impact of a t-shirt message on stutterer stereotypes: A systematic replication. *Journal of Fluency Disorders, 15,* 35–37.

Silverman, F. H., & Paulus, P. G. (1989). Peer reactions to teenagers who substitute /w/ for /r/. *Language, Speech, and Hearing Services in Schools, 20,* 219–221.

Skelly, M., Schinsky, L., Smith, R. W., Donaldson, R., & Griffin, J. (1975). American Indian sign: A gestural communication system for the speechless. *Archives of Physical Medicine and Rehabilitation, 56,* 156–160.

Smith, A. (2005). *Research studies interaction of language and motor processing in stuttering.* The Stuttering Foundation. Retrieved October 3, 2005, from the Stuttering Foundation website: http://www.stutteringhelp.org/Default.aspx?tabid=168

Speaks, C. E. (1999). *Introduction to sound: Acoustics for the hearing and speech sciences* (3rd ed.). San Diego, CA: Singular.

Speech Rehabilitation Institute. (n.d.). *Studies in tachyphemia.* New York: Author.

Stockman, I. J., Boult, J., & Robinson, G. (2004, July 20). Multicultural issues in academic and clinical education: A cultural mosaic. *The ASHA Leader,* pp. 6–7, 20.

Sturm, J. M., & Nelson, N. W. (1997). Formal classroom lessons: New perspectives on a familiar discourse event. *Language, Speech, and Hearing Services in Schools, 18,* 259.

Stuttering Foundation of America (2002). *If your child stutters: A guide for parents* (6th ed.). Memphis, TN: Author.

Tannen, D. (1992). *Gender and discourse.* Toronto: Oxford University Press.

Tanner, D. C. (1980). Loss and grief: Implications for the speech-language pathologist and audiologist. *ASHA, 22,* 916–928.

Task Force on Newborn and Infant Hearing. (1999). Newborn and infant hearing loss: Detection and intervention. *Pediatrics, 103,* 527–530.

Templin, M. C. (1957). *Certain language skills in children, their development and interrelationships.* (Institute of Child Development Monograph Series No. 26). Minneapolis, MN: University of Minnesota Press.

Terrell, B. Y., & Hale, J. E. (1992). Serving a multicultural population. *American Journal of Speech-Language Pathology, 1*(2), 5–8.

Thomas, A. F., & Webster, K. L. (1999). *SLP assistant in the schools.* San Antonio, TX: Communication Skill Builders.

Trace, R. (1992). Musicians no longer turn deaf ear to hearing conversation. *Advance for Speech-Language Pathologists and Audiologists, 2*(19), 9, 11.

Twistleton, E. (1873). *The tongue not essential to speech.* London: Murray.

Tyler, R. (1993). Cochlear implants and deaf culture. *American Journal of Audiology, 2*(1), 26–32.

Tyler, R. (Ed.). (2000). *Tinnitus handbook.* San Diego, CA: Singular.

UCLA Humanities Web Page Portal. (n.d.). *A slow-motion animation of the vocal folds vibrating during speech.* Retrieved October 5, 2005, from: http://www.humnet.ucla.edu/humnet/linguistics/faciliti/demos/vocalfolds/vocalfolds.htm

United States Census Bureau. (2005). *Detailed tables.* Retrieved February 7, 2005, from http://factfinder.census.gov/servlet/DTTable?_bm=y&-geo_id=01000US&-ds_name=DEC_2000_SF1_U&-_lang=en&-state=dt&-mt_name=DEC_2000_SF1_U_P001&-mt_name=DEC_2000_SF1_U_P003&-mt_name=DEC_2000_SF1_U_P004&-mt_name=DEC_2000_SF1_U_P005&-mt_name=DEC_2000_SF1_U_P006&-mt_name=DEC_2000_SF1_U_P007&-mt_name=DEC_2000_SF1_U_P008&-mt_name=DEC_2000_SF1_U_P009&-mt_name=DEC_2000_SF1_U_P010&-mt_name=DEC_2000_SF1_U_P011&-mt_name=DEC_2000_SF1_U_P035&-mt_name=DEC_2000_SF1_U_P036&-format=&-CONTEXT=dt

United States Department of Education. (2002). *ED performance & accountability: Twenty-fourth annual report to Congress on the implementation of the Individuals with Disabilities Education Act.* Retrieved March 3, 2004, from http://www.ed.gov/about/reports/annual/osep/2002/index.html

United States Department of Education. (2004). *The individuals with disabilities education improvement act of 2004* (Section 1414(d)(1)(A)). Retrieved October 5, 2005, from http://frwebgate.access.gpo.gov/cgi-bin/getdoc.cgi?dbname=108_cong_public_laws&docid=f:publ446.108

University of California at Santa Cruz Perceptual Science Laboratory. (2005). *John Bulwer.* Retrieved March 30, 2005, from http://mambo.ucsc.edu/psl/bulwer.html

University of Michigan Health Care System. (2005). *Enhancing your cultural communication skills.* Retrieved April 11, 2005, from http://www.med.umich.edu/pteducation/cultcomp.htm

Utley, B. L. (1993). Facilitating and measuring the team process within inclusive educational settings. *Clinics in Communication Disorders, 3*(2), 71–85.

Van Riper, C. (1971). *The nature of stuttering.* Englewood Cliffs, NJ: Prentice Hall.

Van Riper, C. (1973). *The treatment of stuttering.* Englewood Cliffs, NJ: Prentice Hall.

Van Riper, C. (1979). *A career in speech pathology.* Englewood Cliffs, NJ: Prentice Hall.

Van Riper, C., & Erickson, R. L. (1996). *Speech correction: An introduction to speech pathology and audiology* (9th ed.). Boston, MA: Allyn and Bacon.

Wallace, G. L. (Ed.). (1996). *Adult aphasia rehabilitation.* Boston, MA: Butterworth-Heinemann.

Waltzman, S.B., & Cohen, N.L. (Eds.). (2000). *Cochlear implants.* New York: Thieme.

Watson, M., Murthy, J., & Wadhwa, N. (2003). Phologocial Analysis Practice: An Electronic Workbook [Computer software]. Eau Claire, WI: Thinking Publications.

Weber-Fox, C. (2005). *New research on the roots of stuttering: Language processing and speech motor control: Complex interactions in stuttering.* Retrieved October 3, 2005, from the Stuttering Foundation website: http://www.stutteringhelp.org/Default.aspx?tabid=196

Weiss, D. A. (1964). *Cluttering.* Englewood Cliffs, NH: Prentice Hall.

Westby, C. (1991). Learning to talk—talking to learn: Oral-literate language differences. In C. S. Simon (Ed.), *Communication skills and classroom success: Assessment and therapy methodologies for language- and learning-disabled students* (pp. 334–355). Eau Claire, WI: Thinking Publications.

Wikipedia. (2005). *Demosthenes*. Retrieved March 30, 2005, from http://en.wikipedia.org/wiki/Demosthenes

Wilcock, G. K., Bucks, R. S., & Rockwood, K. (Eds). (1999). *Diagnosis and treatment of dementia: A manual for memory disorders teams.* New York: Oxford University Press.

Williams, A. L. (2003). *Speech disorders: Resource guide for preschool children.* Clifton Park, NY: Thomson Delmar.

Williams, A. L. (2006) SCIP: Sound Contrasts in Phonology [Computer software]. Eau Claire, WI: Thinking Publications.

Wingate, M. (2002). *Foundations of stuttering.* San Diego, CA: Academic Press.

Wood, M. L. (1986). *Private practice in communication disorders.* San Diego, CA: College-Hill Press.

Wright, B. A. (1960). *Physical disability—A psychological approach.* New York: Harper & Row.

Yairi, E., & Ambrose, N. (1992). Onset of stuttering in preschool children: Selected factors. *Journal of Speech and Hearing Research, 35,* 782–788.

Yairi, E., Ambrose, N., & Niermann, R. (1993). The early months of stuttering: A developmental study. *Journal of Speech and Hearing Research, 36,* 521–528.

Yairi, E., & Carrico, D. M. (1992). Early childhood stuttering: Pediatricians' attitudes and practices. *American Journal of Speech-Language Pathology, 1*(3), 54–62.

Zarnoch, J. M. (1982). Hearing disorders: Audiologic manifestations. In N. J. Lass, L. V. McReynolds, J. L. Northern, & D. E. Yoder (Eds.), *Speech, language, and hearing*: *Vol. 3.* Philadelphia: W. B. Saunders.

Zebrowski, P. M., & Schum, R. L. (1993). Counseling parents of children who stutter. *American Journal of Speech-Language Pathology, 2*(2), 65–73.

Zemlin, W. R. (1998). *Speech and hearing science: Anatomy and physiology* (4th ed.). Boston, MA: Allyn and Bacon.

Zraick, R. I., & Boone, D. R. (1991). Spouse attitudes toward the person with aphasia. *Journal of Speech and Hearing Research, 34,* 123–128.

Author Index

Subject Index

f=figure　　　t=table　　　sm=study more　　　ac=audio clip　　　vc=video clip